Intensive nursing care

Intensive nursing care

Zeb L. Burrell, Jr., A.B., M.D.
Lenette Owens Burrell, R.N., B.S.

Baldwin County Hospital
Milledgeville, Georgia

With 75 illustrations

Saint Louis

The C. V. Mosby Company

1969

To those patients
who
made this volume a necessity

and

to those nurses
who
by their eagerness to learn
made it a pleasure

Preface

Beginning in 1966 the medical staff of the Baldwin County Hospital in Milledgeville, Georgia began a series of lectures to our nursing personnel in preparation for the opening of our intensive care unit. In offering this type of in-service training, we have been overawed by the percentage of currently employed nurses who are both interested and willing to give the time and effort necessary to assimilate this material, much of which is new to them. Because of this interest, the program has continued on a regular basis.

In undertaking this type of in-service education, we have been impressed by the absence of textbooks or reference manuals covering intensive care, with the exception of Dr. Meltzer's excellent contribution limited to coronary care.

While physicians vary in their treatment of diseases, we feel that certain cardinal procedures are relative to each disease entity. We have attempted to compile these methods in our book in such a manner that they will aid nursing personnel with various levels of formal training who are assisting in the treatment of patients requiring intensive nursing in a community hospital.

We envision that this volume may be beneficial also for in-service education in hospitals that do not have intensive care units, since critical patients are given this same care in various areas in a general hospital. In addition, we hope it may prove advantageous for medical facilities that may wish to incorporate an intensive care unit in their existing structures.

In compiling this information, we have used a format that will allow easy accessibility at the time of need, with each subject discussed further for clarification. In selecting factual material from the wealth of medical information available, our goal has been to present essential information with succinctness and clarity. Since we believe strongly that directions are followed more accurately when there is understanding, we have attempted to give a brief explanation for the mechanisms involved.

We consider this volume to be an introduction to intensive nursing care of the most frequently seen critical conditions. It is in no way an encyclopedia of all illnesses or methods of treatment that may require this kind of care, but we do hope it will present an approach that will be helpful in the majority of situations. Since the very subject itself necessitates further and continual study, it is hoped that this publication may serve as a stimulus and challenge for further learning.

We wish to acknowledge the help of the following physicians on the medical staff of the Baldwin County Hospital, Milledgeville, Georgia: Doctors Edwin W. Allen, Jr., James E. Baugh, Wilbur E. Baugh, A. M. Boddie, Ronald J. Boyd, David Cardosa, William M. Headley, James Hurst, A. C. Martinez, Perry Moore, Wilbur M. Scott, and Curtis F. Veal.

A separate special thanks goes to Dr. Charles B. Fulghum—associate, teacher, and friend—for his immeasurable help in all areas.

Dr. Ralph G. Newton, Macon, Georgia, was of immense help with the chapter on surgery of the urinary tract.

Appreciation is also expressed to Mr. J. W. Singleton, Administrator, and Mrs. Leone Chambliss, Director of Nurses, for their generous support and encouragement. We are indebted to the following nurses in our Intensive Care Unit: Mrs. Agnes Dent, R.N. (especially for her help with Chapter 37), Miss Janet Dominy, R.N., Mrs. Mildred Edwards, R.N., Mrs. Adair Joiner, R.N., and Mrs. Bertha Sherman, L.P.N.

We are also grateful to Mrs. Mildred Durden, R.N., Mrs. Betty Martin, R.N., Mrs. Nettie Ward, R.N., Miss Jean Williams, R.N., and Mr. David Roberson, C.R.N.A. We also appreciate the help of Mr. Linwood Beck from the Georgia Heart Association. Mrs. Sue Brooks was helpful in ways too numerous to mention.

Appreciation is expressed to Miss Mary Pilcher, R.N. for her valued assistance with Chapter 34.

Gratitude is expressed to Mrs. P. J. Neligan and Dr. Ed Dawson for their help in "undangling" our participles, and to Mrs. Vaness Stripling for reading the entire manuscript for typographical errors.

Special appreciation is extended to Mrs. Weona Wright for her excellent illustrations, which greatly enhance the clarity of the book.

Last but by no means least we are grateful to our four fine children: Lee, Nancy, Valerie, and David for their tolerant understanding during the nights and weekends required to complete this manuscript.

Royalties from the sale of this book will be paid to the Baldwin County Hospital Intensive Care Unit Fund, Milledgeville, Georgia.

Zeb L. Burrell, Jr.
Lenette Owens Burrell

Contents

Introduction

Chapter 1

The intensive care unit: philosophy and personnel

PHILOSOPHY

Intensive care of critically ill patients is based on the fact that although there are thousands of pathologic conditions, the mechanism of death is rather uniformly limited to a fairly small number of physiologic events. Basically all medical practice, including all nursing care, is designed to observe and preserve the vital functions of ventilation, circulation, assimilation, and elimination.

In some instances these vital processes may be amenable to control, at least on a temporary basis. Death can be prevented in many situations if time is gained to perform specific therapeutic measures and to allow the recuperative powers of the body to come into play. Recovery, which would have been impossible otherwise, may then sometimes be achieved.

An intensive care unit groups critically ill patients under the care of specially trained staff members who ideally have both the education and the personality to give attention to minute physiologic variations. Intensive nursing care differs from routine nursing care in that the former requires giving careful consideration to and making detailed observations of the processes necessary to life. Some of the nursing care involves what the nurse *does* for the patient, but most of this care is what she *sees* and *hears* and *feels*. By the nurse's early recognition of the subtle changes that may occur with various illnesses, treatment can be begun early, and serious difficulty thus thwarted in many instances.

Many factors must be taken into consideration when one is planning and equipping a unit, such as the need for a unit, the personnel, physical plan, equipment, and supplies. The personnel will be discussed in this chapter, and information regarding the other factors will be presented in Chapter 37.

TRAINING PROGRAM

The most important element in an intensive care unit is not the hardware but what has been referred to as the "software"; this is personnel, especially nursing personnel. In his excellent book on coronary care, Dr. Meltzer suggests that preferable nursing personnel for this type of unit are youthful nurses with degrees with inservice training for coronary care. Although we agree with this in principle, this type of nurse is usually available in meager numbers in the average community hospital. Therefore, staffing of a unit will depend largely on recruitment from currently employed nursing personnel and should include an intensive training program for them.

Since a training program for already employed nursing personnel may appear to be a formidable undertaking, films and teaching aids that may make the task easier are listed at the end of some of the chapters. Such additional training *is* work and requires extra study and preparation on the part of both the instructor and the student, both of whom already have full schedules. However, the results are gratifying. In addition to improvement of the competence of the nursing personnel and creation of a certain esprit de corps, the overall level of medical and nursing care is elevated in the process.

Considered vital to the learning program and to the intensive care unit are adequate reference books that provide parallel reading for better comprehension. Although the selections will vary according to individual preferences, many of the references used for this volume would be helpful.

INTENSIVE CARE NURSE

Because increasing demands are being made on health care personnel at the present time, some areas of responsibility traditionally reserved for the physician are, of necessity, being delegated to other persons. We have found many capable nurses who are willing and eager to learn the material necessary to enable them to assume some of the responsibility that is required in the intensive care situation.

On the other hand, capable nurses are sometimes hesitant to work in an intensive care unit because of a feeling of inadequate knowledge. As encouragement, they need to be reminded that they have been caring for these critical patients in the past in various areas of the hospital, but that now these patients are grouped together where they can be more closely and accurately observed. Too, basic nursing care is similar for all types of patients; and, with initiative, any capable nurse can obtain the additional knowledge needed for competence.

Several characteristics are essential to the good intensive care nurse. Of paramount importance is the possession of both native intelligence and innate curiosity, enabling her to continue to study and progress in the art and science of medicine, especially in extending her own diagnostic and therapeutic skills. There is little place in an intensive care unit for the so-called good nurse who does exactly what is ordered, no more and no less; therefore initiative is a qualification. Age as such is probably not an important factor; on the other hand, good health is considered essential, because nowhere else in nursing are tasks more arduous.

Factors considered most important by us are the possession of emotional stability and empathy. Ideally the intensive care nurse should be quite stable because her almost continuous care of critically ill patients, many of whom are in a dying state, is bound to take an emotional toll. Her empathy as displayed by her reassuring countenance, soft touch, and kind word of explanation to her patients can make an immense contribution to these individuals. Relatives are frequently distraught and especially concerned at their inability to be with the patient during a period of crisis. This situation can be improved rather promptly and with little effort by the nurse who is thoughtful enough to provide the needed reassurance. Certainly people in the critical or dying situation and their families deserve compassion more than in any other situation in the practice of medicine. Nonetheless, compassion and emotions should not be permitted to interfere with good judgment and logic. The nurse who becomes too deeply involved with the patient may find herself unable to render necessary life-saving service in the moment of crisis.

The key to successful operation of the unit, regardless of the quality of the medical staff, is the kind, intelligent, well-informed, and observant nurse. This is true in no other branch of nursing as it is in the intensive care unit.

RELATED FILMS

Mrs. Reynolds needs a nurse. Black and white, 38 minutes, available from Smith, Kline and French Laboratories, 1500 Spring Garden St., Philadelphia, Pa. 19101.

This very good film shows the importance of personalized nursing and the patient's continual need for emotional support.

Intensive care (M-693). Color, 18 minutes, available from National Medical Audiovisual Center (Annex), Chamblee, Ga. 30005, Attn: Film distribution.

This is an excellent introductory film regarding an intensive care unit.

The patient having cardiovascular disease

Chapter 2

Basic anatomy and physiology of the heart

A comprehensive review of the anatomy and physiology of the heart is beyond the scope of this work, but an understanding of certain basic information is essential to rational management of the cardiac patient. Following is a brief review of the circulatory path, the gross anatomy of the heart, and the basic properties of cardiac muscle cells.

ANATOMY OF HEART AND CIRCULATORY PATH

The heart consists of four chambers: the right and left atria and the right and left ventricles (Fig. 2-1). Valves divide the atria and ventricles on each side of the heart and allow blood to flow in only one direction. A septum forms the division between the two atria and the two ventricles. (The atria are frequently referred to as auricles; but in view of the derivation of the term auricle [ear], atria is the preferable term. The term auricle is sometimes used to describe the conical pouch projecting from the upper anterior portion of each atrium.)

The thin-walled atria are low-pressure collecting chambers. Atrial contraction is rather feeble, resulting only in the last few milliliters of ventricular filling. Deoxygenated blood from the body enters the right atrium from the superior and inferior vena cavae, then passes through the tricuspid valve into the right ventricle. Right ventricular contraction produces an increase in pressure only one fourth to one third as great as left ventricular contraction. The decreased need for contractile force is understood when it is recalled that the only purpose of the right ventricle is to propel the blood, by way of the pulmonary arteries, a relatively short distance to the spongy lungs; this propulsion is done against little resistance. After it goes to the lungs for oxygenation and release of carbon dioxide, the blood returns to the left atrium through four pulmonary veins. The blood then passes through the mitral or biscuspid valve into the left ventricle, the most muscular chamber; its contraction propels the blood through the aortic semilunar valve into the aorta and the systemic circulation at a pressure that approximately equals the systolic blood pressure.

Coronary blood supply. The blood supply for the heart itself comes from the first vessels to branch from the aorta: the right and left coronary arteries (Fig. 2-2). These vessels originate in the root of the aortic valve, and each has two

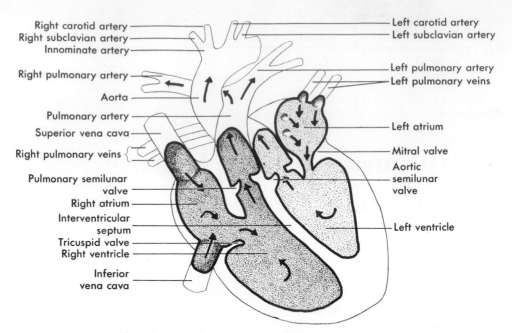

Right carotid artery
Right subclavian artery
Innominate artery

Right pulmonary artery

Aorta

Pulmonary artery
Superior vena cava
Right pulmonary veins {

Pulmonary semilunar valve
Right atrium
Interventricular septum
Tricuspid valve
Right ventricle

Inferior vena cava

Left carotid artery
Left subclavian artery

Left pulmonary artery
Left pulmonary veins

Left atrium

Mitral valve

Aortic semilunar valve

Left ventricle

Fig. 2-1. Schematic representation of heart and great vessel circulation. Blood enters the right atrium from the vena cavae, passes through the tricuspid valve into the right ventricle, then through the pulmonary semilunar valve into the pulmonary artery, and proceeds to the lungs. Blood from the lungs returns to the left artrium through the four pulmonary veins. From the left atrium blood passes through the mitral valve into the left ventricle and then is propelled through the aortic semilunar valve into the aorta and to the body.

Fig. 2-2. Schematic anterior view of the heart.

main branches. The *left coronary artery* divides to form the *anterior descending artery* which supplies arterioles to the left and right ventricles, and the *circumflex artery* which supplies arterioles to the left atrium and left ventricle. The *right coronary artery* divides to form the *posterior descending artery* which supplies arterioles to both left and right ventricles, and the *marginal artery* which supplies arterioles to the right atrium and right ventricle. It is noted that one branch supplies each atrium while three branches supply each ventricle. Although there are few anastomoses between the arteries in the heart, many connections occur between the arterioles. Consequently, if an obstruction occurs in one of the main arteries, blood may still be able to reach the ischemic tissue through this collateral arteriolar circulation. With the passage of time new arterioles develop to provide improved blood supply.

Structure of the heart. Both divisions of the autonomic nervous system have fibers to the heart. The sympathetic or accelerator nerves and parasympathetic or depressor nerves (including vagal fibers) combine to form cardiac plexuses near the aortic arch. These fibers then follow the pathways of the coronary arteries. Most of the fibers terminate in the sino-atrial node, although some end in the atrioventricular node and atrial myocardium.

The *endocardium,* the interior lining of the heart, is composed of a single layer of endothelial cells; these cells are continuous with the arterial and venous intima. The major portion of the heart is composed of cardiac muscle cells or *myocardium.* The exterior surface of the heart is covered with an adherent layer of tissue known as *epicardium,* and the entire heart is enclosed in a loose sac called the *pericardium.* The small space existing between the pericardium and epicardium contains a few drops of lubricating fluid. Since the pericardium is not very extensible, only a small amount of fluid or blood may collect in this space without resulting in cardiac compression or cardiac tamponade.

ABNORMALITIES OF THE HEART

Any abnormality that produces a mechanical interference with the continuity of the chambers produces an additional workload on some portion of the heart. While any valve may be *stenosed,* mitral and aortic stenosis occur most frequently from old rheumatic heart disease. Although any valve may be *regurgitant* or incompetent, again the mitral and aortic valves are far more commonly involved. The former is usually seen as a result of rheumatic heart disease, while the latter is frequently rheumatic or the result of syphilitic aortitis with aneurysmal dilatation. In recent years, however, there has been a marked decline in both rheumatic and syphilitic cardiac damage, a fact due primarily to the control of streptococcal and spirochetal infections resulting from the advent of effective antibiotics in the early 1940's. Because damage was done to their hearts prior to antibiotic therapy, there are still geriatric patients with these conditions.

Certain *congenital abnormalities* may also result in mechanical interference. *Pulmonary stenosis,* a fairly common congenital anomaly, results in hypertrophy of the right ventricle because more work is necessary to force blood through the stenosed valve into the pulmonary artery and then to the lungs. A *defect in the atrial septum* may be asymptomatic, or it may result in a greater workload to ensure adequate oxygenation. An *interventricular septal defect* may result in a leakage of blood from the relatively high-pressure left ventricle to the comparatively low-pressure right ventricle. As a result, the low-pressure ventricle has to propel an extra amount of blood to the lungs repeatedly. This also increases pressure in the pulmonary arterial tree, producing pulmonary hypertension. If the low-pressure right ventricle responds to this strain by hypertrophy to the point of contracting stronger than the left ventricle, a reversal of flow will result so that nonoxygenated blood is mixed with oxygenated blood. The patient will be cyanotic upon exertion.

PROPERTIES OF CARDIAC MUSCLE CELLS

Properties of cardiac muscle cells are such that the cells enable the heart to function in a unique way. These properties include (1) *irritability* or the ability to be stimulated; (2) *contractility* or the ability to shorten when stimulated; (3) *conductivity* or the ability to transmit an impulse; (4) *rhythmicity* or the ability to function with a definite rhythm consisting of stimulation, transmission, contraction, and relaxation; and (5) *automatic action* or a tendency to be self-initiating in the conductivity–contractility–relaxation cycle if no external stimulation is provided.

Certain neuromuscular fibers within the heart are somewhat more specialized for conductivity and automaticity. In the normal heart a very small bundle of fibers, the sino-atrial or *SA node,* is located at the vena caval entrance to the heart. This node is usually the most automatic part of the heart, and the normal cardiac impulse is generated here; hence it is called the pacemaker. From the SA node the impulse is conducted throughout the atrial muscle and the resultant contraction of the atria produces the final few milliliters of ventricular filling. The conducted impulse arrives at the atrioventricular or *AV node*, another small bundle of this same specialized tissue that is somewhat more sensitive to excitation than is adjacent muscle. From this node the impulse is conducted through more specialized fibers that are effective conductors down the *bundle of His*. This bundle divides to form right and left branches and then spreads into a fine network of Purkinje fibers, which underlie the endocardium. These fibers spread into all portions of the ventricles and excite the ventricular myocardium which undergoes a mass contraction, expelling the blood from the heart. The combination of the periods of contraction (depolarization), then rest and recovery (polarization) form the cardiac cycle.

Almost all of the pathologic conditions that give rise to cardiovascular symptoms can be understood in the light of these specialized functions. *Dysfunction of contractility* of the heart muscle produces congestive heart failure that may be either *primary* as myocarditis or inflammation of the cardiac muscle itself, or *secondary* as occlusion to blood flow through a stenosed valve. However, the basic disorder is one of mechanical failure of contractility. The symptoms produced vary greatly, depending on the portion of the heart involved in the dysfunction and the secondary condition contributing to it.

A *dysfunction of irritability,* so that an irritable focus occurs in the heart at some point other than that of normal impulse origin (SA node), accounts for most of the abnormal rhythms. For example, a rapid ectopic focus in the atria may produce atrial flutter, atrial fibrillation (perhaps from multiple ectopic foci), premature atrial contractions, or atrial tachycardia. Nodal extrasystoles and nodal tachycardia result when some portion of the AV node becomes more automatic or irritable than the SA node, so that excitation waves originate from this source before the normal SA impulse. An ectopic focus in an area of ventricular muscle, which has become more irritable than the normal AV node, may produce ventricular extrasystoles, ventricular tachycardia, or ventricular fibrillation, the latter probably from multiple foci.

Failure of conductivity may result in heart block, usually further described by the location of the block. *Sino-atrial block* indicates a blockage at the origin of the impulse and results in standstill. *Atrioventricular block* is a failure of conduction of the impulse from the AV node to the bundle of His and is referred to in degrees, depending basically on the level of the blockage. The so-called *bundle branch block* (BBB) is a failure of conduction in the right or left branch of the bundle of His.

RELATED FILM

Circulation of the blood (EM 211). Color, 8½ minutes, available from state heart association.

This film shows how the heart works, explains the structure of the arteries, and then traces circulation of the blood through the body.

Chapter 3

Acute myocardial infarction

Typical initial orders include

1. Analgesia
2. Slow intravenous infusion
3. Oxygen administration
4. Rest: Fowler's position
5. Frequent check of vital signs
6. Continuous or standby monitoring
7. Hourly check of urine output
8. Administration of tranquilizer
9. Liquid or soft diet
10. Use of anticoagulant
11. Laboratory studies

CLINICAL FINDINGS

The typical patient with a myocardial infarction comes for medical aid with varying degrees of chest pain that is usually described as substernal and perhaps oppressive or squeezing, steady, unrelieved by positional change or eructation, and not fluctuating with respiration. This pain occasionally radiates to the shoulder, elbow, or jaw or seems to go through to the back.

The patient is usually weak, sweaty, and slightly or moderately hypotensive. His color is pale, gray, or cyanotic, and he may be nauseated or vomiting. His pulse is usually rapid, and extrasystoles or other abnormal rhythms may be prominent. Heart sounds may be muffled, and a pericardial friction rub is occasionally present; however the latter is more common several hours after onset. Respiration is usually rapid. The patient is generally quite apprehensive.

PATHOGENESIS

The patient with cardiovascular disease who is most likely to be seen in an intensive care unit is the one suffering from actual acute myocardial infarction or suspected infarction on the basis of coronary artery disease. Since heart disease is the leading cause of death in the United States, a number of epidemiologic and etiologic factors should be mentioned in any review of myocardial infarction.

Some of the elements that have been well documented as playing a role in the etiology of coronary atherosclerosis and subsequent myocardial infarction are the following:

1. The *age* of occurrence of the first coronary occlusion is commonly in the

forties for the male and ten years after menopause for the female, with regular frequency thereafter.

2. A *sex* differential has been noted. The incidence of coronary artery disease is much higher in the male until approximately the sixth or seventh decade, at which time its occurrence in the female approaches that in the male. These differences are thought to be related to the protection afforded the female by estrogenic hormones.

3. *Heredity* seems to be a factor for individuals whose parents or grandparents suffered from arteriosclerotic manifestations, myocardial infarctions, and strokes; they are far more likely to exhibit these maladies than are patients with negative family histories.

4. A *diet* with an abundance of saturated fats and refined sugars has been demonstrated as increasing the incidence of atherosclerosis and subsequent infarction.

5. *Tobacco use,* especially cigarette smoking, has also been rather strongly indicted, while pipe and cigar smoking and tobacco chewing have somewhat less strong positive correlations.

6. A *sedentary occupation* with emphasis on the individual's mental rather than physical activity seems to increase his susceptibility to infarction by comparison with those occupations that require physical labor.

7. *Exercise* seems to protect the individual somewhat from the ravages of this disease when this activity is done on a regular basis, but not when it is done intensely at sporadic intervals. Daily, or almost daily, walking has proven excellent.

8. *Obesity* amounting to 15% or more beyond the ideal weight increases the likelihood of atherosclerotic manifestations; less likely to be affected are those with ideal or slightly lower weight.

9. *Stress,* especially emotional, seems to be a predisposing factor.

10. The presence of *hypertension, diabetes* (even though asymptomatic), and *hyperuricemia* with or without gouty symptoms considerably increases the likelihood of myocardial infarction.

In general usage the terms coronary occlusion, coronary thrombosis, and myocardial infarction are interchanged. Strictly speaking, however, *coronary occlusion* refers to obstruction of the coronary artery, usually by atherosclerosis; *coronary thrombosis* refers to obstruction by thrombus formation. *Myocardial infarction* refers to the necrosis of cardiac muscle deprived of its blood supply that usually, but not always, follows coronary occlusion or coronary thrombosis. The correct term is selected largely on the basis of the location of the damage (whether a main artery or a small tributary) and the collateral circulation. Most infarctions occur in the left ventricle.

Myocardial infarction is an event in a disease continuum rather than a single disease entity. It usually occurs in one of two ways: (1) A patient who has had angina as a symptom of myocardial ischemia experiences a definite change in the pattern of his pain and receives no relief from nitroglycerine or rest or both; or (2) a patient who has had no angina whatsoever typically has sudden persistent chest pain.

The typical patient runs the full gamut in the differential diagnosis of chest pain. Since the thoracic cage and upper abdomen contain many of our vital organs and are innervated by common sources, conditions affecting any of these organs may occasionally mimic myocardial infarction. Examples include spontaneous pneumothorax, pulmonary embolus, perforated peptic ulcer, severe cardiospasm, acute cholecystitis, pericarditis, or pancreatitis. While the physician has the responsibility of making the differental diagnosis, the nurse's keen observations will greatly aid him. When in doubt, the conservative physician usually treats these patients as having had a myocardial infarction until a definite diagnosis can be established.

TREATMENT

1. *Analgesia* is paramount in treatment because the tension and agitation associated with pain also increase the demand for cardiac output and therefore may extend the damage. From 10 to 15 mg. morphine or from 2 to 3 mg. dihydromorphinone (Dilaudid) are usually preferred. These analgesics are generally given in increments at frequent intervals until pain relief is obtained and are then repeated as necessary. If the patient is in excruciating pain, the best mode of administration is intravenous because he may fail to assimilate drugs given by any other route. Recurrence of pain always demands immediate treatment since this discomfort may herald further damage or complications.

Untoward reactions to be noted in regard to analgesia are side effects referable to the digestive tract, such as nausea or vomiting. Since analgesics are depressants, the blood pressure, pulse, and respiration must be watched carefully. This is especially true if a patient in shock begins to assimilate large amounts of the drug; he may then have the symptoms associated with overdosage. Morphine is especially known to be a respiratory depressant; pupils should also be checked for constriction, a sign of increased narcotic effect.

2. *Intravenous fluid* (usually 5% dextrose in water) is begun slowly, primarily to afford ready access to the circulation for medications if abnormal cardiac rhythms or shock or both develop.

3. *Oxygen* is usually given by the most comfortable method available. This alone sometimes significantly reduces the patient's pain; it is generally continued as long as discomfort is present. Although arterial blood is approximately 97% oxygenated, the increase of oxygen in the inspired air may result in 99% oxygenation, which may be enough to make the discomfort and injury less severe. The methods of oxygen administration are discussed on page 97.

4. *Rest* is imperative for reducing cardiac output, and all the patient's movements should be assisted. Fowler's position is usually preferred to aid respiration. Some patients may rest better in the sitting position; chair treatment in the absence of shock is gaining wide acceptance when the patient is lifted in and out of the chair. The use of bedside commodes, when the patient is lifted onto and off the commode, has been demonstrated as requiring less exertion than does use of the bedpan. Stool softeners may be used. The patient should be cautioned against straining during defecation because such straining produces the Valsalva maneuver (forced expiration against a closed glottis). Some patients

have been known to die because this maneuver produces vagal stimulation, and the increased intrathoracic pressure reduces venous return.

The patient is gradually allowed more activity. The nurse should carefully observe the patient's reaction and the effect of activity on his blood pressure, pulse, and respiration. He may begin by doing simple leg exercises, such as flexion and extension of the feet or setting the large leg muscles, to aid in preventing thrombophlebitis. Activity is generally restricted for three months until full scar formation has taken place.

5. *Vital signs* are checked frequently and the pulse observed carefully. Both apical and radial *pulse* should be checked at intervals. The apical beat is usually heard best in the left fifth and sixth intercostal space on a line with the midpoint of the clavicle. Early recognition of changes in the character, rhythm, or rate and prompt treatment may prevent more serious complications. Increasing rate, frequency of abnormal rhythms, premature contractions, or other aberrant rhythms demand prompt therapy.

The *respiratory rate* is watched because an increase may be a forerunner of congestive heart failure fulminating in acute pulmonary edema. A sudden change in rate or character may indicate pulmonary embolism; while decreased respirations may suggest excessive analgesia, as is especially true with morphine.

Blood pressure is checked frequently because it can partially indicate impending shock. While hypotension has been used as the main criterion of shock in the past, it is thought that hypotension in the patient who does not clinically appear to be in shock (skin warm and dry; no tachycardia) probably does not need treatment with pressor agents. Many patients normally have a basal systolic blood pressure of between eighty and ninety. Instead of blood pressure determination alone, fractional hourly urine output may be used as a good criterion for detection of shock as will be mentioned below. However, a gradually declining blood pressure and increasing pulse rate may indicate deterioration and should be reported immediately.

If pressor agents are used, the blood pressure should be checked every 3 to 5 minutes initially, then every 10 to 15 minutes when it appears to be stabilizing. Following this period of initial stabilization, it should be checked at least every hour until these agents are discontinued. Administration of pressor agents should be terminated as soon as the blood pressure is stable, for constriction of renal arterioles may produce renal ischemia.

While *temperature* change is not a major factor in myocardial infarction, there is usually a transient rise on the second or third day. This elevation, ranging from 100° F. to 102° F., is the body's reaction to the toxicity of infarcted muscle. A higher or sustained rise probably indicates complications.

6. *Continuous monitoring* is ordered if the patient appears critically ill, or it may be on a standby basis if the patient seems to be in good condition. Details regarding this subject are presented in Chapter 8.

7. *Hourly urine output* is observed. A gradually falling blood pressure may *suggest* impending shock which may be *confirmed* by decreased urinary output. The rationale is that blood pressure is adequate to prevent cerebral or cardiac damage if the kidneys are able to produce from 20 to 30 ml. of urine per hour.

8. *Tranquilizers* may be helpful since the patient having myocardial infarction is usually quite anxious and frightened. Hydroxyzine (Atarax, Vistaril) may be used for the possible slight protection against arrhythmia that this drug is thought to afford and for the mild tranquilization with little tendency toward inducing hypotension. Tranquilizers may also help to allay the depression usually evident around the third day after the infarction.

9. *Diet* usually begins with low-salt liquids or soft foods to reduce the work load in chewing. It is probably best to limit free salt as an aid in avoiding congestive failure. Hot, iced, and spiced foods are avoided because of the possibility of induction of abnormal rhythms by marked temperature changes in the esophagus or stomach. Stimulants, such as tea and coffee, are usually omitted initially. The marginal patient may require feeding, and care must be taken not to hurry. A diet restricted in calories is ordered if the patient is overweight. Many of these patients with myocardial infarction are also found to be diabetic.

10. Use of *anticoagulants,* which may be begun in the absence of contraindications, is usually initiated and maintained with heparin sodium dosages given at 6- to 8-hour intervals for from 24 to 36 hours or until adequate clotting time prolongation is achieved. Anticoagulation may then be maintained with oral coumarin derivatives or similar types of drugs. The dosage is adjusted so that the patient's prothrombin time is two to three times that of the control.

11. *Laboratory studies* of diagnostic significance usually include serial electrocardiograms, serial SGOT or CPK and LDH or HBD determinations, sedimentation rate, and complete blood count.

Although the *electrocardiogram* may show changes immediately, it may not indicate change for a period of days and may occasionally never show a diagnostic pattern in the presence of certain infarction. The electrocardiogram is also a valuable diagnostic tool in recording evolving changes and may be of assistance in determining the extent of damage; it is also the final authority on abnormal rhythms.

Several enzymes are present in cardiac tissue cells. As a result of cell injury these enzymes may leak into the circulation. Determination of serum levels of some of these enzymes may help to establish the existence of tissue damage. The following enzyme studies have been helpful in confirming the tentative diagnosis of myocardial necrosis:

SGOT (serum glutamic oxalacetic transaminase) has a delay of several hours following tissue death before it appears in the blood in significant levels. A period of 8, 12, or even 24 hours may be necessary for a significant transaminase rise; then it usually returns to normal within three or four days. The *CPK* (creatinine phosphokinase) is another cardiac muscle enzyme with a release pattern similar to that of SGOT.

LDH (lactic dehydrogenase) has a greater time lag and its level tends to remain elevated longer (from two days to one week); therefore, this test may be helpful for the patient who is not seen early in the course of his illness. *HBD* (hydroxybutyric dehydrogenase) is released similarly to LDH.

The *complete blood count* usually shows an elevated white blood cell count with elevation in polymorphonuclear leukocytes, especially when the count is taken several hours after the injury. This reflects the body's reaction to inflammation.

The rise of the *sedimentation rate* after the second day is another nonspecific indication of inflammation and somewhat parallels the temperature curve.

The remainder of treatment consists of watching for complications and treating the patient promptly as well as attempting to prevent extension of damage. Nursing observation is of supreme importance since the early treatment of complications is far more successful than is later therapy.

COMPLICATIONS

The common acute complications of myocardial infarction are *abnormal rhythms, congestive failure, thromboembolism, extension, shock,* and *cardiac rupture.* Treatments of varying efficacy are available for all of these conditions except rupture, which is fatal. The first three complications will be discussed in the following chapters.

Extension of an original infarct may be noted at any time following the initial episode. It may be indicated by recurrence of pain, fever, clinical deterioration, electrocardiographic changes, and recurrence of enzyme abnormalities.

Shock is one of the dreaded complications. Its symptoms include hypotension with reduced pulse pressure; tachycardia with weak, thready pulse; pallor or cyanosis; cold clammy skin; decreasing urinary output; and symptoms of cerebral anoxia. The latter may be manifest as confusion, delirium, anxiety, hypomania, apathy, or unconsciousness.

Shock in the patient with myocardial infarction is probably the result of several factors that may be of varied importance in the individual patient. Therefore, an elastic therapeutic approach lacking the exactness that may be used in other complications is required. Prolonged shock is a poor prognostic sign, and every effort should be undertaken to relieve it promptly. The recovery rate after 12 hours of shock is only approximately 20%.

Shock may originate from the central nervous system as the body's response to pain and may respond to the simple expedient of adequate pain relief. It may result from decreased cardiac output due to the decrease in myocardial contractile power and stroke volume. In this situation, the shock may respond to vasopressor drugs that produce vasoconstriction of peripheral vessels. Because this vasoconstriction is less marked in coronary and cerebral arteries than in other peripheral arteries, coronary and cerebral perfusion is improved. Since vasopressor drugs are similar to epinephrine, they are capable of inducing abnormal cardiac rhythms.

Levarterenol (Levophed) is such a potent vasoconstrictor that it can be given only intravenously. Subcutaneous administration results in ischemic death of tissue due to this same mechanism of vasoconstriction. When an intravenous infusion containing levarterenol inadvertently infiltrates the tissue, prompt multiple injections of phentolamine (Regitine), a vasodilator, into the infiltrated area may neutralize the vasoconstricting effect and prevent development of a necrotic slough.

Myocardial power failure with decreased stroke volume and shock may respond to rapid digitalization or isoproterenol (Isuprel) since both increase contractile force.

Prolonged shock in myocardial infarction may occasionally be the result of acute adrenal insufficiency (adrenal hemorrhage or adrenal anoxia?); therefore, adrenal steroids should be added to the treatment of any patient with acute myocardial infarction and prolonged shock.

RELATED FILMS

Arteriosclerosis. Color, 13½ minutes, available from state heart association.

The film explains atherosclerosis graphically and portrays what happens when it develops.
Myocardial infarction: The nurse's role. Black and white, 42 minutes, available from state heart association.

The film demonstrates nursing care involved for a patient with a myocardial infarction.

Chapter 4

Congestive heart failure

Typical initial orders include

1. Digitalis
2. Diuretic
3. Low-salt diet
4. Rest in bed and chair
5. Fluid intake and output; daily weight
6. Use of anticoagulant
7. Frequent check of vital signs
8. Administration of oxygen if needed

CLINICAL FINDINGS

The typical patient with congestive heart failure or cardiac decompensation is one known to have cardiovascular disease. He gradually notices fatigue, pedal edema, especially toward the end of the day, weight gain, and exertional and nocturnal dyspnea. He may also complain of orthopnea and have a hacking cough with production of mucoid sputum.

On examination the patient may show any or all of the following signs: tachycardia, shortness of breath, engorged veins, pedal or presacral edema, hepatomegaly, and ascites.

PATHOGENESIS

Congestive heart failure can be considered in two categories: (1) acute congestive failure with sudden onset, usually appearing as acute pulmonary edema, which will be discussed separately in Chapter 5; and (2) chronic congestive failure with a more gradual onset.

Chronic congestive heart failure may be seen in any type of heart disease; statistically in the United States it is probably most common in arteriosclerotic or hypertensive heart disease. The patient may have been previously barely compensated and had some unusual strain or load imposed, producing congestive heart failure. For example, he may have additional heart damage, such as a recent myocardial infarction, a mild intercurrent respiratory infection, a febrile illness, or a small pulmonary embolus; or he may have consumed extra salt.

The heart subjected to strain over a period of weeks or months compensates for the extra work load by hypertrophy. If the heart is unable to effectively pump blood from the venous to the arterial circulation, the resulting increased venous pressure causes increased ventricular filling and stretching. This extension

21

of the myocardial fibers results in a stronger contraction, up to a point (Starling's law) at which hypertrophy is effective and compensation is maintained. Beyond this point, increased stretching results in a less strong contraction with the only avenue of increasing cardiac output being to increase the rate. This results in a vicious cycle. The increased rate produces a decreased ventricular diastole with inadequate time for ventricular filling, which is largely a passive process; hence, impaired output.

With venous congestion, extra fluid remains in the interstitial tissues and produces edema which may be noted in the legs, peritoneal cavity, and liver; or it may be generalized and produce anasarca. When the edema is present in the interstitial lung tissues, it produces shortness of breath; if it escapes into the alveoli or bronchioles, it causes a hacking cough productive of mucoid sputum. Extra fluid may also collect in the pleural cavity, producing pleural effusion.

TREATMENT

1. *Digitalis* is the mainstay of treatment for the patient with congestive heart failure in the absence of refractory failure precipitated by digitalis intoxication. If the patient is conversant, he is questioned regarding previous digitalis therapy. If he has not previously been digitalized, the drug is usually administered in fractional doses, full digitalization being achieved in a matter of two or three days, occasionally in 24 hours. Digitalis therapy is generally considered to be satisfactory when the pulse rate ranges in the 80's and 90's in comparison with pretreatment rates of 100+. The decreasing pulse rate is usually associated with diuresis and weight loss.

Administration of digitalis is more leisurely for this patient than for one with acute pulmonary edema. The oral route of administration is frequently used (for example, gitalin [Gitaligin] 0.1 mg. every four hours) with the rhythm and rate checked before each dose. As soon as the pulse rate begins to drop, the frequency of administration is decreased, and the dosage is regulated until a maintenance dose is achieved.

Any time digitalis preparations are given, the nursing personnel should watch for symptoms of toxicity as mentioned on page 271.

2. A *diuretic* medication is usually instituted concurrently with digitalis therapy. Meralluride (Mercuhydrin) is an excellent diuretic for this type patient in the absence of known kidney damage or elevation of blood urea nitrogen. It is usually administered in single 1 ml. intramuscular doses and may be repeated as necessary. The patient should be warned that the drug stings when administered.

The thiazide diuretics function quite adequately when administered by mouth. However, thiazide-induced diuresis and concomitant digitalis administration predispose the patient to the development of digitalis intoxication because the hypokalemia induced by thiazide diuresis potentiates the digitalis. See page 185 for signs of hypokalemia.

Ethacrynic acid (Edecrin) and furosemide (Lasix) are prompt-acting diuretics that may be administered by mouth. In the refractory case, combinations of diuretics may be necessary to achieve adequate reduction of water load.

During her care of the patient, the nurse should note edema, especially in pedal or presacral areas.

3. *Diet* has been a much neglected area in the management of refractory congestive heart failure since the advent of potent diuretics. For the patient whose situation is difficult to control, the addition of a low-sodium diet to the therapeutic regimen is in order. In order to gain the patient's cooperation, it may be wiser to restrict salty foods, such as ham and potato chips, and suggest that he add no salt to his food at the table rather than place him on a very strict low-sodium diet.

4. *Rest* brought about by mild sedation or tranquilization is good treatment for the patient with chronic congestive failure. Rest in bed may be alternated with chair rest with limited ambulation. Initially the patient breathes best in Fowler's position, and he is generally pleased when he is able to gradually lower the head of the bed.

5. *Fluid intake and output* and *daily weight* records are kept to aid in ascertaining diuresis.

6. Use of *anticoagulants* is surrounded by considerable controversy concerning their effectiveness in the prevention of recurrent myocardial infarction. However, their use in the patient with chronic congestive failure is uniformly accepted on the basis of the patient's propensity for venous thrombosis or subsequent embolic episodes because of sluggish venous circulation and venous engorgement. In this situation anticoagulation should be promptly instituted and maintained until adequacy of circulation is well reestablished.

7. *Vital signs* should be checked frequently, especially the pulse and respiration, because they aid in determining the degree of failure. The pulse is also used to indicate digitalis effect. Respiration is noted often to determine the degree of dyspnea. A cough that becomes more frequent or more productive may indicate approaching pulmonary edema. Distention of the neck veins, which should empty when the patient is in the sitting position, should be noted.

8. Administration of *oxygen* may or may not be necessary, depending upon the degree of dyspnea and cyanosis.

Attention must also be paid to the etiologic form of heart disease underlying the failure. For example, hypertensive heart disease demands treatment of the hypertension as well as of the failure; subacute bacterial endocarditis requires antibiotic therapy in addition to treating the failure.

RELATED FILM

Congestive heart failure (EM 266). Color, 8 minutes, available from state heart association. Causes, symptoms, and physiologic background of congestive heart failure are discussed briefly.

Chapter 5

Acute pulmonary edema

Typical initial orders include

1. Analgesia
2. Digitalization
3. Diuretic
4. Fowler's position
5. Oxygen administration
6. Rotating tourniquets
7. Phlebotomy
8. Use of anticoagulant
9. Bronchodilator
10. Respiratory detergents
11. Frequent check of vital signs
12. Low-salt liquids
13. Electrolyte studies

CLINICAL FINDINGS

Acute pulmonary edema is one of the most frequently encountered medical emergencies. The patient, who experiences extreme respiratory distress, may sit with his arms extended away from his body so that he can make maximal use of his accessory muscles of respiration. He is extremely apprehensive and is perspiring profusely, and he may be cyanotic; his neck veins are distended, his blood pressure may be elevated, and his pulse is rapid. There are audible rales, and his rapid respiratory rate is interrupted by frequent episodes of coughing which produces copious amounts of frothy, perhaps blood-tinged, sputum.

PATHOGENESIS

Pulmonary edema is a clinical syndrome rather than a disease entity of itself and is most frequently seen in patients having or suspected of having heart disease. It is congestive heart failure in its extreme. The number of rheumatic and syphilitic patients has declined rather markedly since antibiotic therapy has become available; thus, at the present time, the majority of patients with pulmonary edema are afflicted with arteriosclerotic heart disease. In these patients, the pulmonary edema is more likely to occur at night or in the very early hours of the morning, for the recumbent position serves to mobilize the dependent edema that has previously collected in the lower portions of the body. This extra fluid increases the circulating blood volume; and if the heart is unable to cope with this added fluid so that the left ventricle cannot pump it to the body, the fluid collects in the lungs and then escapes into the spongy tissue.

Frequently, pulmonary edema may be an early manifestation of myocardial infarction or a later evidence of arteriosclerotic heart disease. In the latter, it may be coupled with some other respiratory or cardiac strain, such as influenza or an excessive salt load.

In the absence of demonstrable heart disease, pulmonary edema occurs in the surgical or otherwise traumatized patient whose blood losses have been over-estimated, and whose circulation has been inadvertently overloaded with excessive intravenous fluids during operating room or emergency room treatment. Such edema can also occur with the critically ill obstetric patient. Pulmonary embolism is frequently another factor precipitating acute pulmonary edema, as is the inhalation of irritants.

TREATMENT

1. *Analgesia* is needed for treatment; and morphine in a dose of from 10 to 15 mg. is the drug of choice, for it is effective in reducing anxiety, relieving pain, depressing respiration, and lessening the required cardiac output.

2. In the absence of prior *digitalization,* a full digitalizing dose of a rapid-acting form of digitalis is indicated when pulmonary edema is caused by congestive heart failure. From one half to three fourths of the full digitalizing dose may be administered initially and may be followed by fractional doses at later intervals of from one to three or four hours, depending on the patient's condition. These doses should be administered intravenously, the only reliable way to be certain of effective amount available since some degree of shock may be present.

When any form of digitalis is administered, the nurse should watch for symptoms of toxicity (see page 271).

3. Mercurial *diuretics* have been used for a long time in the treatment of pulmonary edema, and these, too, may be given intravenously. Since onset of diuresis is moderate, one of the newer agents, such as ethacrynic acid (Edecrin), which has a more rapid onset might be preferable.

4. *Fowler's position,* or any upright position, is very important because this patient cannot lie flat. Gravity causes the excessive body fluid to collect in the most dependent portions of the body, and the recumbent position adds to the patient's distress. The upright position also allows gravitational pull on the abdominal contents. Elevating the head of the bed to a 60°, 75°, or even 90° angle gives back support; pillows supporting both arms away from the body may also further aid increased ventilation.

If the patient feels he can breathe better leaning forward with his arms elevated, he could rest his head and arms on the overbed table covered with pillows. If he thinks he can breathe easier while sitting on the side of the bed or in a chair, permit him to do so. Positions in which the legs are dependent may also aid in removing edema from the thoracic area by transferring it to the legs. Any constricting clothing should be loosened.

5. *Oxygen* by any route of administration that will not create further anxiety

Fig. 5-1. The Jobst automatic rotating tourniquet. (Courtesy Jobst Institute, Inc., Toledo, Ohio.)

in an already apprehensive patient is good treatment, for this patient has difficulty in oxygenating blood through the alveolar-capillary membrane when many of the alveoli are filled with fluid. When one is giving oxygen, insisting on a mode of administration that seems to increase the patient's fright probably does more harm than good. In view of the variety of methods of oxygen administration available, several should be tried until the most suitable one is found. Various methods of administration are discussed in Chapter 13.

It is extremely important that the nurse explain to the patient what she is planning to do before she performs a procedure, because he is already frightened and the thought that he is dying is probably uppermost in his mind. Therefore, before administering oxygen by any method, the nurse should quietly tell him what she will be doing and should state that this will make him breathe easier.

6. *Rotating tourniquets* or bloodless phlebotomy serves to decrease the circulating blood volume by entrapment of fluid in the extremities. This may gain time needed for additional definitive measures. A rotating tourniquet machine is ideal (Fig. 5-1). It makes use of four pneumatic cuffs that are inflated; the desired pressure is set at approximately the patient's diastolic pressure. The machine has an automatic timer that releases one cuff and inflates another cuff at set intervals, recommended at five minutes.

Fig. 5-2. Rotating tourniquets showing position of tourniquets with passage of time.

Four sphygmomanometer cuffs are the next best equipment, but four tourniquets and padding, such as abdominal pads, for preventing tissue damage may be used.

The tourniquets are placed as high on each extremity as possible, and initially three (or all four) are tied. In order to produce only venous stasis and not completely occlude the arterial vessels, the tourniquets are tightened so that the nurse's finger can be placed between the tourniquet and the padding. As a further check, the arterial pulse should still be felt in the tied extremity. Within from 5 to 15 minutes the fourth tourniquet is tied and an adjacent one is released; they are subsequently retied and released in the same clockwise or couterclockwise rotating manner.

In order to minimize the release of fluid to the circulatory system, it is advisable to tie off the fourth extremity before releasing the third extremity. As the patient improves and the tourniquets are released, the same caution is observed by releasing only one at a time rather than all three simultaneously (Fig. 5-2).

As was noted, the time for rotation may vary from 5 to 15 minutes, depending on the physician's orders. Some prefer the former because of the patient's increased susceptibility to venous thrombosis and subsequent pulmonary embolism, while others prefer the latter since the personnel are busy performing other duties for the patient.

7. *Phlebotomy* is another physical measure that is of some usefulness. This is specific treatment for pulmonary edema caused by fluid or blood overload and is sometimes quite worthwhile, regardless of the etiology of the pulmonary edema. However, it should be mentioned that this treatment should be used with caution, for it can precipitate circulatory collapse when it is accompanied by profound diuresis.

8. Use of *anticoagulants* is considered by some physicians to be strongly indicated because of the patient's increased susceptibility to venous thrombosis from venous congestion and the use of tourniquets, in addition to the added danger of pulmonary emboli. Anticoagulants may be used on a temporary basis.

Rapid anticoagulation is best obtained by the parenteral administration of heparin sodium with average doses of 10,000 units every six to eight hours as determined by periodic results of the clotting time. Continued anticoagulation is usually achieved with coumarin derivatives in doses controlled by prothrombin time determinations. Note the precautions regarding use of anticoagulants on page 265.

9. A *bronchodilator,* such as theophylline or aminophylline, is sometimes administered very slowly intravenously (not more than 20 mg. per minute due to its hypotensive effect). The effect of theophylline, while rather prompt in onset, is very short lived, but the 15 to 20 minute relief of associated bronchospasm afforded by this agent may be worthwhile.

10. *Respiratory detergents* designed to reduce the surface tension of the bronchial secretions and to decrease the effort required to clear the air passages of these materials may be helpful. The addition of from 20% to 50% ethyl alcohol to the oxygen humidifier in gradually increasing concentrations has proved effective. Other medications may be administered by nebulizer.

11. *Vital signs* should be checked frequently because they reflect the patient's progress or deterioration and his reaction to the various drugs administered.

12. *Low-salt liquids* may be given, for this patient becomes thirsty soon after he begins improving.

13. *Electrolyte studies* should be done because this patient is subjected to both severe metabolic stress and potent diuretic therapy, and electrolyte abnormalities are common.

Treatment of acute pulmonary edema in a patient seen for the first time is one of the most gratifying in medicine. It is frequently possible for a patient near death to progress to reasonably good condition and be well on his way to recovery within a matter of 2 or 3 hours. However, this patient must be watched closely during the later hours for deterioration of his progress, therefore the treatment is tailored from hour to hour.

Chapter 6

Thromboembolism

INTRODUCTION

Thromboembolism is a condition or complication that may frequently afflict patients in the intensive care setting. Although it is occasionally a primary condition with underlying atherosclerosis on the arterial side or varicosities on the venous side, it is most frequently a complication of some primary condition.

The predisposing factors are myriad, including sluggish circulation coincident with any debilitating disease, the febrile state, hypovolemia, or surgical procedures. Traumatic or mechanical factors that impede either venous or arterial circulation, such as abdominal distention, constricting clothing, or tight dressings, may lead to embolism. Other contributing factors may include diabetes, obesity, or any cardiovascular disease.

Critical observation is necessary to detect thromboembolism because the condition may be almost unapparent, or it may be overwhelming and produce intense symptomatology. In the latter situation, the primary origin or condition may be largely obscured.

The symptomatology produced by thromboembolic disease will depend on the location of the obstruction to blood flow and on collateral circulation. Following is a discussion of and treatment rationale for some of the more common thromboembolic disorders.

Pulmonary embolus

Typical initial orders include

1. Analgesia
2. Oxygen administration
3. Use of anticoagulant
4. Antibiotic
5. Antispasmodic
6. Dextran intravenously
7. Sedation
8. Frequent check of vital signs
9. Laboratory studies

CLINICAL FINDINGS

The classic patient having pulmonary embolus will develop sudden knifelike chest pain which produces severe dyspnea. Within a few hours or as long as two or three days later, he usually develops a moderately productive cough and the sputum is frequently blood tinged. Both his temperature and white blood cell count are usually elevated because of the inflammation.

The typical example of pulmonary embolus is the exception rather than the rule. Patients who have been ill from numerous conditions have been seen whose only symptomatology pointing to the pulmonary embolus was a decline in their general condition; they have seemed to be progressing satisfactorily with no apparent cause for their deterioration. Several patients' only manifestation was intense anxiety and slight tachycardia. Pulmonary emboli may be the cause of a temperature spike in a convalescing patient.

PATHOGENESIS

Pulmonary embolism is probably the least frequently diagnosed major complication encountered in general hospital medical and surgical practice, and it is the cause of the sudden death of many patients. Significant pulmonary embolism has been present in as high as 20% of some autopsy series and was frequently unrecognized clinically.

A pulmonary embolus is usually a complication of phlebothrombosis in the deep veins of the leg or pelvis, but the symptomatology may point so overwhelmingly to the chest that the primary site may not be detected even after a diligent search. Fatty emboli from bone marrow may occur during realignment of fractures. The symptoms of a patient with a classic pulmonary embolus closely resemble those of one with a typical myocardial infarction with the exception of a pleuritic component to the chest pain which interferes with normal respiration. In addition, on physical examination abnormal breath sounds may be heard over the involved area of lung. The intensity of symptomatology will vary with the magnitude of pulmonary infarction. The condition should always be considered in the differential diagnosis of chest pain.

The diagnosis of pulmonary embolism associated with the less severe illness taxes the diagnostic acumen of the physician, although the classic case offers no diagnostic problem. Diagnosis is greatly aided by a high index of suspicion if the patient's condition is deteriorating and he is known to be predisposed to the disease. Recognition of pulmonary embolism is important because it is frequently repetitive, and every effort should be made to prevent its recurrence or extension.

Before one considers treatment, a review of prophylactic measures is in order. Early ambulation for the operative and the postpartum patient has probably served to reduce thromboembolic complications more than any other single measure. The use of nonobstructive stirrups for the obstetric and gynecologic patient has also been advantageous. Frequent change of positions and exercise of the legs, even though passive, seems to help in both medical and surgical patients. Because of the danger of emboli, legs should never be massaged and no pillows should be placed directly under the knees, since the popliteal vein is superficial in this area. To reduce the danger of embolism, some surgeons order that their patients who have varicose veins have both legs wrapped to the groin before any surgery.

TREATMENT

1. *Analgesia* with an adequate narcotic seems to relieve a great deal of the associated bronchospasm and arterial spasm.

2. *Oxygen* may be used to increase the concentration of oxygen in the inspired air.

3. *Anticoagulants* should be used immediately for they may limit propagation of thrombosis in the affected pulmonary vasculature and prevent extension or recurrence of thrombosis in the primary site by way of reducing platelet destruction and serotonin release. Sodium heparin is the drug of choice; the usual administration to adults is 10,000 units intravenously. This is followed by intermittent subcutaneous or intravenous administration every six to eight hours, with dosage determined by the clotting time, or until coumarin derivatives adequately prolong prothrombin time.

4. An *antibiotic* is usually given to try to prevent the occurrence of pneumonia at the site of infarction.

5. An *antispasmodic* may aid in the relief of bronchospasm.

6. *Dextran* given intravenously may be used, presumably for altering platelets and intimal adhesion to reduce thrombotic tendency.

7. *Sedation* is necessary to relieve the patient's apprehension and encourage rest.

8. *Vital signs* are checked frequently; their alteration may be the first evidence of deterioration signalling the need for further treatment.

Complications that might occur are similar to those that might follow a myocardial infarction. These include extension of the infarction, shock, congestive heart failure, pulmonary edema, and pneumonia. The treatment regimen is the same as that usually prescribed for each of those conditions.

9. *Laboratory studies* include clotting time determinations to control heparin therapy and prothrombin time measurements to regulate coumarin treatment. The serum enzymes, such as SGOT and LDH, may be helpful for differential diagnosis. A complete blood count, urinalysis, roentgenogram of chest, and electrocardiogram also need to be done. Occasionally special studies are performed, such as lung scans and pulmonary arteriography.

Thrombophlebitis

Typical initial orders include

1. Elevation of patient's leg	4. Use of anticoagulant
2. Analgesia	5. Antibiotic
3. Bed rest	6. Dextran intravenously

Thrombophlebitis is seen in patients in the intensive care unit as a complication of other conditions. The chief concern regarding this condition is that it may be the possible forerunner of pulmonary emboli; however, it is a critical condition in itself in advanced cases.

CLINICAL FINDINGS

The typical patient having thrombophlebitis experiences mild or moderate calf, ankle, and foot discomfort with edema of the leg and warmth over the inflamed area. The leg may appear mottled, and there will be pain on compression or stretching, as with dorsiflexion of the foot (Homan's sign). Systemic reactions include fever, nausea, and anorexia. In severe cases the pain may be extreme if it is associated with arterial spasm; since this spasm decreases the blood supply, the limb may be cool and pale. As a generalization, the more severe the local symptoms, the less likely embolism.

In thrombophlebitis a clot forms which attaches to the intima; as this enlarges it occludes the vessel, thus producing the symptoms just mentioned. If the vein is superficial it is usually palpable, reddened, tender, and usually less likely to produce embolism.

TREATMENT

Treatment is directed toward arresting the condition while the natural fibrolytic forces destroy or recannulate the thrombus.

1. The *leg is elevated* to aid in improving venous return. Some physicians favor the use of a lighted cradle over the leg to improve circulation, while others order warm moist packs. The leg is *never* massaged, and the affected leg or perhaps both legs may be wrapped snugly with elastic bandages.

2. *Analgesia* is used as required; except in severe cases, one-half grain codeine or the equivalent is adequate. Acetyl salicylic acid (aspirin) should not be given with the codeine if the patient is receiving anticoagulants since this drug tends to potentiate the effect of the anticoagulants.

3. *Bed rest* is usually ordered, although physicians disagree on this point. Some think exercise increases the likelihood of producing embolism; others allow exercise in the affected leg to improve circulation and possibly lessen the likelihood of extension.

4. *Anticoagulation* is begun with heparin and followed by coumarin drugs; page 265 provides further reference.

5. An *antibiotic* may be ordered in a few cases in which the phlebitis appears to be precipitated by an infection of a portion of the extremity.

6. *Dextran* may be given intravenously for the purposes mentioned on page 31.

In the rare severe patient, parasympathetic block and large doses of strong analgesics may be required to relieve pain and associated arterial spasm. Surgical interruption of the inferior vena cava may be indicated if conservative treatment fails to prevent recurrent pulmonary emboli. Occasionally thrombectomy is attempted as a direct surgical approach for the patient with severe phlebitis.

Arterial thromboembolic disease

Arterial thromboembolic disease is most commonly seen as a manifestation of arteriosclerotic obstruction to a peripheral artery; this obstruction is the most common mechanism of strokes involving the cerebral or cervical arteries. Thrombotic occlusion of a peripheral artery may occur in any situation in which there is a temporary decrease in blood pressure or blood volume or in which there are factors predisposing one to thrombosis.

With the exception of strokes (see page 148), the most common sites of arterial thrombo-occlusive disease are the lower limbs. The occlusion may be very gradual in its onset as in arteriosclerotic aorto-iliac occlusion, or the Leriche syndrome. When gradual in onset, it is gradual in the production of symptoms.

When occlusion is sudden, there is abrupt production of symptoms. This may result from systemic embolization originating from a mural thrombus following a myocardial infarction. It is also a common complication of abnormal cardiac rhythms, especially chronic atrial fibrillation, because the lack of effective atrial contraction results in poor emptying and stagnation in the auricular appendages, especially the left; this stagnation predisposes the patient to thrombosis.

SYMPTOMS

Symptoms include increasing claudication and decreasing pulsations in the affected lower extremities. The intensity of symptoms is frequently directly related to the rapidity of developing occlusion. The patient who has severe acute onset with pain and pallor in the extremity may be aided by prompt endarterectomy and removal of the thrombus from the affected area. Of interest is the fact that the occlusion is usually at least one segment higher than the symptomatology indicates.

TREATMENT

Typical treatment of the Leriche syndrome is surgical endarterectomy, grafting, or sympathectomy when possible. This surgery is usually followed by long-term use of anticoagulants and vasodilators, although there is still some question as to the efficacy of both forms of drug therapy.

Thromboembolic disease of the mesenteric vessels, usually caused by atherosclerosis, is occasionally recognized when it occurs suddenly with obvious development of an acute surgical abdomen. It is possible for this disease to afflict any patient with the predisposing factors.

The renal arteries may occasionally be involved by thromboembolic occlusive disease, producing an acute situation. If there is complete or almost total occlusion, surgery will be required to accomplish an emergency renal endarterectomy or nephrectomy; this is necessary because of the toxicity and likelihood of producing reflex kidney shutdown in the unaffected kidney.

Thrombotic disease of peripheral arteries originates most commonly in association with arteriosclerotic plaques or subintimal hemorrhage. As mentioned previously, embolic occlusion of peripheral arteries also occurs as a complication of mural thrombosis, or the formation of a clot on the wall of the endocardium in an area of injury to the lining intima of the heart. This is a fairly common complication of myocardial infarction. That surgery and embolectomy are required when the origin is a mural thrombus following a coronary occlusion is a matter of delicate decision. The possibility of subjecting an already critically ill patient to a surgical procedure is weighed against the possible relief of complications by surgical removal.

In summary, the nurse's observations are a key factor as she performs her care of the patient, for she may notice signs that frequently forewarn of serious thromboembolic conditions. Such signs include a rising pulse rate, increasing dyspnea, the occurrence of edema (especially unilateral edema), or the detection of a tender calf during bathing. In addition, the presence of a pulse differential, of small amounts of blood in the sputum, or of slightly bloody or smoky urine are all possible harbingers of danger, and observations made by the astute nurse may lead to early treatment.

Chapter 7

Basic electrocardiography

P Wave: produced by atrial contraction. Normally 0.1 to 0.2 millivolt in amplitude, 0.08 to 0.12 second in duration.

P-R Interval: onset of P wave to onset of QRS, includes atrial depolarization and transmission of impulse through AV node. Isolectric portion drawn during nodal transmission. Normally 0.12 to 0.20 second.

QRS Complex: represents ventricular contraction. Normally the sharpest deflection in the EKG. Q wave normally negative, R wave normally upright; S wave is terminal negative wave. Deflection varies with lead, electrode placement, chest wall thickness, and ventricular muscle mass. Normally 0.04 to 0.10 second duration.

ST Segment: normally isoelectric representing refractory period of ventricular muscle mass.

T Wave: represents ventricular repolarization. Varies considerably in duration and amplitude, usually upright in most leads.

Q-T Interval: measured from onset of QRS complex to end of T wave; represents time of ventricular depolarization and recovery. Normally less than 0.40 second.

U Wave: inconstant deflection following T wave; of little significance.

A detailed review of electrocardiography is not possible in this volume; nevertheless, some understanding of the elements of electrocardiogram production is essential to the electronic monitoring of patients with potential or existing abnormal cardiac rhythms (Fig. 7-1). Since arrhythmias have widely overlapping clinical findings, the electrocardiogram is the final authority in their correct diagnosis.

For the standard diagnostic electrocardiogram, twelve leads are taken which are used to mirror electrical activity of the heart from different spatial locations. From the aspect of study of abnormal rhythms, a single lead is sufficient; lead 2 is customarily used for this study, but any lead that shows the desired components of the electrocardiogram may be used successfully. At times one lead will show various components better than another.

MEASUREMENT

The standard electrocardiogram is a very sensitive voltmeter that records the changes in the electrical activity in the heart. It is calibrated so that a 1 cm. vertical deflection indicates an electrical charge of 1 mv. (ten small squares on standard electrocardiographic paper or two large squares). The tracing is drawn at such a speed that each large division represents 0.20 second and each small division equals 0.04 second. There is a slight time lag between electric activation and muscular contraction.

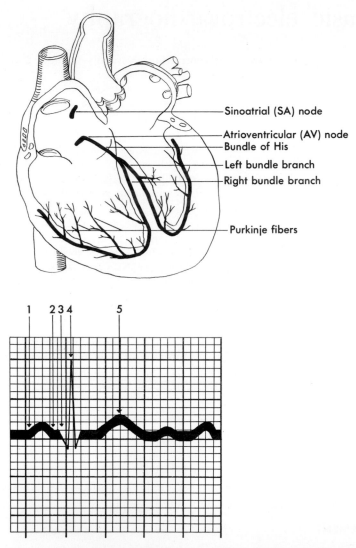

Fig. 7-1. Cardiac conduction system. **1 to 2,** The impulse originates at the SA node and spreads through the atria; atrial contraction produces the **P** wave. **2 to 3,** Impulse arrives at the AV node and is delayed in passage through the bundle of His, producing the isoelectric portion of the P-R interval. **3,** The impulse passing into the bundle branches activates the left portion of the interventricular septum, producing the first negative deflection of the QRS complex. **4,** Ventricular depolarization produces the major portion of the QRS complex. **5,** Ventricular repolarization produces the T wave.

Fig. 7-2. Basic components of the electrocardiogram.

COMPOSITION OF THE NORMAL ELECTROCARDIOGRAM

The normal electrocardiogram is composed of a P wave, P-R interval, QRS complex, ST segment, T wave, and inconstant U wave (Fig. 7-2).

The *P wave*, produced by activation of the atrial muscle, is normally approximately symmetric, usually upright (in lead 2), usually from 0.08 to 0.12 second in duration, and usually only 0.1 or 0.2 mv. in amplitude.

The *P-R interval* includes the P wave and the normally isoelectric interval transcribed during the period of time of activation of the AV node. It is normally more than 0.12 second and less than 0.20 second in duration.

The *QRS complex* is produced by ventricular activation and varies widely in amplitude and basic direction depending on electrical position of the heart, component muscle mass, and other factors. Ordinarily it is from 0.04 to 0.10 second in duration.

The *ST segment* is normally isoelectric and represents the refractory period of the ventricular muscle. It may be depressed by such factors as digitalis or ischemia.

The *T wave* is produced by repolarization or recovery of the ventricular muscle. It varies considerably in amplitude and duration. Although it is usually upright in most leads, it may be inverted due to ischemia or tissue injury. It is also peaked with hyperkalemia.

The *Q-T interval* includes the QRS and T wave and is the period of time required for ventricular depolarization and repolarization. Normally this is less than 0.40 second. Prolongation may occur with electrolyte imbalance, especially potassium deficit.

The *U wave* is an inconstant positive deflection resembling the T wave in form but of less amplitude and duration. It may or may not be identified and has little clinical significance.

RELATED FILM

Disorders of the heartbeat (EM 170). Color, 17 minutes, available from state heart association. This excellent film shows the correlation between the electrocardiogram and the electrical and mechanical activity of the heart; abnormal rhythms are also presented.

Chapter 8

Electronic monitoring

INTRODUCTION

Electronic monitoring as a method of continuing surveillance is being used with increasing frequency. Reduced to its simplest denominator, electronic monitoring provides the advantage of continuous observation of certain vital signs. The type of equipment varies with the vital function to be monitored; more complex machines may assist in monitoring multiple functions.

The increasing reliability and satisfactory use of electronic monitoring equipment is exemplified by the fact that in space explorations of recent decades, numerous vital functions of astronauts in flights are monitored from thousands of miles away, and this information is transferred by radio to ground equipment.

TYPES OF EQUIPMENT

Equipment is available for monitoring almost all body functions including oxygen saturation, central venous pressure, arterial pressure, respiratory rate and depth, respiratory gas content, skin temperature, body temperature, capillary oxygen saturation, and electrocardiographic material. Monitoring of the first two functions is seen with increasing frequency, especially in the teaching- and research-oriented facilities. Electrocardiographic monitoring is the type most often seen in the intensive care unit. Although monitoring of the other body functions is at present more useful to the researcher, the adage that today's research is tomorrow's practice is doubly true in this field.

The distinct advantage of electronic monitoring of cardiac activity is the rapid detection of abnormal rhythms so that they may be further identified and treatment instituted before a serious or critical situation arises. Nurses rapidly become adept at recognizing even minute changes in rhythm from sound or sight.

The simplest type of equipment is a sensitive voltmeter that detects the electrical impulse produced by ventricular activation and translates it into a visible light flash or an audible beep. Most of the equipment of this type has high and low warning devices that can be set to activate an alarm in the event of the passage of a predetermined period of time between impulses, usually from four to six seconds. It may also sound an alarm if the heart rate gets above a certain predetermined setting, usually from 100 to 120 beats per minute, or if the impulses occur closer than every 0.5 second.

The monitoring equipment in general use is slightly more complex and includes an oscilloscope screen that projects the electrical activity of the heart (Fig. 8-1). The electrical impulse, which is produced by cardiac activity and transmitted from electrodes placed on the chest or the extremities, is amplified and transmitted in a form similar to a single lead electrocardiogram. This oscilloscope may be combined with a rate meter that gives a continuous reading of heart rate and also has an alarm. Multiple oscilloscopes may be combined to present monitored information at the nurses station.

The exact pattern produced on the oscilloscope screen will depend somewhat on the position of the heart in the chest, the shape and thickness of the chest, and placement of the electrodes; yet the basic components are essentially the same as those described in the chapter on basic electrocardiography. The continuous presence of an electrocardiogram enables the observing personnel to more readily identify abnormal rhythms and make treatment more specific.

Equipment features. Graphic representation of the electrocardiographic cycle by electronic monitoring equipment is calibrated similar to the electrocardiograph. Some models actually have a graph painted on the oscilloscope so that the deflections correspond in a magnified way to those produced by an electrocardiograph.

Some equipment includes a pacemaker that may be set for either external or internal cardiac pacing. The internal setting requires approximately one-tenth the electric power needed for external pacing. Most of the equipment can be left on standby and may automatically begin pacing after a period of asystole that varies from two to ten seconds. Because of difficulties with electrode con-

Fig. 8-1. The Electrodyne bedside monitor oscilloscope and pacemaker unit. (Courtesy Electrodyne, Westwood, Mass.)

tinuity, it is advisable to leave the electrode switches on internal pacing so that the patient will not be shocked in the event of technical difficulty.

Some machines have a write-out device that produces a strip of tracing automatically when the alarm is sounded. This is helpful in recording electrical events for permanent records and later reference.

Several major companies produce similar electronic equipment at comparable prices. In considering purchase of this equipment, the availability of servicing should be considered in the final selection. If possible, all equipment used in a unit should be purchased from the same manufacturer so that familiarity with controls will be simplified.

Equipment should be checked periodically when it is not in use to ensure that idleness and dust have not interfered with its normal operation. The electrodes should be scrupulously cleaned before storage because the salty paste is corrosive; fine sandpaper may be used.

Since there is considerable variation in controls and the information presented

Fig. 8-2. A typical remote oscilloscope, heart rate meter, alarm, and automatic electro-cardiogram write-out at the nurses' station. Most of these units are of a modular construction so that units may be tailored to need and can be expanded. (Courtesy Electrodyne, Westwood, Mass.)

Fig. 8-3. Typical electrode placement (+) using three-cable system for monitor and pacing standby. Note their relation to nipples.

by various manufacturers, all personnel concerned with using these machines should study thoroughly the manual supplied with each piece of equipment.

ELECTRODE PLACEMENT

Two electrodes are required for pacing, which is the stimulation of the heart by external electric shock. To be effective, these electrodes should be placed so that the current passing from one electrode to the other will pass through the heart in as direct a line as possible. The electrodes should also be as close to the heart as possible to prevent dissipation of the current through other body tissues. This will require that one pacing electrode be placed at approximately the fifth and sixth left intercostal space in the anterior axillary line and the other electrode be placed in the midsternal area.

Monitoring electrodes may be placed in almost any convenient location on the body since the electrical activity of the heart is transmitted throughout the body. Two electrodes are required. As a matter of custom, monitoring electrodes are usually placed near the shoulders or across the chest; however, they might be placed from arm to leg or chest to arm.

Some popular equipment uses the same electrodes for monitoring and pacing (Fig. 8-3). This usually involves a three-electrode arrangement with one electrode doubling for both monitoring and pacing. This electrode would, of necessity, be placed in the left anterior axillary line at approximately the fifth or sixth intercostal space. The other pacing electrode would be placed in the midsternal area. The third electrode, which is used only for monitoring, might be placed on any portion of the right half of the body but is customarily placed in the right anterior axillary line at about the fifth and sixth intercostal space. This results in a monitor pattern resembling lead I in the standard electrocardiogram.

Several types of electrodes are available and none is entirely satisfactory, for each has some disadvantage. Electrodes may be held in place by a wide elastic band encircling the chest for short periods of use, but the presence of this band is somewhat restricting to respiratory activity. Electrode cables are available with Luer-Lok adapters so that an ordinary metal needle may be used for rapid application with the needle acting as the electrode. This is used in the emergency situation for a short time.

Small disposable prepackaged monitoring electrodes, which are commercially available, are on a small piece of adhesive tape. They are attached to the cable by a snap, but these have not been suitable for pacing.

The most satisfactory method of electrode placement in our experience is the use of a three-inch square of moleskin with the electrode placed through a small central hole.

A method for attaching the electrodes should be standardized for each unit. The following procedure is suggested:

1. Explain to the patient that wires will be attached to his chest to closely check his heartbeat and that this will not be painful.
2. If necessary, a four-inch area around the electrode sites is shaved. Room between electrodes is allowed for defibrillator paddles.
3. The sites are cleaned with alcohol sponges, a scrubbing action being used to remove oils and cellular debris. Acetone may be used in the emergency situation because its drying period is practically nil.
4. When cleansing with alcohol, allow the area to dry before painting it with tincture benzoin compound. After the benzoin dries, a small amount of electrode paste is applied to the skin and rubbed in gently. Additional paste is applied to the electrode.
5. The electrode is attached to the skin with moleskin and the contact is checked.

Electrodes applied in this manner have remained that way for several days, but there is a tendency for the skin to become excoriated under the electrode because of the hyperosmolarity of the salt paste. After more than 24 hours most patients will develop some skin excoriation under the electrode; therefore, electrodes should probably be changed at least every 48 to 72 hours.

DETERMINATION OF EQUIPMENT MALFUNCTION

One of the primary functions of personnel using the electronic monitoring equipment is early determination of equipment malfunction. Probably the most likely cause of trouble is a *loose electrode,* preventing reception of electrical impulses by the amplifier. This could occur if adhesive tape became loose, a wire was broken, or the patient turned. In this situation the condition is electrically interpreted as cardiac arrest and the alarm will be sounded. If standby pacing equipment is used, pacing will begin automatically. If set for external voltage pacing, the patient will be shocked unnecessarily. For this reason, the automatic equipment should probably be left on the internal voltage selector; this will result in delivery of approximately one-tenth the external voltage and will produce no harm or discomfort. If the alarm sounds and the nurse determines that cardiac arrest is present, she must only flip the internal-external voltage selector switch to the external position for pacing to begin.

Another likely cause of equipment malfunction is *loss of power* to the equipment, in which case nothing will be transmitted on the screen; it takes a fraction of a second for the operator to realize that the pilot light indicator on the machine is not burning. This differs from the transcription of a straight line which is incident to cardiac arrest.

Disconnection of the cable from the machine will also result in the false alarm of standstill. Wires occasionally become unplugged and after periods of use may become broken or partially frayed, resulting in poor contact or poor conduction. Contact plugs may also become loose fitting. *Incomplete contact of the electrodes with the skin* may result in faulty information, as may *drying of the electrode paste*. If there is a wavy base line, electrodes should be checked to see if one is loose.

Faulty contact has been observed with patients having *pectoris excavatum,* for it is difficult to place the electrodes in their usual position on the chest. In this case the right and left leads may be placed over the triceps muscles. Patients with *large breasts* also present problems for establishing electrode placement and maintaining good contact. Another source of difficulty is the *restless patient* who turns and thrashes in bed; his activity may produce either loss of contact with the electrodes or bizarre patterns wandering vertically over the screen resulting from muscular activity.

RELATED FILM

An introduction to nursing in a coronary care unit (M-1461). Color, 26 minutes, available from National Medical Audiovisual Center (Annex), Chamblee, Ga. 30005, Attn: Film Distribution. This film provides an overview of nursing in a coronary care unit and shows the various types of electronic monitoring devices.

Chapter 9

Abnormalities of heart rhythm

INTRODUCTION

The cardiac rhythms, many of which are referred to as arrhythmias because of their variation from normal rhythm, may be classified in several ways. One effective arrangement is according to those that result from a block to impulse passage and those that occur because of ectopic foci. The grouping may be further extended to indicate the source of the block or foci.

Rhythms may also be classified as normal or abnormal; furthermore, they may be normal or abnormal according to varying circumstances.

Intelligent management of the patient depends on recognition of the type and source of the abnormal rhythm, some of the precipitating causes, its significance, and appropriate treatment.

As is mentioned on page 35 the electrocardiographic tracing is produced by amplification of the electrical current that is produced by cardiac muscle activity. The electrical stimulus usually causes muscular activity that is depicted by the electrocardiogram in a uniform manner. A study of this activity is the most reliable indication of rhythm because the P wave of the electrocardiogram reflects atrial activity, the QRS complex mirrors ventricular activity, and the T wave is the period of repolarization.

The *rate* can be ascertained in the following manner: The paper speed is such that a mark appears at the top every three seconds (or three inches of paper). A convenient way to determine the rate is to count the number of QRS complexes for six seconds and then multiply this number by ten.

INTERPRETATION OF THE ELECTROCARDIOGRAM

The study of rhythms is aided by asking the following questions about each tracing:

1. Are P waves present?
2. Are they normal in appearance?
3. Is the P-R interval normal?
4. Is the P-R consistent?
5. Is the P wave always followed by a QRS complex?
6. Is the QRS complex normal in duration?
7. Is the QRS consistent in form and duration?
8. Is the R-R interval consistent?

9. If inconsistent, is there a pattern of variation in the R-R?

If all questions are answered affirmatively the rhythm is normal, although certain negative answers do not always indicate abnormality. For example, a tracing showing an occasional premature ventricular contraction (PVC) is considered normal; however, questions 4, 6, 8, and 9 would have negative answers. Sinus arrhythmia, a cyclic variation of cardiac activity with respiration, would result in a negative answer to 8, but 9 would be affirmative. A step-by-step study of each electrocardiogram will usually lead to a correct diagnosis of the rhythm.

NORMAL RHYTHMS

This group of normal rhythms includes sinus arrhythmia, sinus bradycardia, and sinus tachycardia. Occasional premature contractions (PVCs) are also usually considered to be normal (Table 9-1).

Sinus arrhythmia. Sinus arrhythmia is a normal rhythm and is important only in differentiation from significant abnormal rhythms. It is the variation of heart rate with respiration; the rate increases with inspiration and slows with expiration.

Electrocardiographically each component of the tracing is normal, and the P-R and Q-T intervals remain constant. However, the R-R interval varies cyclically with respiration (Fig. 9-1).

Sinus bradycardia. Sinus bradycardia is a normal rhythm characterized only by a slow rate of fewer than 60 beats per minute.

Electrocardiographically the origin and transmission of the impulse are nor-

Table 9-1. Rhythms originating at the SA node

	Rate		P wave	P-R interval	QRS complex	R-R interval	Rhythm
	Atrium	*Ventricle*					
Sinus arrhythmia	Normal	Normal	Normal	Normal	Usually normal*	Varies with respiration	"Regularly irregular"
Sinus bradycardia	Under 60	Under 60	Normal	Normal	Usually normal*	Normal	Regular
Sinus tachycardia	100+	100+	Normal	Normal	Usually normal*	Normal	Regular
Dropped beat			Absent for missed beat	Absent for missed beat	Absent for missed beat	Absent for missed beat	Usually regular before and after missed beat
Atrial standstill or cardiac arrest	0	None or few	Absent	Absent	May have occasional ventricular escaped beats	None or irregular	None or irregular

*Any of the supraventricular arrhythmias may be associated with right or left bundle branch block in which case the QRS complex would be abnormal (prolonged).

mal with production of normal P, QRS, and T waves (Fig. 9-2). Sinus arrhythmia and sinus bradycardia are frequently seen together.

Sinus bradycardia is commonly seen in athletes at rest and in others who are in good physical condition, and in the elderly under basal conditions. It may also be produced by any condition or drug that produces vagal stimulation, such as reserpine. It is rarely of significance and requires treatment only when marked or drug-related.

Sinus tachycardia. Sinus tachycardia is a rapid (100 to 150) regular rhythm.

Electrocardiographically the production and conduction of the impulse are normal with formation of normal P, QRS, and T waves (Fig. 9-3). At the more rapid rates it may be impossible to differentiate sinus tachycardia from other rapid regular rhythms.

Sinus tachycardia usually originates from conditions outside the heart, such as excitement, a febrile state, or shock; its significance and treatment depend upon the underlying condition. It may also originate from conditions within the heart, and treatment again depends upon the underlying condition.

Fig. 9-1. Sinus arrhythmia: cyclic variation of the R-R time with respiration. P waves and P-R intervals are normal and constant; QRS and T waves are normal.

Fig. 9-2. Sinus bradycardia: slow normal rhythm, rate 50. Origin and progression of depolarization are normal, resulting in normal P, P-R, QRS, and T's. Rhythm is regular unless sinus arrhythmia producing cyclic variation is also present.

Fig. 9-3. Sinus tachycardia: rate 140, rhythm regular. P waves are normal, P-R is normal and consistent, and QRS complexes are normal. R-R times are consistent.

ABNORMAL RHYTHMS OCCURRING AT SA NODE

The normal cardiac impulse has its origin at the SA node. The only significant abnormal rhythms that originate in this area are atrial standstill occurring for a single beat and sino-atrial block (SA block) (Table 9-1).

Atrial standstill. Atrial standstill occurring for a single beat, usually resulting from vagal stimulation, is generally not significant. It may forewarn of toxicity if the patient is receiving digitalis.

Electrocardiographically this is a totally missed beat with no activity discernible during the period for a usual beat. The rhythm is usually regular before and after the dropped beat.

Sino-atrial block. Sino-atrial block (SA block) is the equivalent of *cardiac arrest* and results in total cardiac standstill unless some other ectopic focus undertakes the function of impulse origination. Commonly the focus will be some portion of the ventricle, which will usually result in idioventricular rhythm. The ectopic beats may be followed by atrial contractions brought about by retrograde conduction of the impulse, or there may be no evidence of atrial contraction. In the situation in which atrial standsill or SA block persists without ventricular escaped beats, death occurs within a matter of from three to five minutes.

Electrocardiographically SA block is represented by a straight base line without evidence of electrical activity (Fig. 9-4).

The cause is usually organic resulting from ischemic involvement of the SA node or intoxication with digitalis or quinidine.

The treatment of SA block includes administration of isoproterenol (Isuprel) or atropine or both. Artificial pacing may be required.

Fig. 9-4. Sino-atrial block: cardiac arrest. No electrical activity is discernible until ventricular escape occurs and causes idioventricular rhythm. This rate will require prompt drug treatment or electrical pacing.

ABNORMAL RHYTHMS ORIGINATING IN ATRIA

Many abnormal rhythms have their origin in the atria. These include premature atrial contractions, atrial tachycardia, atrial fibrillation, atrial flutter, and wandering pacemaker (Table 9-2).

As was mentioned concerning the properties of cardiac muscle cells, all cardiac muscle has the potential of rhythmic activity; yet the pacemaker is normally seated in the SA node because this small tissue discharges its electric potential at a rate more rapid than that of other portions of the heart. The spread of this impulse through the cardiac muscle results in repetitive depolarization of

Table 9-2. Rhythms originating in the atria

	Rate		P wave	P-R interval	QRS complex	R-R interval	Rhythm
	Atrium	*Ventricle*					
Premature atrial contraction (PAC)	Normal	Normal	Abnormal in size, shape, direction	Varies	Normal*	Differs with PAC from other intervals	Slightly irregular due to PAC and compensatory pause
Atrial tachycardia	140 to 240	Same as atria	Abnormal shape and direction, buried in QRS or T	Usually short	Usually normal but may widen with conduction fatigue	Regular	Regular; may begin and end suddenly
Atrial fibrillation	Varies	Varies	No true P waves; wavy base line	Not measurable	Usually normal*	Varies	Totally irregular
Atrial flutter	200 to 400	60 to 150	Sawtooth flutter waves, no baseline, no true P's	Not measurable	Usually normal; may widen with fatigue	Varies	Ventricular rhythm usually regular
Wandering pacemaker	Varies	Varies	Varies as pacemaker wanders	Varies or is absent when AV node is pacemaker	Normal*	Varies	Irregular

*Any of the supraventricular arrhythmias may be associated with right or left bundle branch block, in which case the QRS complex would be abnormal (prolonged).

the muscle so that the impulse never has an opportunity to originate from other areas.

Other areas in the heart may become the pacemaker in either of two general situations: (1) Any factor that reduces the rhythmicity of the SA node to a rate slower than that of other areas may result in impulses originating from other areas and becoming the pacemaker, or (2) any factor that increases the rhythmicity of an ectopic focus to a rate greater than that of the SA node results in this focus becoming the pacemaker.

Premature atrial contraction. A premature atrial contraction (PAC) is characterized by the occurrence of a contraction earlier than would be expected.

Electrocardiographically the rate and rhythm are regular, with the exception of this ectopic beat occurring earlier than expected. This ectopic beat is composed of a P wave abnormal in shape, size, or direction. Frequently the P-R interval may be short; the QRS complex is the same as those appearing with regular beats. It may or may not be followed by a compensatory pause, so that the total of two R-R periods encompassing the PAC is the same as the total of two adjacent R-R periods (Figs. 9-5 and 9-6).

PACs are of varying significance; their presence suggests that an excitable focus exists in the atria. This seems to predispose the patient to the rapid atrial abnormal rhythms that are undesirable, that is, atrial tachycardia, atrial fibrillation, or atrial flutter.

When the significance of the PACs is questionable, the patient may be treated with procaine amide (Pronestyl) by injection if speed of onset is a factor. Quinidine may be given orally when rapidity of action is not critical.

Atrial tachycardia. Atrial tachycardia is a rapid (from 140 to 240 beats per minute) regular rhythm that originates from an ectopic focus in the atria. It is usually a functional arrhythmia mediated by the autonomic nervous system, and it usually starts and stops abruptly (paroxysmal atrial tachycardia, PAT). It may be a manifestation of anxiety and is usually of no clinical significance in an otherwise healthy patient. However, it may be dangerous in a patient having organic heart disease. By not permitting adequate ventricular filling, the rapid rate causes decreased cardiac output with resulting coronary and cerebral insufficiency; congestive heart failure may supervene.

Fig. 9-5. Premature atrial contraction: normal configuration of QRS complex which occurs early (third complex). P wave occurring prematurely is superimposed on preceding T wave. A compensatory pause follows the premature contraction.

Fig. 9-6. Premature atrial contraction: abnormally shaped P wave (indicating abnormal origin) occurs early and is followed by normal QRS and T (fourth complex). A compensatory pause follows the premature beat. Note excessive standardization also.

Fig. 9-7. Atrial bigeminy: rate 80. Alternate beats are premature atrial contractions. A compensatory pause following each PAC results in the alternating R-R's being prolonged and equal.

Electrocardiographically this results in a P wave abnormal in size and shape which may be buried in the QRS complex or T wave. The P-R interval is usually short. The QRS is usually normal but may widen with fatigue of the conduction system (Figs. 9-8 to 9-10).

At slower rates, differentiating atrial from sinus tachycardia may be difficult. In the presence of bundle branch block with wide QRS complexes, the atrial tachycardia may be difficult to differentiate from ventricular tachycardia. Fig. 9-34 has been labeled *Ventricular tachycardia,* but it might just as easily be labeled *Atrial tachycardia with bundle branch block.*

Atrial tachycardia may spontaneously revert to normal. Frequently it may be corrected by measures designed to produce vagal stimulation, such as carotid body pressure in the neck, eyeball compression, painful squeezing of the bridge

Fig. 9-8. Atrial tachycardia: rate 150. Regular rhythm originates in the atria. The QRS is generally normal, and each is preceded by a P wave; P-R interval is within normal limits.

Fig. 9-9. Atrial tachycardia: rate 190; regular. Each QRS is preceded by an abnormal (inverted) P wave. P-R interval is within normal limits confirming normal delay through the AV node. The inverted P wave suggests depolarization proceeding through the atria in a direction the opposite of the usual.

Fig. 9-10. Atrial tachycardia with 3 : 1 block: abnormal (inverted) P waves at rate of 200 per minute. Ventricular rate, 67, is regular. This is a frequent complication of digitalis intoxication.

of the nose, or by having the patient perform the Valsalva maneuver (forced expiration against a closed glottis).

When these measures fail, drug therapy is initiated. The first and least harmful type is sedation or tranquilization or both. The refractory case is usually responsive to propranolol (Inderal), procaine amide (Pronestyl), or digitalis given as a single slightly subdigitalizing dose. Quinidine and procaine amide are both effective agents for terminating this abnormal rhythm, but their use is limited to cases resistant to other types of treatment because of their intrinsic toxicity.

Countershock or cardioversion may be used if the abnormal rhythm is persistent or produces angina or decompensation.

Atrial fibrillation. Atrial fibrillation is characterized clinically by total irregularity with no discernible relation between consecutive beats. This results in variation in rate, and, as the ventricle contracts at various stages of ventricular filling, a variation also occurs in pulse strength.

When atrial fibrillation is more rapid, there is a definite pulse deficit as the ventricle contracts at times when not enough blood is present to result in production of a radial pulse. For this reason a difference in radial and apical rates will be noted, generally directly proportional to the rate of the fibrillation. When listening to the heart sounds, considerable variation will be noted, in both timing and intensity of the sounds.

Electrocardiographically atrial fibrillation is characterized by a wavy base line that is produced by the continuous disorganized depolarization of the atrial muscle without effective atrial contraction; therefore, no P waves are discernible. Although impulses are continuously bombarding the AV node, only a few of these will be of intensity and timing sufficient to be conducted; consequently the wavy base line is interrupted by irregular ventricular contractions. The QRS is usually normal, but it may widen with an increased rate, or it may have been widened previously by conduction defects (Figs. 9-11 to 9-13).

Generally, the more rapid the atrial fibrillation, the more urgent the patient's need for treatment for control of the rapid ventricular rate. A heart rate in normal range with atrial fibrillation will result in a decreased efficiency of cardiac output of from 20% to 30%; at a rate of 150+ the decrease in cardiac output is perhaps 70%.

The etiology of atrial fibrillation is usually organic heart disease, but it may occasionally be functional. It is commonly seen in advanced rheumatic heart disease and ischemic heart disease, and is less frequently manifested in hypertensive disease. It may also result from a metabolic abnormality without demonstrable heart disease, as in hyperthyroidism.

Treatment is determined by several factors, the first being rate. When rate is rapid, the primary need of restoration of a normal rate is usually accomplished by rapid digitalization. The digitalis may be given intravenously followed by fractional doses to lower the ventricular rate to less than 100. If the onset of fibrillation is sudden, simple improvement of coronary perfusion by slowing the ventricular rate will occasionally be sufficient for reversion to normal sinus rhythm.

If it is desirable to convert the rhythm to normal following deceleration (as

Fig. 9-11. Atrial fibrillation: rate 135; grossly irregular. R-R's are inconsistent, no P waves are discernible, and the base line is wavy. QRS is normal.

Fig. 9-12. Atrial fibrillation: rate 80; grossly irregular. R-R's are variable, no P waves are detectable, and the base line is wavy. QRS's are normal.

Fig. 9-13. Atrial fibrillation: slow rate of 55; irregular. R-R's are variable, P waves are absent, and the base line is wavy.

is most certainly true in those cases of short-duration atrial fibrillation), the conversion may be attempted with procaine amide (Pronestyl) by injection. Since this drug produces a significant hypotension, it should be given at a rate less than 50 mg. per minute if administered intravenously. Blood pressure and the EKG should be monitored concurrently. If hypotension becomes a major factor, it may be treated by the administration of small doses of a vasopressor, such as metaraminol (Aramine). The dosage of procaine amide is geared to the amount needed to produce conversion to normal sinus rhythm; however, few physicians administer more than a single injectable dose of 1 gm. over a period of 20 minutes. Once conversion is achieved, procaine amide may be administered in capsule form by mouth, usually 250 mg. every three or four hours, or by intramuscular injection in similar doses.

Lidocaine (Xylocaine) may be used in a manner similar to procaine amide. When the need for conversion is less urgent, the drug of choice is probably quinidine and the dosage varies widely. Except in an extreme emergency, quinidine is usually given orally; several routines seem to be of comparable effectiveness. The usual starting routine is 200 mg. orally every two to four hours under either continuous oscilloscope monitoring or intermittent EKG monitoring, for quinidine toxicity may result in ventricular fibrillation. This catastrophic consequence is usually preceded by a definite widening of the QRS complex that can be determined on the oscilloscope or electrocardiogram. This widening should be adequate indication for discontinuing quinidine therapy. Propranolol (Inderal) has also been used recently in the treatment of atrial fibrillation.

Thromboembolic complications are common in conversion of atrial fibrillation. The inefficiently emptying atria have a tendency to form thrombi, especially in the left auricular appendage. With conversion and the production of normal atrial contractions, these thrombi are frequently dislodged and enter the circulation. For this reason most of these patients receive anticoagulants as a part of their treatment before conversion is attempted.

Atrial flutter. Atrial flutter, another abnormal rhythm usually thought to be produced by a singular ectopic focus in the atria, produces regular rhythmic

Fig. 9-14. Atrial flutter: atrial rate (f waves) 310 per minute with variable ventricular response at 90 per minute. Note sawtooth appearance of base line.

Fig. 9-15. Atrial flutter: atrial rate 340 with sawtooth base line and variable ventricular response of 110 per minute. Ventricular response may be either regular or irregular.

Fig. 9-16. Wandering supraventricular pacemaker: rate 100. Variation in the form of the P wave and P-R interval indicates that the impulse originates in variable areas above the ventricle. QRS complexes are all approximately normal and consistent in duration and direction.

but extremely rapid atrial contractions with a block between the atria and AV node. Therefore, only a fraction of the impulses arriving at the AV node result in stimulation and contraction of the ventricles. The rapidity of the rhythm depends on the degree of AV block .

Atrial flutter can be diagnosed only by use of the oscilloscope or electrocardiograph because it is frequently regular and cannot be differentiated from other rhythms of comparable rates.

Electrocardiographically there is a sawtooth appearance of the flutter waves that results from rapid atrial depolarization occurring at rates of from 200 to 400 per minute. True P waves are absent, and the QRS complexes are usually regular (Figs. 9-14 and 9-15).

Treatment of atrial flutter is essentially the same as for atrial fibrillation. Flutter is generally considered to be a less serious abnormal rhythm, and it is also less frequent than atrial fibrillation.

Table 9-3. Rhythms originating at the AV node

	Rate		P wave	P-R interval	QRS complex	R-R interval	Rhythm
	Atrium	Ventricle					
Premature nodal contraction (PNC)	Normal	Normal	May occur before, after, or be buried in QRS	May be very short if P before QRS	Normal*	Usually regular except for PNC	Regular except for PNC and compensatory pause
AV nodal rhythm	40 to 60	40 to 60	Same as in PNC	Same as in PNC	Normal*	Regular	Regular
AV nodal tachycardia	150 to 200	150 to 200	Same as in PNC	Same as in PNC	Normal*	Regular	Regular
Delayed conduction 1° AV block	Normal	Normal	Normal	Greater than 0.20 second	Usually normal	Regular	Regular
2° AV block (2 : 1 or 3 : 1 block)	Normal	½ or ⅓ atrial rate	Normal. Ratio of P to QRS of 2 : 1 or 3 : 1	May be consistent when P followed by QRS	Usually normal	Usually regular	P-P interval and R-R interval both regular
Wenckebach	Normal or slow	Slightly slower	Normal	Progressive lengthening	Normal except for dropped beat	Irregular	P-P interval regular, R-R interval varies
Complete AV block (3° block)	Usually 60 to 80	30 to 40	Normal if originates in SA node	Continuously changes	Shape depends on ectopic focus, usually wide	Irregular	Two separate pacemakers, both usually have independent rhythm

*Any of the supraventricular arrhythmias may be associated with right or left bundle branch block, in which case the QRS complex would be abnormal (prolonged).

Wandering pacemaker. Wandering pacemaker is a rhythm produced by varying supraventricular pacemakers.

Electrocardiographically the P waves usually vary in form and duration, and the P-R likewise varies. The QRS is usually normal unless some type of intraventricular block is present. The R-R interval is irregular (Fig. 9-16).

This arrhythmia usually indicates organic disease.

If the rate is rapid, digitalis, procaine amide, propranolol, or quinidine may be indicated. If the rate is slow, atropine or potassium may be given, or digitalis withdrawal may be necessary.

ABNORMAL RHYTHMS ORIGINATING AT AV NODE

Abnormal rhythms originating at the AV node include premature nodal contractions, AV nodal rhythm, AV nodal tachycardia, and various degrees of AV nodal block (Table 9-3).

Premature nodal contraction. A premature nodal contraction (PNC) occurs when an ectopic focus in the AV node stimulates the ventricle to contract, thus forming a normal QRS complex.

Electrocardiographically the P wave associated with this premature nodal contraction occurs either in its normal place with a very short P-R interval or immediately following the QRS complex because of retrograde conduction since atrial depolarization occurs somewhat slower than ventricular depolarization. The QRS complex is normal, and the rate is usually unaffected (Figs. 9-17 and 9-18).

Fig. 9-17. Premature nodal contraction. Origin of the impulse is low in AV node, with ventricular activation following generally normal pathway and retrograde atrial activation being delayed so that P wave follows QRS (superimposed on ST segment). There is a compensatory pause before next normal cycle.

Fig. 9-18. Premature nodal contraction. Origin of the impulse high in AV node results in retrograde atrial activation (inverted P wave) and short P-R interval (0.10 second).

The etiology may be nodal ischemia, drug effect, or the result of autonomic nervous system activity.

The only significance of nodal extrasystoles is their tendency to predispose the patient to nodal tachycardia.

Treatment includes sedation or administration of quinidine or procaine amide (Pronestyl).

AV nodal rhythm. AV nodal rhythm occurs when the AV node is more rhythmic than the SA node; it is usually a slow rhythm.

Electrocardiographically a P wave occurs because of the retrograde conduction of the impulse from the AV node; it may be located before, after, or hidden in the QRS complex. If it occurs before the QRS complex, the P wave is usually abnormal in shape or direction or both and is followed by a short P-R interval. The QRS complex is usually normal.

Nodal rhythm may indicate organic interference at the SA node. If the rate is unduly slow, atropine or isoproterenol (Isuprel) may be used. If digitalis toxicity is suspected, this drug is withdrawn and supplemental potassium is given.

AV nodal tachycardia. AV nodal tachycardia occurs when an irritable focus in the AV node discharges impulses more rapidly than the SA node and assumes the role of pacemaker.

Electrocardiographically the rate is rapid. An abnormal (usually inverted) P wave is produced since this retrograde impulse does not follow a normal path. This P wave may occur immediately before, be buried in, or follow the QRS complex, depending on whether the point of origin is high or low in the node. The QRS complex is normal. This rhythm resembles atrial tachycardia in form except that the P waves are not as discernible (Fig. 9-19).

This abnormal rhythm may indicate nodal ischemia or disease, or it may be functional and mediated by the nervous system.

Treatment is directed at reduction of the rapid (from 150 to 200) rate to relieve poor cardiac filling. It is similar to the treatment of atrial tachycardia which includes digitalis if it has not been ordered previously, procaine amide (Pronestyl), and propranolol (Inderal).

AV nodal block. AV nodal block occurs in several degrees. It is usually a manifestation of organic heart disease in the AV node but can also be caused by drugs, such as digitalis.

Electrocardiographically the impulse originates in the SA node and a P wave

Fig. 9-19. Nodal tachycardia: rate 100. QRS is followed by an inverted P wave, indicating retrograde atrial activation; ventricular activation follows normal pathway.

is formed. There may be a delay in conduction through the AV node that produces a prolonged P-R interval; then the QRS complexes are normal *(first degree block)*. Occasionally every second beat (2:1 block) is completely blocked at the AV node so that only a P wave is present on this beat. With 3:1 block each third P wave is followed by a QRS complex. The 2:1 and 3:1 blocks are examples of *second degree block*.

In more severe cases there is complete block at the AV node so that the P waves occur at regular intervals but they are not followed by QRS complexes. However, an ectopic focus in the ventricles usually stimulates it to beat at a rhythm and rate independent of the atrial rhythm *(third degree block)*.

First degree AV block. First degree AV block is not clinically detectable.

Electrocardiographically the P wave is normal. The P-R interval is prolonged greater than 0.2 second resulting from a delay of passage of the atrial impulse through the AV node into the bundle of His. The subsequent ventricular contraction is delayed; the QRS complex is normal (Fig. 9-20).

Treatment is not required, but AV block is frequently an early manifestation of digitalis intoxication. Its presence should alert one to the possible subsequent occurrence of greater degrees of AV block.

Second degree AV block. Second degree AV block reduces heart efficiency. It occurs when a certain number of the P waves are not followed by ventricular contractions because of failure of conduction of some, but not all, of the P waves into the ventricular excitation system. Both atrial and ventricular rates are frequently slow. Atrial tachycardia with block, as shown in Fig. 9-10 does occur.

Two types of second degree AV blocks are commonly recognized: 2:1 or 3:1 block and the Wenckebach phenomenon.

Electrocardiographically in *2:1 AV block* the P wave is normal and the QRS

Fig. 9-20. First degree AV block. Prolongation of P-R interval greater than 0.20 second (0.28 second) indicates delay in passage of impulse through the AV node.

Fig. 9-21. Second degree AV block: 2 : 1 block; atrial rate 60; ventricular rate 30. Alternate impulses arrive at the AV node during the refractory period so that no ventricular response occurs.

complex is normal; however every other P wave is not followed by a QRS complex (Fig. 9-21). In *3:1 AV block* only every third P wave is followed by a QRS complex.

Electrocardiographically in the *Wenckebach phenomenon* the P wave and QRS complex are both normal. There is a progressive lengthening of the P-R interval with each beat until a QRS complex is eventually dropped. In this situation the P-P interval is regular, but the R-R intervals vary (Fig. 9-22).

Treatment of this group of blocked abnormal rhythms, common manifestations of digitalis intoxication, consists of checking digitalis status. They can sometimes be relieved by administration of potassium ions, isoproterenol (Isuprel), or atropine-like drugs.

The greatest consideration given this group of abnormal rhythms is the fact that they usually appear prior to the onset of more complete blocks for which electronic pacing may be required. The presence of one of these blocks is a positive indication for continuous electronic monitoring and the immediate availability of standby pacing equipment.

Third degree AV block. Complete AV block or third degree block results when no atrial impulses are transmitted through the AV node into the ventricular conduction system. This may result in temporary ventricular standstill (Adams-Stokes syncope), a situation that demands electronic pacing (Fig. 9-23).

Most commonly the presence of complete AV block is followed by spontaneous resumption of ventricular contraction at a slower idioventricular rate, usually at a regular rhythm. If the ventricular rate is less than from 35 to 40 beats per minute, it may be inadequate to support consciousness or adequate coronary, cerebral, and renal perfusion.

Fig. 9-22. Second degree AV block: Wenckebach phenomenon. The P-R interval is progressively prolonged with impulse periodically arriving at the AV node during the refractory period so that no ventricular response is produced.

Fig. 9-23. AV dissociation: atrial rate 80; regular; ventricular rate 35. There is no consistent relation between P waves and QRS complexes. Ventricular complexes originate from a single focus.

Fig. 9-24. AV dissociation: third degree AV block; atrial rate 80; regular; ventricular rate 30 to 40 and irregular. There is no relation between P waves and QRS impulses except when an atrial impulse arrives at the AV node at exactly the right time to produce a conducted response. The first and fourth QRS complexes in this strip are such so-called captured beats. The ventricular rhythm originates from multiple foci, producing variations in the shape of QRS complexes.

Electrocardiographically normal P waves occur at regular intervals, and QRS complexes occur at regular intervals; but they are independent of each other, for the impulse is completely blocked at the AV node. Occasionally a QRS may follow a P wave when the two rhythms coincide so that the transmitted atrial wave arrives at the AV node when the node is capable of depolarization. This is known as a *captured beat* (Fig. 9-24).

Treatment with drug therapy includes administering isoproterenol (Isuprel) or atropine as a temporary measure. Atropine is administered in very large doses parenterally with doses of 2.5 mg. given repetitively. Isoproterenol is usually administered as a diluted intravenous drip. It has the advantage of an almost instantaneous effect, but this requires that the patient receiving the drip be continuously monitored.

External or internal pacing may be required if drug treatment is ineffective. When AV block results in ventricular standstill, external pacing is the most prompt and effective treatment available for the emergency situation.

The pacing should be at a rate of from 60 to 70 beats per minute with the voltage on the pacemaker adjusted to produce a definite pulse and return of consciousness. If prolonged pacing seems imperative, internal pacing using either transjugular internal pacing or needle electrodes should be used since external pacing in the conscious patient is quite painful.

Several efficient implantable pacemakers are available for the patient who requires permanent pacing. If patients have to be transferred to an area where thoracic surgery is available for the permanent implantation, a portable battery-powered pacemaker with either internal or external electrodes may be used. Isoproterenol (Isuprel) drip may maintain the ventricular rate at an adequate level during the transfer. The method for applying needle electrodes and pacing is explained on page 42. These patients may also require support of respiration (page 92).

ABNORMAL RHYTHMS ORIGINATING IN VENTRICLES

Abnormal rhythms originating in the ventricles are classified as left or right bundle branch block and ectopic ventricular rhythms including premature ven-

Table 9-4. Rhythms originating in the ventricles

	Rate		P wave	P-R interval	QRS complex	R-R interval	Rhythm
	Atrium	Ventricle					
Bundle branch block (left or right)	Normal	Normal	Normal	Normal	Prolonged or distorted M- or W-shaped complexes	Usually regular*	Regular if basic rhythm regular
Premature ventricular contraction (PVC)	Usually normal except for PVC		Not identified with extra beat	Not identified with extra beat	Wide distorted complex with compensatory pause	Usually regular except for PVC	Previous beat + PVC + compensatory pause = 2 normal beats; regular otherwise
Coupled rhythm (bigeminy)	Slow	Twice the atrial rate	Alternate P waves are obscured	Normal or prolonged with alternate beats	Wide distorted complexes	Alternate R-R's are consistent	"Regular irregularity"
Ventricular tachycardia	Varies	150 to 200	Normal or obscured by QRS, conduction retrograde to atria	Not identified	Widened slurred complexes	Regular or nearly regular	Rapid and regular or nearly regular
Ventricular fibrillation	Not discernible	Rapid	None discernible	Not discernible	Wavy chaotic lines; no definite complexes	Grossly regular	Erratic; no effective beat

*Bundle branch block may occur with any supraventricular arrhythmia, in which case the consistency of the R-R interval depends on the basic rhythm.

tricular contractions, ventricular tachycardia, and ventricular fibrillation (Table 9-4).

Blocks are produced by interference with the conduction system within the ventricle. These are generally right and left bundle branch blocks (RBBB and LBBB) of varying degrees, peri-infarction blocks, and intraventricular blocks.

The ectopic ventricular rhythms result from an irritable focus within the ventricle. This may be of no significance, as the occasional PVC; or it may be the result of organic disease resulting in an electric difference between adjacent normal and ischemic tissue. The ectopic foci are also rather frequently influenced by metabolic, chemical, and medicinal agents.

Generally, abnormal ventricular rhythms are of greater significance than abnormal supraventricular rhythms because ventricular activity is responsible for the major portion of effective circulation, while atrial activity only serves to assist in ventricular filling.

Ventricular blocks. The ventricular blocks are usually seen as blocks of the right or left branch of the bundle of His. They are produced by a block in the ventricular conduction system so that the transit time of depolarization is decreased to that portion of the ventricular muscle affected by the block.

The cause is usually organic, such as a myocardial infarction, hypertrophy, or scarring. It may also result from ischemia or drugs, such as quinidine.

Electrocardiographically the P wave and P-R interval are usually not affected because the block is in a branch of the AV conduction system. However, bundle branch block may occur with any basic supraventricular rhythm; the rate and rhythm are not related to bundle branch block.

There is a prolonged ventricular complex (longer than 0.12 second). The ventricles contract asynchronously, perhaps causing an M- or W-shaped ventricular complex, depending on the relation of the electrodes to the forces of depolarization. This form of block produces very little functional interference and requires no treatment.

Left bundle branch block (LBBB) is always thought to indicate heart disease (Figs. 9-25 and 9-26). Right bundle branch block (RBBB) is occasionally seen in normal hearts (Figs. 9-27 and 9-28). The real importance of these findings is their interference with the interpretation of the changes indicating myocardial infarction. It is difficult or impossible to diagnose myocardial infarction electrocardiographically in the presence of left bundle branch block.

Premature ventricular contraction. A premature ventricular contraction (PVC) or ventricular extrasystole is the most common ventricular abnormal rhythm. It originates from a focus somewhere in the ventricle and may be considered normal, or it may result from an irritated or ischemic area, or be produced by drugs, such as digitalis.

Electrocardiographically the P wave may not be discernible. The abnormal

Fig. 9-25. Left bundle branch block: leads I and III; wide QRS (greater than 0.12 second). In LBBB the major QRS deflections in leads I and III go away from each other, that is, up in I and down in III.

Fig. 9-26. Left bundle branch block with atrial fibrillation as basic rhythm. LBBB almost always indicates organic heart disease.

Fig. 9-27. Right bundle branch block: leads I and III; wide QRS with major portion down in I and up in III. RBBB may be seen in the absence of organic heart disease. This tracing also shows first degree AV block (P-R 0.22 second).

Fig. 9-28. Right bundle branch block; QRS 0.13 second; deflection in I and III toward each other. Because of position variation, it is frequently not possible to differentiate RBBB and LBBB from single leads.

Fig. 9-29. Premature ventricular contractions: abnormal (prolonged 0.10 second or greater) QRS without a preceding P wave, followed by T wave in a direction opposite the QRS. A compensatory pause is evident.

Fig. 9-30. Premature ventricular contractions originating from multiple foci in the ventricle. Three different foci result in variable QRS–T patterns on this strip.

QRS is prolonged and occurs before time for the normal QRS. There is usually a compensatory pause after the PVC so that two R-R intervals with the abnormal beat and the compensatory pause equal two normal R-R intervals. Because the ventricular depolarization does not follow the usual conduction system pathway, it is considerably slower than normal, resulting in a ventricular complex of longer than 0.12 second wide. The direction of the complex is determined by the relation of the point of origin to the electrodes (Figs. 9-29 and 9-30).

An occasional PVC is of no significance. If it occurs with increasing frequency, the presence of an irritable focus is indicated and it may be a forerunner of ventricular tachycardia or ventricular fibrillation. Generally speaking, the more frequent, the more ominous. Extrasystoles occurring on the descending side of the normal T wave are particularly foreboding as precursors of ventricular tachycardia.

Treatment is usually based on the use of procaine amide (Pronestyl) or quinidine if the PVC is not caused by digitalis toxicity.

Ventricular bigeminy. Ventricular bigeminy is an abnormal rhythm in which the regular beats are normal in every respect, but the alternate beats have all the characteristics of PVC's. This rhythm usually indicates digitalis intoxication (Fig. 9-31).

Ventricular trigeminy. Ventricular trigeminy, which is usually indicative of digitalis intoxication, occurs when two normal beats are followed by a PVC; then this abnormal pattern repeats itself.

Ventricular tachycardia. Ventricular tachycardia is a rapid rate resulting from ventricular irritability or ischemia, digitalis intoxication, or anoxia (Fig. 9-32).

Electrocardiographically there is no associated P wave; however unrelated P waves may be seen. The QRS complexes are longer than 0.12 second in duration. They are approximately but not exactly regular; for example, they may vary from 150 to 154 to 156 in consecutive full-minute counts (Figs. 9-33 to 9-35).

This is an ominous rhythm for two reasons. (1) It predisposes the patient to ventricular fibrillation which is almost always fatal. This dreaded arrhythmia is always a possibility in the presence of ventricular tachycardia. The patient suspected of having or demonstrated to have ventricular tachycardia should always be continuously monitored. (2) The rapid rate does not allow adequate time for ventricular filling; this results in decreased cardiac output which may culminate in congestive heart failure.

Treatment is the prompt use of procaine amide (Pronestyl) intravenously or quinidine intramuscularly.

Ventricular fibrillation. Ventricular fibrillation is the result of random contractions of small myocardial fiber groups without any effective concerted ventricular contraction (Figs. 9-36 and 9-37).

Electrocardiographically ventricular fibrillation appears as a wavy, totally erratic base line with no discernible, definite complexes. It resembles no other pattern of abnormal rhythm. The only other possibility for a similar pattern is an artifact due to malfunction of the monitor; in this case the patient's appearance would not suggest an alarming condition (Figs. 9-38 to 9-40).

Fig. 9-31. Ventricular bigeminy. Alternate complexes are premature ventricular contractions. This is a common manifestation of digitalis intoxication.

Fig. 9-32. Premature ventricular contractions. A run of several consecutive PVC's as in this strip should alert personnel to the possibility of more serious impending arrhythmias, such as ventricular tachycardia or ventricular fibrillation.

Fig. 9-33. Ventricular tachycardia: rate 130; grossly regular, wide QRS, slight variation in R-R intervals, slight variation in form of QRS. T wave is in direction opposite to major QRS deflection. P waves are discernible apparently at a much slower rate and are unrelated to QRS.

Fig. 9-34. Ventricular tachycardia: rate 180; wide QRS, nearly regular and uniform. The regularity and uniformity of this strip are such that absolute differentiation between ventricular tachycardia and supraventricular tachycardia with intraventricular block is not possible without esophageal leads or a record of onset or termination.

Fig. 9-35. Disorganizing ventricular tachycardia: rate 250; moderate variation in QRS and R-R; much more erratic than in preceding strips. This activity produces very little circulation and is likely to completely disorganize into ventricular fibrillation.

Fig. 9-36. Ventricular fibrillation: total disorganization of ventricular activity. No circulation takes place.

Fig. 9-37. Ventricular fibrillation: total disorganization of ventricular activity. No circulation takes place.

Fig. 9-38. Artifact: poor electrode contact because of dry paste. Basic rhythm is apparently atrial fibrillation with rate 100.

Fig. 9-39. Artifact: alarm sounding. The difficulty is a loose electrode.

Fig. 9-40. Artifact: somatic movement and patient's moaning. High rate would trigger alarm.

Treatment by defibrillation. The only effective treatment is prompt electrical defibrillation performed by means of an electric shock of short duration accomplished through the use of an electric coil that increases the available current and can be discharged rapidly. On most equipment the amount of shock can be varied from 45 to 400 joules or watt seconds.

Upon recognition of ventricular fibrillation, the nursing personnel should perform the following:

When the alarm sounds, the oscilloscope should be checked for a quick, tentative appraisal. If a strip recorder is available, it should be turned on and then one should go quickly to the patient's bedside. If he responds to one's presence or call, a false alarm has sounded because of technical difficulty. The source should be detected and the trouble corrected.

If ventricular fibrillation has occurred, the patient will be unconscious or convulsing. This is followed immediately by respiratory arrest.

The exact time should be noted or an automatic timer started if available. Auxiliary personnel should call the physician.

The emergency cart is brought to the bedside, the defibrillator is connected, and power is set at maximum wattage. Power is turned on; most defibrillators have a flashing light that is activated when the coil is charged, indicating that the machine is ready. This usually takes about 10 or 20 seconds. If the defibrillator is equipped with a synchronizer for use in cardioversion, this should be in the *off* position (Fig. 9-41).

Electrode paste is generously applied to the defibrillator paddles, but none should extend beyond the electrodes or on any portion of the electrode handles.

Fig. 9-41. Direct current defibrillator. This particular model may be paired with the PMS-5 (see Fig. 8-1) bedside unit for synchronized cardioversion. (Courtesy Electrodyne, Westwood, Mass.)

Skin burns occur at the site of the entry of the current if there is a high resistance, but electrode paste reduces this resistance. The paddles have a large diameter to increase the area of skin shock and reduce the likelihood of skin burn. Since foreign matter reduces the area of uniformity of the shock, the paddles should be kept scrupulously clean. A fine grade of sandpaper may be used for this purpose.

Electrode paste is applied generously to the chest wall where the paddles will be placed. Preferred electrode placement varies; however, any position that permits the electric shock to pass through the ventricular muscle mass will suffice. The paddles may be placed midanterior (just to right of sternum below the clavicle) and left lateral (in anterior axillary line at fifth intercostal space), midanterior (to left of sternum in second or third interspace) and posterior (area immediately below the left scapula, avoiding the spinal column), or bilaterally at the level of the fifth intercostal space in anterior axillary line.

The decision as to who will do the actual defibrillation will need to be made at each medical facility. In larger areas where resident physicians are available at all times, it may be done by them; however nurses may also perform this treatment when they have been properly instructed. Since time is of the essence in attempting to save the life of the patient, it is recommended that the nurse perform the defibrillation if a physician has not arrived by the time the equipment is in readiness.

For the actual defibrillation, some machines are constructed so that one person can defibrillate through use of a switch on the handle of one of the electrode paddles or through a foot pedal. Other machines require two persons: one to place and hold the electrodes while the other pushes the shock button. During the shock the paddles should be held tightly against the chest wall, and all personnel should stand away from the bed while the shock is being given. The operator should have dry hands and be certain no part of his body touches the uninsulated electrodes, which could prove fatal.

The patient usually responds with ventricular arrest for a second or so; this is transmitted as a straight line on the oscilloscope. A normal or ectopic rhythm then resumes spontaneously, or external pacing may be required. If fibrillation persists, repeated efforts should be performed at approximately 30-second intervals. If the patient has not responded within four or five minutes, permanent brain damage is likely to occur after this period.

During the few seconds or minutes required for reestablishment of adequate circulation and respiration, it may be necessary to perform external cardiac massage (page 71) and artificial ventilation (page 92).

Any short period of circulatory arrest, as with ventricular asystole or ventricular fibrillation, results in a rapidly advancing metabolic acidosis that must be treated with parenteral alkalis, such as sodium bicarbonate or sodium lactate. Following this sodium administration, the patient should be watched carefully for signs of congestive heart failure or pulmonary edema.

Epinephrine may also be injected intravenously or directly into the heart to improve cardiac tone. Antiarrhythmic drugs, such as procaine amide (Pronestyl), may also be given to prevent recurrence of ventricular fibrillation.

There have been reported cases of spontaneous conversion of ventricular fibrillation; therefore, some physicians recommend that the first act when ventricular fibrillation is noted is to strike a forceful blow to the patient's chest. Since the patient is being monitored, it could be immediately ascertained if this converted his rhythm. If so, the physician should still be immediately notified and the defibrillator put in readiness in case of a recurrence.

In the post-resuscitation period the patient should be observed extremely closely. An intravenous infusion should be maintained for ready access to the circulation, and an indwelling catheter may be inserted to assess any degree of shock as indicated by decreased urinary output. If the rhythm converts to approximately normal but the patient remains unconscious or stuporous, mannitol may be given on the supposition that this depression of the central nervous system may be due to cerebral edema.

There may be some hesitation on the part of both physicians and nurses regarding the nurse's performing pacing and defibrillating procedures. A portion of this reticence may be on the grounds of liability. By reasoning that the nurse is most readily available at the onset of the fibrillation, time is critical, and if she has been properly instructed, the more negligent course for her to follow would be to fail to attempt defibrillation.

The attorney general of the state of Georgia was requested by the Georgia Hospital Association through the Georgia Department of Public Health to render an opinion. Although the opinion is applicable only to Georgia, it should approximate that for other areas. Following is a summary of his ruling dated December 29, 1967.

> The nurse administering emergency care in the intensive care unit is not practicing medicine illegally. The existence of an emergency and the fact that services are rendered gratuitously absolve nurse and hospital of civil liability. The ruling is based on a Georgia statute that permits persons without medical licenses to give emergency medical treatment where such services are rendered gratuitously and notes that the nurse-patient relationship in a hospital is consensual rather than contractual.

In summary, the role of the nurse in ventricular fibrillation is as follows:

1. When the alarm sounds, she quickly glances at the oscilloscope screen and turns on the strip recorder.

2. She goes to the patient's bedside to assess the situation.

3. If the patient is convulsing or unconscious and the oscilloscope pattern is ventricular fibrillation, she starts the automatic timer or notes the exact time and instructs auxiliary personnel to call the physician.

4. The emergency cart is brought to the bedside, the defibrillator is plugged in and turned on. Electrode paste is applied to the paddles.

5. She applies electrode paste to the patient's chest where the paddles will be placed.

6. If the physician has not arrived by the time the defibrillator is charged, the defibrillation is performed.

7. The oscilloscope screen is observed to see if normal rhythm is established. If not, the defibrillation is repeated at 30-second intervals, or until the physician arrives.

8. If spontaneous circulation and respiration are not established after the first defibrillation, external cardiac massage and artificial ventilation between defibrillations are performed.

9. Other nursing personnel will have drugs ready for the physician's immediate use, such as epinephrine, sodium bicarbonate, and calcium chloride.

EXTERNAL CARDIAC MASSAGE

External cardiac massage, the rhythmic compression of the heart between the lower sternum and the thoracic vertebral column, is used as a method of circulatory support when effective circulation is not present. Combined with artificial respiration, it can provide an emergency oxygen supply to vital organs in the body.

Difference between clinical death and fainting. The nurse must be able to quickly recognize the need for this emergency therapy. There are distinguishing points between clinical death, or the cessation of functional circulation and respiration, and fainting. Both patients may have a deathlike appearance and both are unconscious. However, in cardiac arrest the patient has apnea, dilated pupils, no detectable heart sounds, and no palpable carotid or femoral pulsations. In contrast, a person who has fainted has shallow breathing, major pulsations, and lack of pupillary dilatation. Additional signs of death in the monitored patient are minimal systole, cardiac standstill, or ventricular fibrillation.

Procedure. When palpating the carotid artery, one should palpate lightly below the area of the carotid artery bifurcation (inferior to the angle of the jaw). Pressure over the carotid sinus, which is located in this area, may stimulate vagal response which could depress any cardiac activity present (see Fig. 13-3, page 91).

To prepare the patient for cardiac massage, a bedboard or diet tray is quickly placed under his thorax since massage is more effective against a firm rather than yielding surface. The head is hyperextended to facilitate airway patency.

The rescuer either stands or kneels at the patient's side while leaning over the patient in such a manner that he can use the weight of the upper portion of his body to add to the necessary force. It is not advisable to straddle the patient since the heel of the hand is more likely to press the ribs in addition to compressing the sternum. The rescuer, with both arms extended, places the heel of one hand over the central portion of the lower half of the sternum with the heel of the hand parallel with the long axis of the patient's body. The heel of the other hand is placed atop the first hand to add more pressure, since considerable effort is necessary to perform adequate cardiac massage. *Only* the heel of the hand is used to avoid pressure over a large area of the chest. Applying vertical pressure, the rescuer quickly depresses the patient's sternum about 1½ to 2 inches for about one-half second and then abruptly releases this pressure. The hands are not removed from the patient's sternal area so they will be in position for the next compression. A rhythm of one compression a second or a little faster is established. The main point of motion is the lower portion of the sternum and the costal cartilages (Fig. 9-42).

This maneuver compresses the heart between the sternum and spinal column and forces blood from the heart; with removal of pressure, the heart again fills

Fig. 9-42. External cardiac compression. Note that the heel of the hand is over the lower half of the sternum and parallel with the sternum.

with blood. Elevating the legs may improve venous return. The Trendelenburg position is not recommended since the abdominal organs would increase the pressure against the lungs and further impede ventilation.

In order for any significant effect to be derived from cardiac resuscitation, adequate ventilation *must* be sustained. Methods of artificial respiration are discussed on page 92. If two rescuers are present, one interposes a quick deep lung inflation in the ratio of one inflation following every five compressions. If the rescuer is alone, she inflates the lungs two to three times and then feels for a pulse. If it is absent, she then begins cardiac massage. She alternates 15 sternal compressions with two deep rapid lung inflations, quickly changing from the compression to the ventilation position. If there is a question of adequate respiration, cardiac compression should be temporarily halted after 30 compressions to ensure that the chest is expanding adequately during artificial respiration.

The adequacy of effort can be determined by improved color, occasional gasping respirations, or spontaneous movement. A second person can check for pulsations in the femoral or carotid arteries or see if the pupils have constricted. The pupils give a good index of cerebral oxygenation; they begin dilating within 45 seconds following anoxia and constrict just as rapidly with adequate circulation and ventilation.

If it is necessary to move a patient needing cardiopulmonary resuscitation, it is imperative that the resuscitation be continued during the transfer.

Complications. Complications can occur from cardiac massage. If the hands are too close to the diaphragm, the liver, spleen, and pancreas may be contused and may possibly rupture since they are more or less immobile organs. Additionally, the xiphoid process may be broken from the tip of the sternum. Pressure too high on the sternum may cause it to fracture or may produce separation of the costosternal cartilages. If pressure is placed over them, the ribs may fracture, which can lead to fatty embolism from the rib marrow (symptoms, page 107). Pneumothorax can result from a tear of the pleura or lungs from fractured ribs, or it may occur following rupture of an emphysematous bleb.

While cardiac massage is being performed, auxiliary personnel should quickly obtain needed equipment so that it will be in readiness when the physician arrives. The first drug of choice is epinephrine which may be given directly into the heart as a myocardial stimulant; it is diluted to 10 ml. and given with a $3\frac{1}{2}$ inch 22-gauge needle. Sodium bicarbonate is given intravenously to combat acidosis, while calcium chloride intravenously improves myocardial tone. Atropine may be given for marked bradycardia, and vasoconstrictors such as levarterenol (Levophed) may also be necessary. The defibrillator and pacemaker should be immediately available, as well as equipment for supporting respiration. Supplies for an intravenous infusion and possibly a venous cutdown are also necessary.

Following successful resuscitation, the patient should be monitored for from 48 to 72 hours and observed closely. The vital signs should be checked frequently and any signs that might indicate acid-base or electrolyte imbalances (page 181) noted. He should be observed for evidence of brain damage, fractured ribs or sternum, signs of fat embolism, and especially signs of pneumothorax if any injections have been given into the heart. The patient should have a chest x-ray as soon as is feasible.

RELATED FILMS

Cardiac arrhythmias. Color, 23 minutes, available from Abbott Laboratories, North Chicago, Ill. 60064.

This excellent film shows abnormal cardiac rhythms as they occur in a dog's heart.

Nurse in emergency cardiopulmonary resuscitation (EM 394). Color, 15 minutes, available from state heart association.

The functions and responsibilities of the nursing personnel in cardiopulmonary resuscitation are illustrated.

Chapter 10

Hypertensive encephalopathy

Typical initial orders may include

1. Maintenance of adequate ventilation
2. Reserpine intramuscularly
3. Magnesium sulfate intravenously
4. Mannitol or urea intravenously
5. Sedation
6. Laboratory studies

CLINICAL FINDINGS

The typical patient having hypertensive encephalopathy or hypertensive crisis will come for medical treatment complaining of a severe, incapacitating, pounding headache. His symptoms of dizziness, confusion, and blurred vision may suggest central nervous system disease; and he may also have generalized twitchings, usually first noted in the facial musculature. There may also be localizing central nervous system signs, such as cranial nerve palsies, hemiparesis, or hemiplegia. In addition to facial flushing, the blood pressure is usually greater than 200 mm. mercury systolic and 120 diastolic. The diastolic reading is the more significant figure since it represents peripheral resistance during the resting phase of the cardiac cycle. When hypertension has progressed from normal to an elevated figure within a short period of time, hypertensive encephalopathy may appear at somewhat lower levels.

PATHOGENESIS

This syndrome is generally considered to be the result of cerebral edema secondary to the hypertension. Since the brain is enclosed in the nonexpansile cranium, even the slightest increase in interstitial fluid in the brain produces a sizable increase in intracranial pressure, thus compressing the intracranial structures.

Hypertensive encephalopathy may accompany a number of primary conditions, such as malignant hypertension, a sudden exacerbation of essential hypertension produced by a severe emotional experience, extra salt consumption, abrupt withdrawal of antihypertensive medications, acute nephritis with generalized anasarca, or chronic nephritis with nephrosclerosis. It may accompany toxemia of pregnancy or coarctation of the aorta, complicate pheochromocytoma, or occasionally accompany other endocrinopathies.

74

Regardless of the etiology of the hypertensive encephalopathy, treatment is designed to promptly reduce systemic hypertension and relieve the cerebral compression.

TREATMENT

1. *Adequate ventilation* must be maintained, for this patient may not be fully conscious and the airway may become obstructed (page 89).

2. *Reserpine* administered intramuscularly has proven to be an excellent drug for prompt reduction of systemic hypertension; its onset of action is usually within minutes when it is administered parenterally. For some unexplained reason, the dose required parenterally is considerably greater that the usual oral dose, and it is not uncommon for doses to range from 0.5 mg. to 5 mg. by injection. The blood pressure should be monitored very closely when this potent drug is used and the dosage carefully regulated. Since many of these patients also have some arteriosclerotic and circulatory problems, they do not tolerate hypotension.

3. *Magnesium sulfate* may be given intravenously if the patient shows signs of cerebral irritation, such as twitching, convulsions, or coma. In addition to being a good cortical depressant and producing sedation, it also has a prompt hypotensive and diuretic effect.

4. *Mannitol or urea* administered intravenously may also be used to reduce intracranial pressure if the patient is resistant to other modes of therapy (page 272).

5. *Sedation* by injectable barbiturates may be used if the patient is convulsing. Sodium amytal is usually given intravenously in whatever dosage is required to control the seizures.

6. *Laboratory studies* are undertaken to ascertain the degree of damage to other organs produced by the hypertension and to search for the primary etiology. Significant elevation of the blood urea nitrogen may suggest kidney disease, either as a cause or as a result of the hypertension. An intravenous pyelogram or renal arteriography may suggest unilateral renal disease. Electrolyte studies may indicate renal disease or hormonal difficulty, such as the elevated sodium and depressed potassium associated with aldosteronism or the depressed carbon dioxide frequently seen in chronic renal disease.

Urinalysis and phenolsulfonphthalein excretion may help to ascertain renal status. Twenty-four hour urine excretion studies may be performed for 17 ketosteroids (an excess suggests adrenal hyperplasia or adrenocortical adenoma) or catecholamines (an excess suggests the presence of pheochromocytoma).

A chest x-ray may identify associated congestive heart failure, cardiac hypertrophy, or the typical notched ribs seen with coarctation of the aorta. An electrocardiogram may also suggest associated cardiac hypertrophy or ischemia.

In the event that treatable specific causes of the hypertension are found, therapy is initiated. Examples of correctable conditions include excision of a unilaterally diseased kidney, surgical reconstruction of diseased renal arteries, or surgical removal of hormone-producing tumors, such as pheochromocytoma or adrenal adenoma. Management of fluid and electrolyte difficulties usually helps tremendously. Chronic kidney disease associated with hypertension frequently produces chronic acidosis which responds somewhat to treatment.

Water intoxication (page 184) is similar to hypertensive encephalopathy in its manifestations; specific correction of electrolyte imbalance is therapeutic in this situation.

In most cases of hypertensive encephalopathy, no specific treatable condition will be found. Once the blood pressure has been lowered for a few hours by the injectable measures, the majority of patients will require some form of maintenance therapy. This may be achieved in many cases by the use of individual or combinations of oral diuretic and antihypertensive drugs. Patients must be encouraged to continue treatment with regular follow-up because long-standing hypertension produces systemic damage that is sometimes irreversible. Prolonged hypertension may produce strain, hypertrophy, and failure in the heart; edema, hemorrhage, and increased arteriosclerosis in the vessels of the brain; and increased atherosclerosis in the coronary and renal vessels.

RELATED FILM

High blood pressure (EM 172). Color, 7 minutes, available from state heart association.

Briefly outlined are facts about hypertension, and this film proves to be an excellent introduction to a discussion regarding high blood pressure.

Chapter 11

Vascular surgery

During the past three decades tremendous advances in the direct surgical attack on pathologic conditions of the cardiovascular system have been made. Whereas cardiac surgery is limited primarily to the larger medical centers and teaching institutions, surgical procedures on the peripheral vascular tree are becoming commonplace as larger numbers of surgeons are trained in this field. Consequently the postoperative vascular patient is being seen with increasing frequency in smaller hospitals' recovery rooms and intensive care suites as well as in the major medical centers.

By definition vascular surgery refers to surgery on any blood vessel; but this discussion will be limited primarily to arterial surgery of the aorta and its major branches, since venous surgery rarely produces critical illness.

PATHOGENESIS

Except for surgery for the occasional patient with severe trauma, surgery on the great vessels is usually directed toward relief of occlusive arterial disease or major vessel aneurysms. The etiology of occlusive arterial disease is essentially the same regardless of the location, whether coronary, carotid, or aorto-iliac arteries; for the occlusion is basically atherosclerotic, thrombotic, embolic, or a combination of these factors. Atherosclerotic plaques are more common at the bifurcation, or branching, of an artery because the arterial intima in this area is subject to injury from the high pressure currents produced by major change in direction of blood flow.

DIAGNOSTIC STUDIES

The symptom complex produced by occlusive arterial disease is entirely dependent on the area of the body involved, and several definite syndromes are well recognized. Patients having the disease will frequently appear in the intensive care unit during the immediate preoperative period when special diagnostic studies, especially arteriography, are being performed and again in the immediate postoperative period.

More precise diagnosis of arterial difficulty is possible by the injection of contrast media into the arterial tree. The approach will vary considerably with the portion of the arterial tree to be studied; however, the preferred method for study of the cervical, brachial, and vertebral trees at the present time is power injection of contrast media through a catheter threaded through a femoral artery up to the aortic arch, for this allows study of the great vessels arising from the arch of the aorta. When use of this route is not possible because of peripheral arterial disease, a catheter may be inserted through one of the brachial arteries into the aortic arch. Use of the intra-arterial catheter permits simultaneous visualization of the entire carotid-vertebral system and other portions of the arterial tree. The carotid system may be studied by direct injection of the dye into the carotid artery in the neck below the bifurcation when the catheter approach is not possible.

The femoral approach is also excellent for study of the thoracic and abdominal aorta and the renal arteries. Again, iliac or ileo-femoral disease may prevent this approach, and direct puncture of the aorta through the lumbar area may be performed.

Related nursing care. Before arteriography, food is withheld from the patient, and he is usually given a premedication such as meperidine (Demerol) and atropine. An antihistamine may be ordered in an attempt to lessen any untoward reaction to the contrast media.

Following arteriography, the patient will frequently have exacerbations of his symptomatology for a short period. In addition to watching for these symptoms, the nurse also notes any evidence of toxicity to the contrast medium through responses such as skin reactions, hypotension, nausea and vomiting, respiratory difficulty, convulsions, or anaphylactic shock. Leakage with hematoma formation in the area of the arterial puncture should be noted, as well as any signs of inflammation. Since the contrast medium may produce arterial spasm, the pulse distal to the arterial puncture should be checked. If no pulse can be detected, the physician should be notified immediately.

Since this patient usually has diffuse vascular disease, symptoms may be precipitated by fairly small changes in hemodynamics; thus vital signs should be checked frequently. It is necessary to observe the patient for evidence of myocardial insufficiency, arrhythmias, and congestive heart failure. Each patient should probably be electrocardiographically monitored during arterial studies and the immediate post-study period. The urinary output should be checked for 24 hours since the dye being excreted may cause temporary renal insufficiency.

Carotid insufficiency is among the more common syndromes of occlusive arterial disease; much of the symptomatology referable to the central nervous system actually has its point of maximum pathology in the great vessels in the neck. These areas are amenable to direct surgical approach if the pathology is located outside the cranium. The patient so affected typically is a middle-aged or elderly individual who has been having symptoms suggesting a transient stroke.

In addition to the usual frequent observations, the patient undergoing cerebral arteriography and other studies preparatory to carotid artery surgery must be watched for evidence of arterial insufficiency to the cerebral hemisphere. Visual disturbances, episodic weakness or numbness of an extremity, varying degrees of facial weakness, aphasia, intermittent confusion—all will be noted only by close observation and careful questioning of the patient.

Following carotid surgery the temporal arterial pulse on the affected side should be closely checked each time vital signs are checked. It is also advisable to check the radial pulse and blood pressure on the same side as the surgery or arteriogram or both. The status of vision and of the cranial nerves on the affected side is important; a brief review of the method for checking most of the cranial nerves is presented on page 143. Signs suggesting increasing thrombosis following either arteriogram or surgery demand prompt notification of the surgeon; these include decreasing temporal pulse on the affected side or decreasing blood pressure and radial pulse on the affected side, especially the right side. This is true because the right carotid and subclavian arteries are formed by the bifurcation of the innominate artery, whereas the carotid and subclavian arteries on the left originate directly from the aortic arch (see Fig. 2-1, page 10). The nurse should also check to see that all extremities can be moved and whether speech has been affected.

VERTEBROBASILAR ARTERIAL OCCLUSIVE DISEASE

Vertebrobasilar arterial occlusive disease is also frequently approached surgically. The symptoms usually give evidence of affection of either balance or the cranial nerves, since the brain stem is more directly supplied from the vertebral than the carotid arteries (cranial nerve signs, page 143). Because the vertebrobasilar arterial systems arise from the subclavian arteries, the symptoms previously mentioned may be associated with diminished pulsations and lowered blood pressure in the arm on the same side.

BRACHIAL ARTERY SURGERY

Axillary or brachial artery surgery or arteriogram is somewhat less common than carotid; however, the best method for following patients so afflicted is according to the pulse on the affected side. Skin color and temperature of the limb also give good clues to arterial competence, especially by comparison with the opposite extremity. Diminished temperature and pulsations or increased pallor should be reported.

AORTIC SURGERY

Aortic surgery may be required for repair of an *aneurysm* or for restoration of continuity in occlusive disease (Leriche syndrome). An aneurysm, caused by weakening of the middle muscular layer of the artery, may be of several types. The *fusiform* aneurysm affects the entire circumference of a segment of the artery, the *sacculated* aneurysm is a herniation of only one area of the vessel, while a *dissecting* aneurysm occurs when blood makes its way between the intimal lining and the muscular layer of the artery.

A very large thoracic aortic aneurysm may be an incidental finding upon chest x-ray if it has not encroached on the lumen of an artery resulting in ischemic symptoms or if it has not caused symptoms by exerting pressure on adjacent structures such as the spine, great veins, or tracheobronchial tree. The asymptomatic aneurysm discovered incidentally is more common than the symptomatic aneurysm, in both the chest and abdomen. An abdominal aortic aneurysm may interfere with blood flow through the renal arteries, producing ischemic renal disease.

Since an aneurysmal dilatation is usually filled with thrombus, this may extend to produce thrombotic obstruction of major vessels. The abdominal aneurysm commonly originates below the level of the renal arteries so that ischemic symptoms may be referable to the legs.

Occlusive aorto-iliac disease produces a definite symptom complex, the Leriche syndrome. There is pain on walking (intermittent claudication) that may be of a severity to demand cessation of effort until it has subsided. Unless collateral circulation is good, this is progressive. Trophic changes occur as demonstrated by thick nails and poor skin texture of the feet. There is a definite and persistent pallor and decrease in skin temperature with progressive changes peripherally. Pulsations checked in the femoral, popliteal, posterior tibial, and dorsal pedis arteries are diminished or absent. Poor healing follows minor trauma or infection and may progress to frank gangrene. Impotence is an important early symptom in the male. Commonly this type of aorto-iliac disease is bilateral but usually more severe on one side.

Surgical approaches. There are numerous approaches to surgery for arterial obstruction. The simplest is *endarterectomy,* which involves a simple peeling and removal of the atheromatous material lining the vessel, thus reestablishing circulation. This procedure is frequently adequate if only short areas of vessels are affected and if such areas are accessible to the direct surgical approach.

When endarterectomy is not possible, *grafting* with a synthetic material of low sensitivity potential, such as teflon, may be done. There are infinite variations to these procedures. Occasionally the graft is used to replace the affected vessel when it would be technically simple and would not add to the operative time. Another method is to anastomose the graft to the vessel proximal to the area of occlusion and to the same vessel or one of its major branches distal to the occlusion. The graft then serves as a bypass for blood flow.

A *venous graft* is occasionally used for vessels the size of the carotid, popliteal, femoral, or brachial arteries. In this situation a strip of vein is removed under standard surgical conditions and is inserted or used as an onlay or bypass graft. Since a vein has valves, the direction of the vein has to be reversed when it is used as a graft so that the valves will remain open.

Postoperative care. Following aortic surgery it is imperative that the temperature and pulse of the patient's affected extremities be noted. The patient is also observed for signs at the graft of occult hemorrhage that may be signified by increasing back pain. The physician should be notified of leg pain that might indicate arterial spasm, embolism, or thrombosis. A continuous assessment of urinary output is vitally significant. Decreased urinary output, after being reestablished following surgery, suggests the possibility of thrombosis of the renal arteries and may indicate the need for immediate reexploration. Decreased urinary output may also be evidence of the lower nephron syndrome following prolonged periods of renal ischemia. A test dose of several hundred milliliters of 20% mannitol intravenously will usually produce diuresis if the circulation is not impaired. Impairment of the renal circulation would be almost absolute indication for reoperation.

These patients usually have distention and paralytic ileus due to intestinal mobilization incident to the surgery and may require nasogastric suction until effective peristalsis returns.

POSTOPERATIVE ORDERS FOR ANY VASCULAR SURGERY PATIENT

Initial postoperative orders for any vascular patient might include the following:

1. The patient should turn, breathe deeply, and cough frequently.
2. Temporal pulses should be checked frequently (in carotid surgery).
3. Pulse, color, and temperature of affected extremities (in aorto-iliac surgery) should be checked and any areas of anesthesia or cramping noted.
4. Urinary output and specific gravity should be recorded at hourly intervals.
5. Monitoring should be continuous and onset of abnormal rhythms noted.
6. Antibiotics should be administered.

There is a tendency for the nurse to think of these surgical patients as being very delicate and to fear that performing routine nursing care including suction, turning, and so forth may rupture the anastomosis. It should be pointed out that the anastomosis is continuously subjected to the physiologic variations in arterial blood pressure and that no routine nursing procedure is likely to cause pressures greater than the physiologic variations.

During the course of surgery, fairly large doses of heparin are injected intermittently into the distal segment of the arterial tree beyond the occlusion. At the end of the procedure the heparin is theoretically neutralized by the injection of protamine in a dose of 1 mg. for each 100 units of heparin used. Since this is only an approximate neutralization, this patient should be watched closely for signs of wound oozing that might foretell of anastomosis oozing. Occasionally orders are written that the circumference of the operative area be checked hourly. This is only necessary for the first few hours, for the patient's natural homeostatic mechanism then becomes effective and the patient may even receive anticoagulants therapeutically after the first 72 hours if it is indicated.

Although the surgery is sterile, antibiotics are usually given because of the severe complications, morbidity, and mortality that can follow infection at the surgical site.

The patient having respiratory disease

Chapter 12

Basic anatomy and physiology
of the respiratory system

FUNCTION OF RESPIRATION

The function of respiration is to transfer oxygen from the external air to the blood for transport through the body and also to rid the body of carbon dioxide. Other metabolites, such as ketone bodies, are also discharged in the expired air under certain conditions.

FACTORS IN NORMAL RESPIRATION

Respiratory function depends upon the integrated activity of component parts of the respiratory system, namely (1) brain and nerves, (2) thoracic cage, (3) alveolar-capillary membrane integrity, (4) lung elasticity, and (5) an intact airway.

The *first* factor in normal respiration is *nervous control of respiration* which is seated in the respiratory centers in the brain stem. Under normal conditions these centers are primarily regulated either directly or reflexly by the concentration of carbon dioxide in the blood. Chemoreceptors located in the carotid arteries and aortic arch also supply the brain stem with information. These chemoreceptors are generally more sensitive to excess carbon dioxide than to oxygen deprivation; however, they are also sensitive to the oxygen state and blood pH. Under certain circumstances, either the carbon dioxide or the oxygen state or blood pH may serve as the primary stimulus to respiratory activity. An example of this is metabolic acidosis as seen in the diabetic or uremic patient, or the patient after short periods of respiratory failure. Kussmaul breathing results from the body's attempt to elevate pH by blowing off excess carbon dioxide.

The motor innervation for respiratory activity is transmitted by the phrenic, spinal accessory, and thoracic intercostal nerves.

The *second* factor in normal respiration is an *intact thoracic cage,* often referred to as the respiratory bellows because of its ability to change shape and volume. This cage consists of the ribs, intercostal muscles, sternum, and diaphragm and is partially formed posteriorly by the stationary spine. Inspiration involves contraction and descent of the diaphragm at the same time the internal diameter of the chest is increased by elevation of the rib cage; these are primarily musculoskeletal functions. This chest expansion creates a negative pressure

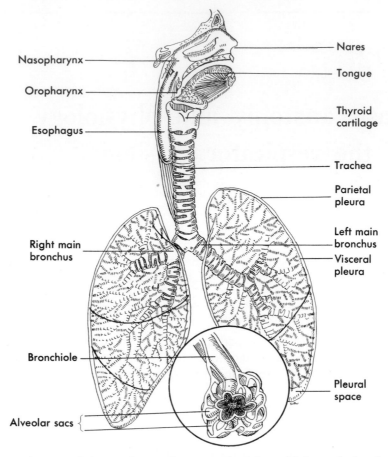

Nasopharynx

Oropharynx

Esophagus

Right main
bronchus

Bronchiole

Alveolar sacs

Nares

Tongue

Thyroid
cartilage

Trachea

Parietal
pleura

Left main
bronchus

Visceral
pleura

Pleural
space

Fig. 12-1. Airway and lungs. Insert shows terminal bronchiole and alveolar sac with related alveolar capillaries.

allowing air to rush into the respiratory tree until the pressure differential is equalized. Normally expiration is a passive function that results in expulsion of air when the components of the thoracic cage are permitted to relax. In certain types of airway obstruction, such as asthma, expiration may also become an active process.

The *third* factor in respiration depends upon the *integrity of the alveolar-capillary membranes* across which oxygen is transferred from the inspired air to the blood, and carbon dioxide and other metabolites are transferred from the blood to the alveolar air in expiration.

The *fourth* factor affecting respiration is *lung compliance* or *elasticity*. This involves the ability of the lung to expand to fill the increased volume created by the thoracic cage during inspiration, thus transferring the air into the alveolar system.

The *fifth* feature of respiration is an *intact airway* that involves patency of the nose (or mouth), pharynx, larynx, trachea, bronchi, and bronchioles.

PLEURA

The *pleura* is a moist, serous membrane that covers the lung (visceral pleura) and the inner surface of the thoracic cage (parietal pleura). Normally these surfaces are kept moist by a few milliliters of serous fluid which reduces the friction with respiratory motion. The area between the membranes is normally only a potential space because the visceral pleura is in contact with the parietal pleura. However, in abnormal conditions, this potential space may fill with air (pneumothorax), pus (empyema), blood (hemothorax), or fluid (hydrothorax).

RESPIRATORY DIFFICULTY

From the foregoing paragraphs it is evident that adequate respiration may be prohibited at several areas. Paralysis of the respiratory center is seen in bulbar poliomyelitis, occasionally in basilar artery thrombosis, and in cerebral hemorrhage that involves the brain stem. Purely nervous interference may occasionally accompany trauma involving the spinal cord.

Respiratory difficulty is encountered at the neuromuscular level in myasthenia gravis because of failure of transmission of the impulse from nerve to muscle. Respiratory paralysis at this site is frequently produced with drugs by the anesthetist to provide total muscle relaxation for the purpose of intubation and assisting in surgical exposure.

Interference with adequate respiration is seen in a number of abnormal conditions affecting the thoracic cage, such as kyphoscoliosis with a fixed rib cage. Hindrance also occurs with limited expansion of the chest from chest wall trauma, especially when steering wheel injuries separate the sternum from the ribs bilaterally. In this case there may be paradoxical motion of the chest wall; on descent of the diaphragm, at the time when the internal diameter of the chest should be increasing, it is decreased by the retraction of the sternum.

It is difficult to distinguish clinically between abnormalities of lung compliance and alveolar-capillary block, but features of both are commonly seen in the patient with severe pulmonary fibrosis and emphysema. Respiratory difficulty at the alveolar-capillary level is also seen in alveolar congestion in pulmonary edema or in the patient recovering from salt water drowning. The filled alveoli do not provide gas exchange although they may be adequately perfused with blood.

Loss of airway patency is the most common form of respiratory system failure; it is also the most easily reversible. Maintaining this patency in the critical patient is one of the most important functions of the nurse. This is especially true if the patient is also unconscious and his head is allowed to flex upon his chest. The relaxed muscles of the jaw permit the mandible to drop back, and the relaxed tongue plugs the airway. Airway obstruction is probably the most common preventable cause of accidental death. Partial airway obstruction frequently occurs in any situation in which there is interference with the cough reflex or an increase in mucus production, such as anesthesia, sedation, or bronchitis. Normal nervous stimulation, strenuous activity of the thoracic cage, integrity of the alveolar-capillary membranes, and lung compliance are all of no avail unless there is a patent connection to the atmosphere.

Chapter 13

Supporting respiration

NEED FOR ASSISTED VENTILATION

Regardless of the type of illness, the need for respiratory support or assisted ventilation is one of the more frequent requirements of the critically ill patient. The kind of respiratory support required will depend entirely on the condition of the patient; therefore, a brief review of pathologic situations that may necessitate assisted ventilation will give some indication of the type of support needed.

Assisted ventilation will be necessary for the patient whose *airway is obstructed* due to muscle relaxation, regurgitation, aspiration, asphyxiation, or bronchial asthma. It may also be needed if there is *inadequate gaseous diffusion* as might be seen during extensive pneumonia or chronic pulmonary insufficiency. Assisted ventilation may also be necessary when there is *inadequate respiratory muscular activity* as in chest injuries, so-called flail chest, or myasthenia gravis; or *inadequate nervous system control* as might occur in oversedation, brain stem injury, poliomyelitis, or increased intracranial pressure.

Not directly related to respiration but needed for adequate respiratory function is *sufficient pulmonary vascular perfusion,* which might be absent in certain heart conditions or shock. Also unrelated to the respiratory system but essential to its function are *environmental factors,* such as oxygen content of inspired air which might be inadequate at high altitudes.

The need for respiratory support is emphasized by the fact that the leading cause of death of obstetric patients is aspiration and asphyxiation rather than the more dreaded complications of hemorrhage, toxemia, and infection. If this is the leading cause of death of relatively healthy patients, it is certainly a major factor in critically ill patients. It has also been estimated that considerably more damage occurs to the patient with a head injury from the effects of anoxia than from the trauma itself.

SIGNS OF ADEQUATE RESPIRATION

Certain conditions ensure adequacy of respiration. These include (1) presence of a patent airway, (2) chest wall or abdominal movement with each respiration, (3) air flow at the mouth or nose, and (4) good skin color.

Patent airway. Presence of a patent airway includes maintaining an open airway by means of *positioning* and any *mechanical maneuvers* designed to ensure patency, such as adjunctive airways or suctioning.

The unconscious or semiconscious patient will frequently assume a position with the head flexed upon the chest with the tongue occluding the oropharyngeal area. An example of this type of airway obstruction in a healthy person is snoring, and an occasional person in normal sleep will completely obstruct his airway in this manner. Most people who "wake themselves up snoring" are actually awakened by respiratory obstruction.

Positioning. Positioning for airway patency includes such maneuvers as hyperextension of the head or anterior displacement of the mandible or both. *Hyperextension of the head* is accomplished by lifting the back of the neck with one hand while simultaneously tilting the head back by applying firm pressure over the forehead with the other hand. This maneuver pulls the angle of the jaw forward and may allow resumption of spontaneous respiration. Folded sheets or blankets 2 or 3 inches thick may be placed under the patient's shoulders to maintain this position (Fig. 13-1).

Anterior displacement of the mandible will also correct obstruction by the tongue and may be accomplished by one of two methods: (1) The mandible is *pushed* forward by pressure applied bilaterally at the angles of the jaw. (2) It is *pulled* forward by grasping the chin with an index finger under the chin and the thumb under the lower lip; it may be necessary to put the thumb into the

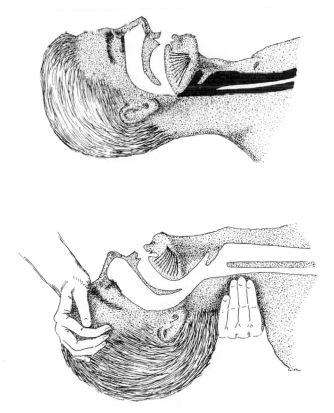

Fig. 13-1. Hyperextension of the neck for maintaining a patent airway.

Fig. 13-2. Anterior displacement of the mandible from the mandibular angle or at the chin for airway maintenance.

patient's mouth along the side of the cheek to pull the mandible forward. This positioning is helpful with obese patients. The maneuver alone may relieve the obstruction, or hyperextension of the head may also be necessary. Anterior displacement must be held constantly until either the patient recovers or some other form of airway patency is established (Fig. 13-2).

The carotid sinuses and carotid bodies aid in reflex control of blood pressure, heart rate, and respiratory rate and depth. They are located bilaterally where the common carotid artery bifurcates to form the internal and external carotid arteries. This bifurcation underlies the sternocleidomastoid muscle slightly inferior to the angle of the mandible (Fig. 13-3). For this reason anterior displacement of the mandible should be done with the fingertips placed at the angle of the jaw; for excessive deep pressure at the mandibular angle may result in compression of these sensitive structures just mentioned. This could result in bradycardia, occasionally to the point of cardiac arrest.

Mechanical maneuvers. An *adjunctive airway* may be inserted. One selects the right size and makes certain that it lies over the tongue and does not push the tongue into the pharynx. Even when an airway is inserted, it may be necessary that the head be hyperextended. An airway may be needed if there is partial obstruction during expiration due to the valvelike action of the soft palate. The increased pressure during inspiration separates the base of the tongue and the posterior pharyngeal wall, but the pressure is minimal during passive exhalation. If partial obstruction continues the air trapped in the respiratory tract is forced into the stomach, leading to regurgitation and the danger of aspiration.

Suctioning may be necessary to remove excessive secretions. It is most important to remove vomitus before attempting inflation, for acid material can be forcefully blown from the tracheobronchial tree into the lungs and can produce chemical necrosis and bronchopneumonia. The airway can be cleared by suctioning the nasopharynx or oropharynx.

Endotracheal suctioning may also be necessary. The suction catheter is inserted through the nose or mouth and is rapidly advanced simultaneously with

Fig. 13-3. Approximate relationship of carotid artery bifurcation to the angle of the mandible and anterior border of the sternocleidomastoid muscle. Sensory receptors affecting reflex control of blood pressure, pulse, and respiration are located in this area.

the onset of inspiration (if the patient is breathing) since this is the time at which the epiglottis is open the widest. Entrance of the catheter into the larynx will be signalled by a violent paroxysm of coughing and some degree of laryngospasm. The catheter is quickly moved up and down the trachea for only a few seconds because the patient may become quite hypoxic while the foreign body, the catheter, is in the larynx.

A Y valve should be placed in the aspirating system as is mentioned on page 102. The method of care of the catheter between periods of use is described on page 102.

Movement of chest wall or abdomen. Chest wall or abdominal movement should be noted with each respiration. In all methods of ventilation, absence of chest wall or abdominal movement indicates inadequate ventilation.

Air flow. Air flow at the mouth or nose may be checked by feeling or listening for it. The dorsum of the nurse's hand almost touching the nose and mouth is an excellent and readily accessible flow meter. With a little practice, the nurse is able to detect the flow of even small amounts of air from the nose and mouth during expiration. One can listen for breath sounds over the lung fields if there is doubt about the adequacy of ventilation.

Labored breathing may be encountered in a patient who appears to have adequate chest wall movement or even exaggerated respiratory effort yet who experiences relatively little gas exchange. Probably the most common example of this type of difficulty is the crowing respiration of the child with croup; his physical activity of respiration is quite exaggerated, but there is little airflow. If there is marked continued laryngospasm, an emergency tracheostomy or cricothyroid puncture is necessary.

Difficulty in breathing may also attend partial obstruction due to positioning. Increased hyperextension of the patient's head corrects this in many cases.

Skin color. Good skin color may be used as an index to the adequacy of respiration. Cyanosis is an excellent indication of anoxia except in two situations.

Fairly commonly the anemic patient with a hemoglobin less than 8 or 9 gm. percent will not have enough hemoglobin to impart the blue color of cyanosis to the skin or nailbeds; therefore this patient remains pale in spite of inadequate ventilation. Certain poisonings that permanently oxidize hemoglobin may also prevent the bluish color of cyanosis. The most common example of this is carbon monoxide poisoning whereby the patient may be totally anoxic and still be quite pink.

Cyanosis in the deeply tanned or nonwhite person may be detected by noting the bluish discoloration of the fingernails, toenails, and the palms of the hands. The sclera become pale and the gums and conjunctiva are cyanotic.

METHODS OF ASSISTING VENTILATION

Assisted ventilation may be necessary if there is inadequate respiratory effort in spite of an open airway. This may be accomplished by use of (1) expired air ventilation, (2) a portable resuscitator, or (3) intermittent positive pressure breathing.

Expired air ventilation. Expired air ventilation includes *mouth-to-mouth* and *mouth-to-nose resuscitation*. This may be the first maneuver used for a patient who has experienced sudden respiratory failure, such as that accompanying electric shock or cardiac arrest. This type of resuscitation involves three salient points: (1) hyperextension of the head, (2) maintenance of an adequate seal between the operator's mouth and the patient's airway, and then (3) inflation of the patient's lungs with the resuscitator's expired air.

The following method is used for *mouth-to-mouth resuscitation:*
1. The *head is hyperextended* as described on page 89. In addition, the patient's nostrils are occluded with the thumb and index finger of the hand that is creating pressure against the forehead. The patient's lips need to be slightly separated to allow influx of air.
2. An *adequate seal* must be maintained between the operator's mouth and the patient's mouth. The nurse takes a deep breath, opens her mouth widely, and then completely seals it over the patient's mouth.
3. The *patient's lungs are inflated* with the operator's expired air. The operator blows until the chest rises; then she removes her mouth to allow passive exhalation, listens to breath sounds from the mouth, and observes the descent of the chest.

The rescuer needs to double her tidal volume with each ventilation. Initial inflations are as rapid as possible to oxygenate the lungs; thereafter the patient's lungs are inflated from 12 to 16 times per minute. The inflations should be delivered smoothly rather than with a rapid force, for the latter approach has a tendency to also inflate the stomach.

Resuscitation attempts are usually initiated immediately if there is no obvious obstructing material in the mouth; however, if secretions or foreign materials are present, they may be cleared by a quick swabbing of the mouth with a cloth, such as a sheet or part of the patient's clothing, wrapped around the rescuer's fingers. A "bubbly" sound at expiration usually indicates that fluid is in the respiratory tree and suctioning is needed.

If the operator thinks that she is blowing into an obstructed area, further hyperextension of the head usually corrects this difficulty. If the resistance continues, the mouth should be quickly inspected for any evidence of obstruction.

The procedure is practically the same for *mouth-to-nose ventilation* except that the patient's nose is used for the airway and his mouth is closed during inspiration. The patient's mouth is allowed to open during passive expiration, for there is usually a valvelike obstruction by the soft palate to expiration through the nose. The force of inspiration must be greater than for mouth-to-mouth resuscitation because the nasal passages are smaller.

The mouth-to-nose method is preferred by some resuscitators since it may be easier to attain a seal, especially if cardiac compression is also being performed. It is simpler for the operator with a small mouth to obtain a seal and may be preferred if there are extensive injuries of the oral region. It may also be necessary if the patient develops rigid muscle tone that prevents opening the mouth.

Expired air resuscitation requires that the operator become hyperventilated so that she has twice her usual tidal volume because she is blowing against the resistance of a flaccid chest. This is hard work and is especially difficult if the patient is obese. She should not be particularly alarmed at the occurrence of symptoms of dizziness and tingling after several minutes of this hyperventilation. These symptoms can be controlled by slowing the ventilatory rate slightly or by exchanging places with another available member of the team, if possible. The use of a bag and mask can be initiated as soon as the device is available.

There may be a question as to the value of expired air for resuscitation. Measurements have been made which determine that a person can elevate the oxygen content of his expired air to 18% when he doubles his usual tidal volume; he simultaneously reduces his expired carbon dioxide concentration to 2%. When it is remembered that the usual oxygen concentration of ambient air is approximately 20%, the value of this method of resuscitation is evident.

A *pair of* **S** *tubes,* or double oral airways, may be used for mouth-to-mouth ventilation. The appropriate airway (that is, neither so long that it pushes the epiglottis against the larynx nor so short that it does not reach the back of the pharynx) is inserted until the flange of the tube covers the lips; then it is pressed firmly against the lips to effect a seal. The advantages of this method are that it allows better observation of the chest as the lungs are inflated and it is more esthetically acceptable. The disadvantage is that it is difficult to maintain a seal around the flange.

Portable resuscitator. A *portable resuscitator,* or bag and mask, may suffice for a short period of time (Fig. 13-4). This piece of equipment has distinct advantages, for it is safe, efficient, and simple to use, and allows more direct observation of the patient's chest during inspiration. It is accepted by personnel who dislike the close contact of expired air resuscitation, an aversion perhaps due to esthetics or to fear of cross infection.

There are two distinct disadvantages to the use of the bag and mask: (1) The mask must fit the contour of the patient's face or there will be leakage of air. (2) Practice and strength are necessary to master the technique of using one hand

Fig. 13-4. Artificial ventilation using bag and mask. Note hyperextension of head, the folded sheet under the patient's shoulders, and the nurse's little finger pulling the jaw forward.

to hold the mask tightly and hyperextend the head while simultaneously squeezing the bag with the other hand.

Use of this equipment involves cardinal principles: there must be a patent airway and a properly fitting mask.

A *patent airway* must be maintained for this method to be effective. The methods previously mentioned include hyperextension of the head or anterior displacement of the mandible or both. Insertion of an adjunctive airway is not mandatory in all cases, but it is helpful for the edentulous or obese patient.

A *properly fitting mask* prevents leakage. An assortment of sizes that will conform to most facial features should be available. After the head is hyperextended, the mask may be first fitted to the top or bottom of the face. To be fitted from the top of the face first, the mask is applied to the bridge of the nose by the thumb and index finger of one hand. As the mask is placed over the mouth, the lips can be separated before pressure is applied over the lower part of the mask to effect a seal. The lower border of the mask is beneath the lower lip. The fourth and fifth fingers are used to pull forward on the mandible. A reverse procedure may be simpler for some operators.

The other hand is free to squeeze the bag. If the operator's hand is small, she can compress the bag against the patient's head to increase the volume. Each deflation of the bag delivers about 800 ml. of tidal volume which will support the respiratory needs. If the resuscitator stands at the patient's head, it may be easier to maintain upward pull on the mandible and downward pressure over the bridge of the nose.

One can check the adequacy of ventilatory efforts by observing the patient's bare chest and upper abdomen. Regardless of the method used, the chest or abdomen or both should increase in diameter. Artificial respiration of any type is inadequate unless movement of one part or the other takes place.

The airway is obstructed if the chest or abdomen does not rise or the bag does not empty; hyperextending the head even more corrects the condition in most cases. If the bag empties but the chest does not rise, there is leakage around the mask and it needs to be refitted. The face and mask are quickly dried before the mask is reapplied.

Oxygen should be added to the inhaled air as soon as it is available. It can be given while using the bag and mask for resuscitation by attaching the tubing from the oxygen to the adaptor on the portable resuscitator.

Intermittent positive pressure breathing. Intermittent positive pressure breathing (IPPB) machines may be used as aids to respiration although they are not satisfactory for use in the emergency phases of artificial respiration. This is especially true if external cardiac compression is necessary, for the inspiratory phase of the cycle terminates prematurely due to sternal compression, resulting in shallow and insufficient ventilation. These machines are necessary for continued ventilation when the patient does not resume spontaneous breathing.

Two types of machines are available. One type provides a fixed *pressure* while the other presents a fixed *volume* of gas.

The Bird and Bennett respirators are commonly used pressure-cycled instruments (Fig. 13-5). The detailed operation of these machines, as of other technical

Fig. 13-5. The Bird pressure-cycled respirator. Note (1) adjustable pressure control, (2) air mixture, (3) expiratory time, (5) inspiratory time. Sensitivity control (4) is on the ring on the left and is not identified in this photograph. (Courtesy Bird Corporation, Palm Springs, Calif.

instruments, is best explained in the instruction manual furnished by the manu-facturer; however, several generalizations are possible.

These machines deliver oxygen-gas mixtures to the lungs under pressure. This aids in increasing the saturation of the arterial oxygen and the removal of carbon dioxide, thus assisting in regulating the respiratory acid-base levels.

These machines may be used in two ways: (1) to assist inadequate ventilatory effort and (2) to provide artificial ventilation when there is no ventilatory effort.

Assisting inadequate ventilation. When the respirator is used to assist inade-quate ventilation, it is set so that it is triggered by the patient's feeble respiratory effort. When triggered, the machine provides the oxygen-gas mixture under an increasing pressure until it reaches a preset pressure level. During this pressure phase, the oxygen-gas mixture is forced into the airway, filling the lungs and expanding the chest if the airway is patent and if there is no leak in the system. When the preset pressure is reached, a valve opens to release this pressure, permitting expiration to take place because of the normal elasticity of the lungs and chest wall.

When used in this manner three controls are significant.

1. *Oxygen dilution.* This is adjustable on all models. Gas mixtures possible include atmospheric air or various oxygen dilutions with air or other gases, such as helium. These gas mixtures need to be humidified to counteract the drying effect of the gas.

2. *Sensitivity control.* The amount of patient effort necessary to trigger the pressure cycle is adjusted with this control.

3. *Pressure control.* This control is adjusted to the amount of pressure present at the mask or airway connection. This pressure will then be forced into the chest providing that the airway is patent and that there is no leak in the system, such as in the tubing or where the mask fits the patient's face.

This pressure control is usually adjusted to 15 to 20 ml. of water pressure. Initially the pressure may be lower if the patient is conscious until he becomes accustomed to the machine and may then be raised to the ordered level. With large individuals or increased chest wall resistance, higher pressure may be required.

When used for assisting ventilation, these respirators may be used supportively over a period of hours or days. They may also be used intermittently, such as for 15 or 20 minutes four times daily, to improve the exchange of oxygen and carbon dioxide and to prevent or treat atelectasis. The number of times used decreases as the patient improves.

Providing artificial respiration. When these machines are used to provide artificial respiration, oxygen-gas mixture under pressure is provided to the air-way at regular periods. The respirator continues to inflate the patient's lungs until the preset pressure is attained. The pressure is then released, and expiration occurs because of the elasticity of the lungs and chest. Some models must be cycled manually, but most models can be set to cycle automatically.

Several factors can be controlled with use of this equipment for artificial respiration. The *oxygen dilution* regulates the oxygen percentage presented at the airway. *Sensitivity* is set on the automatic cycle. The *pressure control* varies the pressure presented during the inflationary phase. Pressure required for adequate artificial ventilation is usually greater than for assisted ventilation (usually around 25 ml.).

Frequency or *rate control* permits variation in the number of complete cycles activated per minute. This control is usually set within usual respiratory range of 15 to 20 per minute. Hyperventilation might be desirable when functional lung tissue is reduced or toxins, such as carbon monoxide, are excreted in the expired air. Decreased rate might be desirable when one is checking for return of spontaneous respiratory effort.

In addition, certain models can be set to cycle automatically following the lapse of a preset period of time without spontaneous respiratory effort. In this use the equipment might be said to be providing both assisted and artificial respiration.

Intermittent positive pressure breathing may be accomplished with machines that present a fixed volume of oxygen-gas mixture. This type is preferred by some physicians who think there is less variability in the oxygen-gas mixture that the patient receives.

Problems attending assisted ventilation. When controlled ventilation is used, it is recommended that the patient *sigh* or inspire deeply at regular intervals to aid in preventing atelectasis. To accomplish this in the unconscious patient, the pressure control is turned to the prescribed increased pressure for the instructed number of breaths. This procedure is usually repeated hourly, or as ordered by the physician.

In all types of assisted ventilation, abdominal distention due to air entering the esophagus is a problem. Gentle pressure applied to the upper abdomen will help to expel air from the inflated stomach. If regurgitation occurs, the patient's head is quickly turned to the side before the vomitus is aspirated. If prolonged assisted ventilation seems likely, this problem of gastric insufflation can be corrected by insertion of a nasogastric tube or endotracheal tube.

A tracheostomy will also prevent gastric distention from air. In addition, it provides an adequate seal for mechanical respirators when an adaptive cuff is used, affords ready access to the tracheobronchial tree for suctioning, and reduces the dead space in the respiratory tree.

Drug treatment. Drugs have a very minor place in supporting respiration with three possible exceptions. Methylphenidate (Ritalin) is used in barbiturate overdosage, and nalorphine (Nalline) is used in morphine intoxication; both are fairly effective respiratory stimulants. Another possible exception is caffeine, which stimulates the respiratory center during Cheyne-Stokes respiration. No time should be lost from artificial ventilation to search for effective drug treatment, for immediate mechanical support of respiration is necessary until adequate respiration is achieved.

OXYGEN THERAPY

Oxygen therapy is needed for a wide variety of disease conditions. Basically, increased oxygenation of the inspired air assists the essential respiratory function of oxygenation in the presence of impaired ventilation, circulation, or diffusion. While it improves oxygenation, one must remember that oxygen therapy does not improve the other major respiratory function: carbon dioxide removal. The increased oxygen content of the inspired air may actually be detrimental in some disease conditions (page 123).

Precautionary measures are necessary when oxygen is administered. Materials that produce static electricity, sparks, or flames are potentially dangerous since oxygen supports combustion and are therefore restricted. Smoking is not allowed in the area while oxygen is in use, and all lighters, matches, and smoking materials are removed from the patient's room. A sign should be displayed that oxygen is in use as a further reminder to both family and personnel.

Oxygen should be administered in a manner agreeable to an already apprehensive patient. Some patients tolerate a face mask, while others have a feeling of choking when they use it; some are comfortable in an oxygen tent, while others experience claustrophobia. Because there are many methods of oxygen administration available, one can try several until the most suitable is discovered. Before administration, one should explain the procedure to the patient and reassure him concerning its efficacy.

Oxygen may be administered by means of a canopy tent, face tent, facial mask, nasal cannulae, or nasal catheter.

When a *canopy tent* is in use, the concentration of oxygen around the patient is greater; therefore further safety measures are instituted. Woolen blankets are not used since they produce static electricity, and a hand bell is substituted for the electric signal bell because of the danger of sparks. Although a mattress protector is usually standard equipment, one should check to see that it is in place; since oxygen is heavier than air, the protector is necessary to conserve the oxygen and prevent its absorption into the mattress.

When the tent is used initially, the temperature is set to 70° F., but later it may be regulated as the patient desires. After the tent is flushed with oxygen the gauge is set around 10 to 12 liters per minute. The tent is tucked under the mattress on both sides and at the top; a folded bath blanket enveloping the bottom of the tent may be used to prevent leakage from this area.

The *face tent,* a cuplike device that fits around the patient's cheeks and chin, may be most suitable for extremely anxious patients, for there are fewer mechanical restraints that might further agitate a person who is already apprehenesive. After the patient becomes accustomed to it, fasten the strap that holds the face tent in place. The usual range of flow is from five to eight liters per minute.

When a *facial mask* is used, the oxygen flow is turned on and then the patient is allowed to position the mask and become accustomed to it before the retaining straps are fastened. The setting for oxygen flow is usually eight to ten liters until the patient becomes used to the mask; then the flow is decreased to six to eight liters. The reservoir bag expands and partially collapses with each respiration; if it collapses completely, the oxygen flow should be increased. If oxygen is needed for an extended period of time, the skin under the mask will need attention. The skin should be washed, dried, and lightly powdered at least every two hours, as should the mask.

Nasal cannulae may be used if the patient breathes through his nose; he must be cautioned against mouth breathing since this dilutes the oxygen concentration. The cannulae are repositioned at least every two hours so the direct flow of oxygen does not irritate the nasal mucosa. A water-soluble lubricant should be used as a protective covering for the nasal mucous membranes. The oxygen flow is usually set from four to six liters per minute.

Nasal catheters come in varying sizes and have many small holes encircling the distal end. The approximate distance for insertion is determined by measuring from the tip of the nose to the tip of the ear with the nasal catheter. The natural droop of the catheter is determined by rotating it between the fingers, and then the catheter is inserted so that this curvature follows that of the nasopharynx. Before being inserted, the tip is lubricated with a water-soluble material. Lubricants with oil bases are not recommended because they pose the danger of causing lipoid pneumonia.

A word of caution is worthwhile here. We have seen at least two patients whose already critical condition was made even more acute by severe gastric distention. This was due to their swallowing oxygen administered by a nasal catheter that was inserted too far in the pharynx. For this reason, the pharynx should be inspected after the catheter is inserted. If the tip of the catheter is visible, it is withdrawn approximately 1 to 2 cm. ($\frac{1}{2}$ to 1 inch).

RELATED FILM

Prescription for life (EM 101). Color, 48 minutes, available from state heart association.

This film provides physiologic and clinical information covering the ABC's of emergency resuscitation.

Chapter 14

Tracheostomy

> **Typical initial orders include**
>
> 1. Suctioning as needed
> 2. Removal and cleaning of inner cannula
> 3. Instillation of sterile saline drops in tracheostomy tube
> 4. Humidity
> 5. Conversation assistance
> 6. Semi-Fowler's position
> 7. Encourage coughing and deep breathing; turn every two hours
> 8. Encourage fluids
> 9. Dressing and tape changes as needed

Tracheostomy, or the production of an artificial opening through the neck into the trachea, is performed for a number of reasons and in many different situations.

REASONS FOR PERFORMING TRACHEOSTOMY

Probably the most common reason for a tracheostomy is to maintain a patent airway, as is frequently necessary when there is injury and soft tissue–swelling about the head and neck or occasionally following a thyroidectomy. It may be performed when a patient is expected to be unconscious or unable to assist in expectorating secretions for a period of time, such as following a craniotomy.

A tracheostomy is sometimes performed to eliminate approximately 150 ml. of dead space in the respiratory tree. The procedure might be effective in any situation in which there is a severe decrease in tidal volume. It will be recalled that for respiration to be effective, the external air must come into contact with the alveolar-capillary membranes. If only a few milliliters of air are moved during each respiratory effort, the inspired air is grossly diluted by the relatively large volume of expired air in the nasal, oral, pharyngeal, tracheal, and bronchial passages. A tracheostomy is frequently done to reduce the dead space in a patient with an acute exacerbation of chronic respiratory insufficiency, usually brought about by pulmonary fibrosis and emphysema.

Tracheostomy may occasionally be required for a patient with severe obstructive asthma or status asthmaticus or when laryngeal edema is present from a severe allergic reaction. It is sometimes indicated in cases of chest injury with marked impairment or insufficiency of the respiratory bellows.

Tracheostomy provides ready access to the airway for cleansing which may be advantageous in any patient who has an impaired cough reflex and also requires tracheobronchial aspiration, such as a comatose patient. It may be beneficial for any patient in poor general condition who is producing large quantities of sputum, such as the critically ill patient who also has superimposed pulmonary edema or one with overwhelming pulmonary infection, such as multiple lung abscesses or bronchiectasis. The tracheostomy provides a means for prompt and efficient cleansing of the tracheobronchial tree.

A tracheostomy may be helpful in simplifying assisted ventilation. All of the mechanical respirators are equipped with an adaptive cuff that is easily attached to a tracheostomy; this lessens the chance of the leakage that is more likely to take place when a face mask is used. A cuffed tracheostomy tube further decreases the possibility of leakage when it is coupled with a mechanical device for artificial ventilation.

A tracheostomy also obviates the rather strenuous task of keeping the upper airway patent in an unconscious patient.

RECOGNITION OF NEED FOR TRACHEOSTOMY

Nursing personnel may recognize the need for a tracheostomy from changes indicating respiratory distress. These signs include increasing respiratory difficulty signified by an increasing rate or a change in the breathing pattern so that it becomes gasping. Severe dyspnea may also be manifested by increased muscular effort during breathing signified by the patient's using the accessory muscles of respiration, and finally by sternal retraction.

If there is trauma to the soft tissues of the neck, edema may increase to the point that it compresses the trachea. Measuring the circumference of the neck at frequent intervals immediately after the injury may aid in determining the extent of swelling.

Other signs of respiratory distress include an increasing tachycardia, cyanosis, and the patient's purposeful change from a recumbent to an upright position to aid his breathing. He will also be quite apprehensive and will speak in phrases between labored breaths.

The physician is immediately notified, and the nursing personnel gather the needed equipment which includes a tracheostomy tray, sterile gloves, disinfectant, local anesthetic, a towel or blanket roll to place under the shoulders to hyperextend the neck, and suction equipment.

TRACHEOSTOMY CARE

Tracheostomy care is not particularly complicated although it requires meticulousness and is individualized for each patient. Techniques vary considerably in different institutions; some doctors believe that aseptic technique should be followed by use of a sterile disposable catheter and sterile gloves for each suctioning, whereas others think that a scrupulously clean technique is acceptable since the area is normally contaminated by air inspired with each breath. In view of the fact that it seems more practical, nursing care relating to the latter technique will be described. Personnel should remember to wash their hands frequently with a germicidal soap.

1. *Suctioning* of the tube should be done as needed; this will vary greatly with each patient. Most patients require very frequent suctioning during the first 24 to 48 hours because the trachea responds to the foreign body (tracheostomy tube) by producing copious secretions. In addition to emergency suctioning to maintain a patent airway, some physicians prefer that the patient be suctioned at least every 2 hours for the first 24 to 48 hours to remove mucus before it becomes hardened. This care also reduces the possibility of infection from these secretions, an excellent culture medium for bacteria.

The whistle-tip catheter has a smooth, rounded end that allows more effective removal of mucus plugs than does a urinary-type French catheter with its opening on the side. The diameter of the suction catheter should be no more than two-thirds the diameter of the lumen of the tracheostomy tube to allow entrance of air to facilitate suctioning. Although the suction catheter does not completely occlude the lumen of the tube, its presence tends to stimulate bronchial spasm and coughing so that the patient will receive very little oxygen while being suctioned. For this reason suctioning should be intermittent, and the nurse should form the habit of holding her breath while suctioning her patient as an aid in determining when it should be discontinued.

The catheter, which should be attached to the suctioning equipment with a T or Y valve, can be placed in the trachea without suction which lessens damage to the tracheobronchial membranes. By placing a finger over the open valve, one can create suction and apply it intermittently.

Suctioning should be deep enough to clear the airway of secretions so that the patient can breathe quietly. Immediately after a tracheostomy, it is desirable to enter both bronchi to remove secretions in order to maintain patency and reduce the possibility of infection. As the patient improves and secretions become minimal, deep suctioning may cause trauma to the membranes and be more harmful than helpful. Because of the anatomic structure of the neck and thorax, rotating the head to the right and elevating the left shoulder makes the left main bronchus more accessible to suction; turning the head to the left and raising the right shoulder makes the right main stem bronchus more readily available.

The catheter should be rotated as it is withdrawn; intermittent suction during withdrawal lessens the possibility of damage to the tracheal membranes. After the patient has been suctioned, clean water should be suctioned through the catheter to remove secretions inside the instrument, and then the outside of the catheter is wiped to remove external secretions; it is placed in an antiseptic or disinfectant solution to soak between uses to reduce the possibility of contamination. Solutions used might be aqueous benzalkonium chloride (Zephiran) 1:750 or sodium bicarbonate solution 5%. If it is necessary that the upper respiratory tract be suctioned, separate catheters should be used.

2. *The inner cannula should be removed and cleaned* thoroughly periodically. A suggested method is to rinse it under cool running water to remove most of the mucus and then use double pipe cleaners in the lumen to remove mucus by friction. Encrusted mucus may be loosened by soaking the inner tube in hydrogen peroxide, a mild antiseptic, for a *brief* period of time, such as from three to five minutes. This briefness is emphasized because the removable inner

cannula permits secretions to be evacuated more readily; if the inner cannula is not in place, secretions become encrusted in the lumen of the outer tube and may occlude the patient's airway. While the inner tube is soaking in hydrogen peroxide the lumen of the outer cannula can be suctioned to remove any secretions present.

The inner cannula should be handled carefully since those made from silver dent easily. Before its reinsertion, it should be inspected to see that no foreign particles which could be aspirated, such as string or lint, are present. The outer tube should be held during insertion and removal of the inner cannula; this lessens trauma at the operative site and decreases irritation of the trachea around the lower opening of the outer cannula. After reinsertion one should make sure that the inner tube is locked in place.

3. *Sterile normal saline drops* instilled directly into the tracheostomy tube immediately prior to routine suctioning aid in loosening secretions and stimulating the patient's cough reflex. The number of drops will vary according to the order of the physician, usually from 3 to 5 or maybe as many as from 10 to 15.

4. *Humidity* is needed since one of the functions of the nasopharynx is to moisten the inspired air. One of the common complications with a tracheostomy is the development of inspissated material within the tracheobronchial tree. A steam or cold water vaporizer used near the patient will help to prevent drying of mucosal secretions.

An alternative procedure is the light placement over the tracheostomy of a half thickness 4 by 4 inch gauze compress which is moistened frequently with water. One must make certain that no loose threads or bits of cotton can be inspired.

Detergents or mucolytic agents may be used with the tracheostomy; however, care must be taken that the concentration reaching the tracheobronchial tree is not excessive because none of the material is diluted by secretions from the nasopharynx.

5. *Communication methods* must be explained to the patient with a tracheostomy tube. When the larynx is otherwise intact, the nurse should remember to show the patient that he is able to speak by the simple expedient of covering the tracheostomy tube, thus permitting air to flow out over the vocal cords. If the patient is unable to cover the tube the nurse can do this for him, and other methods of communication must also be established, as with hand or eye signals. If the patient is able to write his messages, the use of a child's magic slate is recommended.

6-8. *Semi-Fowler's position* is usually preferred for most efficient breathing. *Coughing and deep breathing* are important in preventing lung complications since the body's normal defense of filtering the air through the upper respiratory passages has been eliminated. The patient should be instructed to hold the sides of the tube as he coughs to lessen the irritation caused by the tube's movement; this also lessens his fear of expelling it. *Turning* is important in preventing hypostatic pneumonia, for the turning causes movement of secretions which are then expectorated more easily. *Adequate fluid intake* will aid in liquefying secretions.

Fig. 14-1. A tracheostomy dressing that requires no cutting.

9. *The dressing* under the tracheostomy tube should be changed when it becomes soiled because dried blood and other secretions near the surgical incision encourage bacterial growth. The operative site should be checked frequently for bleeding. The skin may be cleansed with hydrogen peroxide when a new dressing is applied. The suitable dressing shown in Fig. 14-1 has no loose strings that might be aspirated.

When changing the tapes, one nurse holds the tube in place while another nurse replaces the old tapes. A slit is cut about one inch from the end of the tape, and this slit end is placed through the flange of the tube; the tape is threaded through the slit, and the two tapes are tied securely with a square knot placed on one side of the patient's neck (Fig. 14-1).

Several other points should be mentioned concerning care of a patient with a tracheostomy. Reassurance of the patient and his family is of primary importance because both are apprehensive and fearful that the patient may die from asphyxia. One can allay anxiety by explaining procedures and making the call button easily and instantly accessible if the nurse must leave the patient's bedside. The patient also needs encouragement when he first attempts to swallow or eat because he is fearful that food and liquids may enter the tracheostomy tube when he swallows.

The obturator fits inside the outer tube and has a smooth, rounded end which protrudes beyond the outer tube and permits easy insertion. It accompanies the individual tracheostomy tube and should be resterilized after its initial use and then always be kept at the bedside for ready accessibility. Occasionally a patient will cough violently and expel the tube; rarely one will panic and remove the outer tube. The immediate availability of the obturator which fits the tube then in use greatly facilitates replacement of the tube. The obturator is also used to plug the tracheostomy tube when the physician wishes to check the normal respiratory passageway prior to removal of the tube. Another precautionary measure includes the availability at the bedside of another sterile tube of the same size as the one worn by the patient and of a pair of sterile tracheal forceps which could be used to hold the trachea open in the event that the tube was expelled and immediate replacement could not be accomplished.

CUFFED TRACHEOSTOMY TUBE

A cuffed tracheostomy tube is occasionally used, primarily in conjunction with a positive pressure respirator to form a closed system or to reduce the possibility of aspiration from lack of laryngeal and pharyngeal protective reflexes. The care of the patient fitted with this tube is similar to that previously described and includes a few additional observations and points of care.

When this tube is used, the area around the trachea is sealed by the inflation of an encircling balloon around the lower portion of the outer cannula. This prevents air from entering or escaping from the upper passageway and also reduces the possibility of aspiration of secretions from the upper respiratory tract into the lower trachea. The cuff, which is usually made of soft rubber, is inflated by injecting air into a fine bore tubing that leads to the balloon. A small pilot balloon is located distally in the inflating tubing; inflation of this balloon signifies that the cuff balloon is also inflated.

Equipment needed to inflate the cuff includes a 10-ml. syringe and a hemostat whose ends are padded with rubber tubing to prevent damage to the small bore tubing. To inflate the cuff, the syringe is filled with from 5 to 10 ml. of air. The fine bore tubing may be equipped with a flanged end to accommodate the syringe, or it may be sealed, in which case air is injected by needle. The least amount of air is injected that will adequately seal the trachea.

The nurse may assume that a seal has been made if there is no audible escape of air from the patient's mouth or nose or around the tracheostomy tube or if air cannot be felt in these areas when the patient exhales. The amount of resistance of the trachea against the cuff when the tube is gently tugged is also a suitable indication of a seal. If the patient is conscious he may attempt to speak; if the cuff is properly inflated he will be aphonic, since there is no escape of air over the vocal cords.

After the balloon is inflated the hemostat is clamped over the tubing to prevent air leakage, and the syringe is removed. At this time the pilot balloon should be partially inflated. With each inflation the amount of air required should be recorded, and any appreciable increase in the amount needed should be reported to the physician since it might indicate tracheal dilatation.

The physician should also be notified immediately if difficulty is encountered in inflating the cuff. These cuffs occasionally develop a leak that can be detected when the pilot balloon deflates while the tubing is still clamped. Rupture of the cuff balloon will be apparent under the following conditions: (1) Large amounts of air will not inflate the pilot balloon, and no resistance to this increased volume of air is met; (2) more air can be withdrawn from the fine bore tubing than was injected originally; (3) the patient continues to be able to speak; or (4) the positive pressure respirator is unable to maintain adequate respiratory movement with pressures or volumes that were previously adequate.

Since the patient's only route for air exchange is through the patent tracheostomy tube, the tube must be kept meticulously clean. If a respirator is being used, some method of manual ventilation must be immediately available, should a mechanical failure occur. In the event of an emergency, the face mask should be removed from the mechanical ventilator and replaced with the adaptive tracheostomy cuff.

The air inspired through the respirator needs adequate humidification, which is usually achieved with sterile water. The nebulizer and connecting tubing should be resterilized at least every 48 hours since this equipment may be a source of infection. Placing the nebulizer below the level of the trachea will prevent nebulizer condensate from entering the trachea.

Since secretions from the upper respiratory passageway tend to accumulate in the trachea immediately above the cuff, they should be removed by suction immediately before deflation of the cuff to prevent their passage into the lower respiratory tree. It is *very important* that the cuff be periodically deflated to reduce the possibility of tracheal ischemia and necrosis, complications resulting from use of a cuffed tube. A suggested period of deflation is five minutes every hour.

To lessen the possibility of tracheal necrosis, some physicians recommend that the cuff be inflated only to a point at which the leak from the positive pressure ventilation is minimal. They also believe that this slight passage of air will aid in removing secretions through the larynx.

Chapter 15

Chest injuries

Chest injuries are particularly hazardous since the chest contains the organs concerned with the vital functions of circulation and respiration, both of which must continue without interruption for even short periods of time. Also, chest injuries are becoming increasingly common, principally because of automotive transportation and the relationship of the steering wheel to the automobile driver's chest.

Chest wounds may involve the bony framework of the chest, the heart, lungs, or great vessels; and combined injuries are frequent. The liver and the spleen may also be damaged.

INJURY TO CHEST FRAMEWORK

Rib fracture. Uncomplicated fractured ribs pose little problem in care other than pain relief; however fractured ribs occurring in a patient with impaired pulmonary function may result in voluntary splinting to the point of inadequate ventilation. This situation can usually be managed by adequate pain relief, careful attention to bronchial cleansing, frequent deep breathing and coughing, and suctioning when necessary. Assisted ventilation may be required.

Fractured ribs may result in torn blood vessels producing hemothorax; pneumothorax results if the pleura and lung tissue are lacerated. If rib fracture is complicated by external communication, there is the added danger of infection. Primary management of these conditions will be mentioned later in this chapter.

Sternum fracture. Fracture of the sternum is not ordinarily hazardous of itself. On the other hand, because of the rather marked amount of bone marrow contained in the sternum, the patient is somewhat more prone to developing fatty embolism from a sternal fracture than from other comparable-sized injuries. The fatty embolization syndrome, which also attends major fractures of long bones, is characterized by the production of sputum containing fat, by microscopic hematuria with occasional fatty droplets in the urine, and possibly by delirium. These findings are due to microembolism in the lungs, kidneys, and central nervous system. Usually fever results from the inflammatory process, and pain may occur at the site of embolism because of local ischemia and vasospasm. Fatty embolism does not require specific treatment other than antibiotics and supportive therapy. By refraining from additional orthopedic manipulation, further embolism may be avoided and these patients can be expected to recover.

Flail chest. Of more functional significance than a fractured sternum is the so-called flail chest. This is produced by a blow to the anterior chest wall which results in fracture or separation of the costochondral cartilages so that the sternum is largely free floating. The injury produces rather severe pain that causes the patient to voluntarily limit respiratory effort. In addition, it greatly interferes with adequate ventilation since the anterior chest wall is nonfixed or free floating; the chest loses its bellows function, and paradoxical motion of the anterior chest wall may be noted. During inspiration when the diaphragm is descending and the chest internal diameter expanding, the sternum moves paradoxically, that is, retracts. This greatly reduces the effective ventilation, perhaps cutting tidal volume by as much as from 50% to 75%.

Treatment. Immobilization of the sternum and assisted ventilation comprise the primary management of flail chest. Immobilization is sometimes accomplished by putting indwelling screws in the body of the sternum; traction with pulleys and weights is then applied to these screws to prevent the paradoxical motion of the sternum during inspiration, thus permitting adequate ventilation. Since this and other definitive treatments, such as open fixation of the interrupted cartilages, are time-consuming operative procedures, it is usually necessary to support respiration with assisted ventilation until the surgery can be performed. The ventilation may be accomplished by means of a portable resuscitator until endotracheal intubation can be done.

INJURY TO HEART

Myocardial contusion. Because of the position of the heart between the bony spinal column and the sternum, severe chest compression may result in myocardial contusion as the heart is compressed between these bony structures. The area of damaged myocardium may produce a condition similar to myocardial infarction, both electrocardiographically and clinically. Therefore, the patient must be watched for all of the complications to which patients with myocardial infarction are susceptible, including abnormal rhythms, shock, heart failure, and thromboembolism. Except for use of anticoagulants, which would be contraindicated, the management of these complications is essentially the same as for those arising from a myocardial infarction (page 19).

Hemopericardium. Resembling the event of myocardial rupture following infarction is hemopericardium following myocardial contusion; however, it differs from rupture in that the prognosis is considerably less grave. Hemopericardium usually results from blood oozing from injured myocardium into the pericardial sac. The gradual compression of the heart by the collection of pericardial blood results in a number of signs that may be recognized by the observant nurse. These symptoms are largely produced by decreased diastolic filling as the atria are progressively compressed by the accumulation of pericardial fluid. This will result in a gradual increase in pulse rate and a gradual narrowing of pulse pressure (with or without a drop in systolic pressure). Moreover, the jugular veins will be distended since the vena cavae are unable to empty effectively.

The same effect of poor drainage of the pulmonary blood into the left atrium will result in failure of diastolic filling of the left ventricle, and a paradoxical pulse may be felt. In this situation the pulse disappears during the inspiratory phase of respiration; the combination of negative intrathoracic pressure and increased intrapericardial pressure causes a few beats during which no left-ventricular filling occurs, and this situation, if unrelieved, will bring about rather prompt pulmonary edema and death.

The electrocardiographic voltages may progressively decrease as the hemo-pericardium increases, for the blood in the pericardial sac acts as insulation between the myocardium and the electrocardiograph electrodes.

Definitive treatment is directed toward alleviating the collection of peri-cardial blood by means of a pericardicentesis. A large caliber (16 to 18 gauge) needle is inserted into the pericardium, and the occluding blood is withdrawn. If this procedure is effective, there will be a prompt loss of the paradoxical pulse, a temporary drop in the pulse rate and blood pressure as a result of return of diastolic filling to normal, and then prompt improvement in circulatory status. Patients should be watched closely for recurrence of hemopericardium. Its reappearance might signal the necessity for exploration and the possibility of suture of a myocardial tear.

INJURY TO LUNG

Contusion of lung. Chest injury may also result in contusion of the lung, pro-ducing an area of traumatic pneumonitis. In addition, communication of a bronchiole with the pleural cavity can lead to pneumothorax.

Pneumothorax. Pneumothorax is produced when there is communication between the atmosphere and the pleural space so that the intrapleural negative pressure is lost. This can occur either from a free communication through the chest wall or a channel into the bronchial tree.

Tension pneumothorax. Tension pneumothorax results when the communi-cation between the pleural space and the atmosphere is not free but has a ball valve or flutter valve type of opening. Through this opening, air is drawn into the pleural cavity by the negative pressure of inspiration, but on expiration the change in the chest wall or lung results in closing of the communicating space so that the intrapleural air cannot escape. With each respiratory cycle the entrapped air increases, thus progressively compressing the adjoining lung tissue.

Clinically, tension pneumothorax is heralded by increasing respiratory dis-tress, cyanosis, tachycardia, and a definite unilateral effect of respiration, the affected side being almost fixed in a relative inspiratory position and moving little with respiratory effort. A chest x-ray confirms this, for the mediastinal structures and trachea may be shifted away from the affected side.

Treatment. The treatment for pneumothorax is prompt thoracentesis and removal of the trapped air. If a tension pneumothorax is present with continuous leakage, a thoracotomy catheter must be inserted and connected to a closed drainage system.

Hemothorax. Another complication of chest injury is hemothorax, in which either an intercostal or a lung vessel is torn so that blood leaks into the pleural cavity. This is particularly serious since the chest cavity is capable of holding an astounding amount of blood; exsanguination into the chest cavity without evidence of external blood loss may result. Here again, in addition to the decreased blood volume and decreased cardiac efficiency with shock, the patient is further impeded by decreased respiratory efficiency from the associated collapsed lung. Furthermore, since the mediastinum is mobile rather than rigid, it may shift, thus perhaps decreasing the expansibility of the uninvolved lung and also interfering with venous return.

The presence of hemothorax is suggested by increasing dyspnea, unilateral respiratory lag, tachycardia, hypotension, and perhaps frank shock. Respiratory dullness and decreased breath sounds are elicited over the affected side, produced by the fluid (blood) in the pleural space.

This condition is promptly relieved by thoracentesis with removal of the blood and adequate replacement of the lost blood volume. If the hemothorax recurs, it is best treated by closed chest drainage or perhaps even by exploration in an effort to alleviate the source of blood loss.

Treatment. In all of these situations—hemopericardium, pneumothorax, hemothorax—an immediate chest x-ray by means of a portable machine will help to elucidate the exact nature of the problem; but the nurse can be extremely helpful in suspecting them, noting minute variations in the patient, and notifying the physician of these changes.

Closed chest drainage. Closed chest drainage is an arrangement by which fluid, blood or air may be drained from the pleural space while the negative pressure of the intrapleural space is maintained. This continues to be a source of wonderment to many nurses; but if one recalls the function of a thoracotomy, it is relatively easy to understand.

A catheter is placed within the chest cavity in the pleural space either through a trocar or by open surgery, and then the catheter is affixed to the skin so that no air may enter or leave from around the incision. The patient may leave the emergency room or operating room, where this procedure is usually done, with this catheter clamped, or it may be attached to the closed chest drainage system.

Closed chest (or water seal) drainage equipment consists of a gallon bottle fitted with a two-hole rubber stopper through which two tightly fitting glass tubes extend. Both tubes are patent; one is short and allows air to escape from the bottle. The other tube, which is connected to the drainage tubing proximally, has its distal end submerged one to two inches in sterile water in the drainage bottle (Fig. 15-1). Convenient disposable sets are also available.

The purpose of the water trap is to permit drainage of air, fluid, or blood while simultaneously maintaining the constant negative pressure within the pleural space. In this manner, excess air may bubble from the pleural cavity; yet when the pressure within the pleural space becomes negative, air is not allowed to enter from the tube because it is sealed by the water in the bottle being sucked up into the tube. Therefore, the negative pressure is maintained by the force of gravity on this column of water. The excess air that escapes from the pleural space into the bottle can then leave the bottle through the short glass tube in the stopper. In addition, material collecting in the pleural space is permitted to drain and is collected in the bottle.

Occasionally the first thoracotomy bottle is attached to a second bottle that

Fig. 15-1. Closed chest drainage. Note that two clamps are on bed readily available if the thoracotomy catheter requires clamping.

serves as a double safety valve for protecting the sterility and vacuum of the system. The vacuum in this system may be maintained by the effect of gravity; or, if air leakage is fairly significant or drainage great, it may be facilitated by low intensity suction attached to the second thoracotomy bottle.

In cases of increased damage, surgeons sometimes insert two thoracotomy catheters with two separate closed chest drainage systems. One is usually high in the pleural cavity while the other is lower, or they may be anterior and posterior. The upper tube removes air that rises because of its light nature, while the lower tube expedites drainage of heavier secretions. Multiple tubes might also be used in individuals with pleural scarring or loculated collections of fluid.

Related nursing care. To maintain gravity drainage, the bottles must remain lower than the patient. Regardless of the care with which the nursing service uses thoracotomy bottles, other ancillary personnel, especially housekeepers, may elevate the bottles for the purpose of housecleaning or bed moving. Therefore care should be taken that the bottles be either firmly affixed to the floor or placed in some type of stand that is lower than the patient.

If it is necessary that the patient be moved for the purpose of x-ray or other procedures, the thoracotomy tube may be disconnected *after* the catheter is double clamped, thus preventing air from entering the pleural space. If it is necessary to continue the drainage while such procedures are done, the patient and the closed chest drainage equipment are transferred to the facility. During the transfer the catheter is double clamped; then the bottles may be placed on the same level with the patient on the stretcher. After arrival, the bottles are lowered and the clamps removed.

Observation of a patient undergoing closed chest drainage includes several points. The system is airtight, so care must be taken that no pins are placed in the tubing and that all connections are taped to decrease the possibility of air leaks. The long glass tube in the drainage bottle must *always* be under water.

After the thoracotomy catheter is connected to the closed chest drainage system, a strip of adhesive tape should be placed vertically on the bottle with the water level indicated. If there is excessive drainage, the level at each hour can be marked on this tape.

The character of the drainage should be noted as to whether it appears grossly bloody or diluted with serum or exudate. If the drainage is only pinkish but then becomes a bright red, the physician should be notified immediately.

Fluctuation of the water in the tube in the drainage bottle should be watched. Initially there is usually great fluctuation as the pressure in the pleural space changes with respiration. As the lung reexpands, this pressure gradation diminishes and there is little fluctuation. Failure of the occurrence of at least minimal fluctuation indicates difficulty, as when the tube is occluded with a blood clot; such occlusion prevents drainage and does not allow for changes in pressure. One must be sure that drainage is not obstructed by blood clots or kinks in the tubing. If the drainage is great, an order may be given to periodically milk or strip the tubing. This is always done *toward* the drainage bottle.

As a precautionary measure two clamps are immediately available at the bedside in the event that the bottles are broken. If the clamps are not accessible, the catheter is simply bent to occlude air flow until help can be obtained. Forceps used should have no teeth that might damage the tubing.

The function of measuring the drainage and refilling the bottle with the measured amount of sterile water may be the responsibility of either the physician or the nurse. Whatever the case, the catheter must be double clamped before the stopper is removed from the bottle. Aseptic technique is used and one must work quickly.

The patient is always initially placed in semi-Fowler's position. Surgeons vary in their attitude regarding turning their patients. Some wish that their patients be turned from side to side every two hours, while others prefer that their patients lie on the affected side most of the time. Adherents of the latter believe this lessens pain, permits better expansion of the unaffected lung, facilitates drainage, and helps to prevent spread of any possible infection to the mediastinum and unaffected lung. When the patient is lying on the operated side, folded towels may be placed on either side of the tubing, or the tubing may fit inside a rubber ring to increase the comfort.

The dressings should be checked for drainage and the patient watched for shock or hemorrhage. Any increasing dyspnea or cyanosis should be reported. The patient is encouraged to cough, and splinting of the wound may make the coughing less painful. The dose of analgesia may be decreased so that the drug can be given more frequently. Fluid intake should be forced so that sputum will be liquefied; a vaporizer may also help achieve liquefaction.

RUPTURE OF GREAT VESSELS

Rupture of great vessels can result from chest injury. If the vessels are veins, the symptoms depend on the blood loss and the area into which the blood drains, whether mediastinal, pericardial, or pleural. Rupture of a major intra-thoracic artery results in prompt exsanguination. However, if the tear is small, the blood loss might be slower and the clinical picture might resemble a dissecting aneurysm.

Definitive treatment is surgical repair and replacement of blood volume. Additional supportive therapy may include drainage of compressing collections by means of closed chest drainage.

INJURY TO ABDOMEN

Although the liver and spleen are located in the abdominal cavity, they are largely protected by the lower thoracic cage. Therefore, any patient with a chest injury should be closely observed for signs of a surgical abdomen.

Contusion of liver. Contusion of the liver with bleeding is usually heralded by abdominal tenderness, distention, and evidence of occult blood loss although the chest remains clear. This condition usually requires blood replacement as well as surgical exploration for hemostasis.

Contusion of spleen. Contusion of the spleen followed by splenic rupture is especially insidious since the capsule of the spleen is quite elastic and the splenic pulp may sustain quite a significant injury without rupture of the capsule. This condition results in bleeding into the spleen and its gradual enlargement so that it may attain a tremendous size before it suddenly ruptures. The rupture is heralded by the immediate onset of profound shock, abdominal rigidity, and signs of peritoneal irritation. Rupture is most likely to occur from one to three days following injury, and its detection requires careful observation; this condition requires immediate surgery.

Chapter 16

Status asthmaticus

Typical initial orders include

1. Adrenergic agent
2. Sedation or tranquilization
3. Bronchodilator
4. Steroid
5. Antibiotic
6. Oxygen administration
7. Respiratory detergent
8. Fluids
9. Expectorant
10. Laboratory studies

CLINICAL FINDINGS

The typical asthmatic patient in an intensive care unit is one who has had severe asthma for more than 24 hours. At the time he arrives he has usually had nearly the maximum doses of his usual asthmatic remedies. Since the major component of these medications is usually ephedrine or some epinephrine-like agent, he may require treatment for epinephrine intoxication (adrenergic crisis, page 259) as well as treatment for severe asthma.

Typically the patient is seated and is pale, perspiring profusely, leaning forward with arms rotated inward, and using all his accessory muscles of respiration. He is slightly to moderately cyanotic, and the respiratory rate may be increased, his wheezing audible without aid of a stethoscope. Some patients' respiratory rate is not increased because the extreme prolongation of the expiratory phase prohibits a rapid rate. The pulse is usually rapid, and the blood pressure may be depressed. Generally the patient appears exhausted from the extreme effort necessary to breathe and from contributing factors of insomnia and anorexia.

If the patient is approaching adrenergic crisis, his pupils will be widely dilated, he will be unusually apprehensive, and he will be experiencing extreme tachycardia, 150 beats or more per minute. The blood pressure is likely to be elevated initially; then as toxicity increases, a drop in pressure may result from incomplete diastolic filling (from the short diastole of rapid rate) and exhaustion. However, this has considerable variation.

PATHOGENESIS

The basic etiologic factor involved in asthma is usually allergy, but there are usually other major contributing factors in the patient in status asthmaticus. These include unusually hot or cold or extremely dusty immediate surroundings, recent contact with other inhaled antigens, or a respiratory infection; emotional factors are also frequently important.

The normal physiologic protective mechanisms may become exaggerated to the point of contributing to the pathology in the patient with severe asthma. Bronchi become constricted to decrease inhalation of the foreign antigen, thereby producing bronchospasm. Copious amounts of thick, tenacious mucus are secreted to dilute and entrap the foreign material being inhaled. There is also dilatation of blood vessels and hypertrophy of the bronchial walls. Because of all these factors and a cough reflex weakened by exhaustion, diffuse small areas of atelectasis are likely to occur secondary to bronchiolar obstruction. If this condition is widespread and prevents gas exchange, the patient can die of asphyxia.

Since bronchi dilate during inspiration and tend to constrict during expiration, there is a tendency for air to be trapped peripherally during expiration by obstruction from stenosis and edema; therefore, the primary efforts of the patient are in expiration.

TREATMENT

1. An *adrenergic agent* is used if the patient has not been treated with these agents for this episode. Aqueous epinephrine 1:1,000 in small doses may be administered for immediate effect; then epinephrine in oil 1 ml. of 1:500 solution may be given intramuscularly at eight hourly intervals after the acute phase has subsided.

2. *Sedation or tranquilization* or both are required, for these patients are extremely anxious because of the nature of the illness. Moreover, their apprehension may be increased by the use of adrenergic agents. The sedation must be definitely limited, however, to preclude the possibility of respiratory depression. Small doses of meperidine (Demerol), such as from 35 to 50 mg., from 50 to 100 mg. hydroxyzine pamoate (Vistaril), or from 15 to 30 mg. phenobarbital at three- to four-hour intervals with or without ephedrine-like agents may be indicated. Again it must be noted that respiratory depression is not present before subsequent doses are administered. Because of its depressing effect on respiration, morphine is *not* used.

3. A *bronchodilating agent* is used, and most are pharmacologically akin to epinephrine. Ephedrine may be used by mouth for prolonged maintenance or for supplementing injectable or inhaled bronchodilators. Because of the anxiety and tachycardia produced by these drugs, they are frequently combined with mild sedatives or tranquilizers.

Intravenous theophylline (aminophylline), a nonadrenergic agent, is a good bronchodilator although the effect is of very short duration. Theophylline may be administered in intravenous fluids up to 1 gm. over a two- to three-hour period of time. Isoproterenol (Isuprel) is a good bronchodilator and is usually administered by nebulization although it is available for parenteral use and in tablets for buccal use. It is not effective if swallowed.

4. A *steroid,* such as dexamethasone (Decadron) or hydrocortisone (Cortef) may be given intravenously initially. A steroid is used in the severe asthmatic patient for two purposes: (1) to decrease inflammation and (2) to block allergic reactions. Any patient with severe asthma probably needs administration of this drug over a short period of time, the dose and type of drug varying somewhat according to the severity of the situation.

For immediate effect, intravenous administration of the drugs just listed is quite helpful; corticotropin (ACTH) gel can be given intramuscularly for a more prolonged effect. Prednisone or another similar drug may be given by mouth for longer effect.

A typical patient might initially receive 4 mg. of dexamethasone in the intravenous fluid in conjunction with theophylline with an order for maintenance doses of prednisone, 5 mg. by mouth four times daily.

5. An *antibiotic* is given almost routinely because infection frequently affects the patient with status asthmaticus. A throat or sputum culture should be done *prior to the first dose* of the antibiotic. For routine treatment while one is awaiting culture reports, the erythromycin-penicillin group of antibiotics is probably preferred because they are more likely to influence the usual respiratory infections than are some of the broader spectrum antibiotics. As an example, 250 mg. erythromycin or 250 mg. penicillin may be ordered orally every six hours.

Because of the patient's increased tendency toward experiencing allergic reactions, he should be questioned carefully regarding any previous reactions to antibiotics.

6. *Oxygen* may be given if the patient is cyanotic or in extreme respiratory difficulty. However, with the presence of fairly long-standing respiratory insufficiency, oxygen deficit may be the driving force for respiratory exchange; and the patient must be evaluated carefully for respiratory depression with improved oxygenation, for this may lead to the occurrence of respiratory acidosis.

7. A *respiratory detergent* may occasionally be quite helpful in enabling the patient to get rid of much of the inspissated bronchial mucus. A good route of administration is open face tent with oxygen being used as the carrier. It may also be administered by positive pressure machine, but few patients with a severe case of status asthmaticus will tolerate that machine. The detergent and this mode of treatment are more effective for the patient with chronic asthma.

Ethyl alcohol in gradually increasing concentrations may considerably decrease the surface tension of the bronchial secretions and also aid in expectoration. The treatment may be started by bubbling oxygen through a 10% to 20% solution of alcohol placed in the container that humidifies the oxygen. The flow can be set at a low rate, such as from 2 to 3 liters per minute; gradually increments of alcohol are added until a 40% to 50% solution is reached. The patient may also absorb the alcohol given in this manner to assist in tranquilization, but he should be closely observed to avoid oversedation with accompanying hypotension. The humidifier containing oxygen should be clearly labeled while in use, and the solution should be discarded after the acute episode has passed because the solution is clear and cannot be distinguished from water.

It is again stressed that when oxygen is used as the vehicle for either alcohol or a respiratory detergent, one should watch for increased carbon dioxide retention, which will lead to carbon dioxide narcosis and respiratory depression. If the depression becomes too severe, assisted mechanical ventilation may be necessary.

8. *Fluid intake is encouraged,* for the patient who has had severe asthma for several days has probably created a fluid and electrolyte deficit due to the poor fluid intake and extreme diaphoresis. Since this dehydration also contributes to the tenaciousness of the bronchial secretions, adequate hydration usually aids in better sputum production.

A hematocrit greater than 50 or hemoglobin greater than 15 gm. usually indicates the need for additional hydration. Intravenous fluids are generally given initially to serve as the vehicle for medication and to aid in correcting dehydration.

The patient usually initially prefers a soft or bland diet and can progress to a diet as desired. He should be questioned regarding any food allergies and these noted prominently on his chart.

If the patient is nauseated or vomiting, usually from excessive adrenergic agents, it is best to limit oral fluids until these symptoms subside rather than risk more fluid loss from the oral route plus the danger of aspiration.

9. An *expectorant,* such as ammonium chloride, may be ordered to aid in liquefying the bronchial secretions. Antihistaminics are usually not used because of their drying effect.

10. *Laboratory studies* include *electrolyte studies* to detect any abnormalities. A *chest x-ray* should be taken because unsuspected areas of pneumonic consolidation, pulmonary infarction, or pulmonary effusion may be completely obscured during physical examination by the extremely noisy and active respiratory effort. Spontaneous pneumothorax may also occur if dilated alveoli at the surface of the lung rupture into the pleural space. The chronic entrapment of air peripherally in the lungs from frequent and severe asthma may lead to chronic pulmonary emphysema.

An *electrocardiogram* should be used to aid in the detection of pulmonary infarction, cor pulmonale, or electrolyte imbalances, especially hypokalemia.

In extreme cases it may be necessary to perform a tracheostomy to decrease the respiratory dead space.

RELATED FILM

Cold light endoscopy. Color, 30 minutes, availble from the Upjohn Company Film Library, 7000 Portage Road, Kalamazoo, Mich.

This excellent film shows examinations of many of the body's internal organs during their normal and abnormal conditions, including bronchial asthma as it is occurring.

Chapter 17

Pneumonia

Typical initial orders include

1. Antibiotic
2. Adequate fluids: intravenous and oral
3. Oxygen administration
4. Humidity
5. Expectorants
6. Analgesics and antipyretics
7. Endotracheal suctioning if necessary
8. Respiratory isolation
9. Turn, breathe deeply, and cough frequently
10. Laboratory studies

CLINICAL FINDINGS

The patient with pneumonia in the intensive care unit usually has this illness either (1) as a complication of some other serious or debilitating disease or (2) as an overwhelming infection with one of the organisms less sensitive to the commonly administered antibiotics.

The patient, who is quite febrile, flushed, and short of breath, usually experiences severe coughing which may produce moderate amounts of blood-tinged sputum. There may be a visible lag in respiratory motion on the side most severely involved, especially if extensive consolidation is present. The patient may be somewhat cyanotic.

PATHOGENESIS

Pneumonia, or inflammation of lung tissue, may be due to infection (bacterial, rickettsial, fungal, or viral) or chemicals (lipoid or kerosene). Concurrent with this inflammation, there is exudation, filling and stretching of some alveoli, and collapse of adjacent alveoli. The nonfunctional areas may coalesce into a solid area of lobular or lobar distribution, producing lobar pneumonia. The inflamed areas may be multiple, patchy, and distributed along the terminal bronchioles, producing bronchopneumonia.

These consolidated areas of lung tissue are unable to bring inspired air into contact with blood for gas exchange; therefore, blood brought to these areas by the pulmonary circulation is returned to the systemic circulation in a sub-oxygenated state.

As bacteria multiply in the alveoli, they cause the following pathologic changes to occur:

1. *Red hepatization,* in which state blood serum and cells escape from the capillaries and enter the alveoli;
2. *Gray hepatization,* in which state the alveoli are filled with cells and fibrinous exudate so that the alveoli contain no air;
3. *Resolution,* finally occurring when the exudates are removed by phagocytosis.

TREATMENT

Treatment for pneumonia is both specific and supportive.

1. *Antibiotics* to which the organism producing the condition is sensitive are administered. (The initial dose is given *after* the sputum culture has been obtained.) If the patient has not received prior treatment, the organism is likely to be either a streptococcus or a pneumococcus, both of which are highly sensitive to penicillin; this drug, then, is usually the first to be administered. More recently there has been a tendency toward initial treatment with ampicillin because it has a somewhat broader spectrum than penicillin and seems to be less likely to produce resistant strains.

If the patient has received prior antibiotic treatment, the organism is most likely to be either staphylococcus coagulase-positive or Friedländer's bacillus (*Klebsiella pneumoniae*). These organisms are usually sensitive to less wide variety of antibiotics, and administration of either chloramphenicol (Chloromycetin), methicillin sodium (Staphcillin), or erythromycin is usually initiated.

2. *Adequate fluids,* administered either intravenously or orally, are usually needed by the patient with extremely high fever who is dehydrated because the increased metabolic rate incident to fever greatly increases the body's need for fluid. If the critical condition is prolonged, the type and amount of fluid will have to be tailored to the patient's blood electrolyte studies.

Taking liquids orally is encouraged to aid in adequate hydration; however, the patient with pneumonia may have adynamic ileus as a part of general toxicity. In this case oral intake of fluid is withheld because of the likelihood of gastric distention and vomiting, and hydration is maintained with intravenous fluids until peristalsis returns.

A urinary output of 1,000 ml. or more each 24 hours usually indicates adequate hydration; therefore, urinary output of from 300 to 400 ml. at each change of nursing shifts suggests sufficient fluid intake.

3. Additional *oxygen* may help to relieve the patient's dyspnea. It is administered by the method most satisfactory for each patient (page 97).

4. *Humidity* should be increased in the patient's immediate surroundings by the use of a steam or cool water vaporizer. The humidified air assists in preventing inspissation of large amounts of mucus, thus aiding in cleansing of the tracheobronchial tree.

5. *Expectorants* may be necessary to relieve the frequent and inefficient coughing.

6. *Analgesics,* such as codeine, may be necessary to suppress the central

nervous system cough reflex; *antipyretics,* such as salicylates, are needed to reduce the fever. If the patient is too ill to take oral medications, it may be necessary that an injectable preparation be prescribed. If the patient is febrile to the point of experiencing central nervous system irritability, mild sedation may be necessary.

7. *Endotracheal suctioning* may be required if the sputum is particularly tenacious. Although this procedure is usually performed by the physician, it may be done by the nurse in an emergency (page 90).

8. *Respiratory isolation* is effected in an effort to prevent cross infection with other patients who are also seriously ill. The patient having pneumonia should not be placed in an intensive care unit unless the physical facilities are such that adequate isolation technique can be provided.

9. The patient should be instructed to *turn, breathe deeply, and cough frequently.* Although these are routine orders for most patients, they are very important for the patient with pneumonia since they aid in removal of exudates from the respiratory tree. The patient's side is splinted to reduce the pain associated with coughing. Frequently he will expectorate sputum that is tinged with bright red blood early in his illness. As the disease progresses and resolution begins, the sputum becomes rust colored.

10. *Laboratory studies* generally include a complete blood count, sputum culture, blood culture, and roentgenogram of the chest. Both cultures are obtained before administration of the antibiotic. A direct smear of the sputum for gram stain may give a rather good hint as to the type of organism involved, especially if it looks like a pure culture of staphylococcus on direct smear. The blood culture may indicate that the patient has bacteremia; some patients have a true septicemia.

Tracheostomy. Occasionally a patient will require a tracheostomy for the purpose of adequate tracheobronchial suction. This is especially true in the debilitated patient who lacks the energy for adequate coughing or who has an inefficient cough reflex. A tracheostomy will also lessen the work of breathing by reducing the respiratory tract dead space.

COMPLICATIONS

Complications of pneumonia are *systemic* or *local* or both. Systemic complications include *circulatory collapse, septicemia, meningitis,* and *acute bacterial endocarditis.* Local complications include *respiratory insufficiency* from necrosis of lung tissue, *lung abscess, empyema,* and *atelectasis.*

Circulatory collapse may be heralded by a drop in blood pressure and a pulse elevation in excess of that indicated by fever. Certain bacterial toxins are capable of producing rather severe hypotension; the advent of shock and hypotension in the patient having pneumonia is a bad prognostic sign. This shock is usually treated with pressor agents and large doses of adrenal steroids, usually administered intravenously.

Septicemia may begin by recurrence of a spiking fever, occurrence of petechiae, and a positive blood culture in addition to the manifestations of pneumonia. The occurrence of septicemia once definitive treatment has been initiated suggests that the organism is resistant to the treatment being used. A change of antibiotics or use of an additional antibiotic is usually indicated until a sensitivity study is confirmed by the laboratory.

Meningitis is heralded by physical signs of delirium; nuchal rigidity; and evidence of central nervous system irritability, such as tremors or convulsions and abnormal signs, such as Kernig's and Brudzinski's signs (see Glossary). The presence of meningitis is confirmed by spinal fluid findings.

A somewhat less common complication is *acute bacterial endocarditis* with changing murmurs and evidence of cardiac involvement in addition to those of pneumonia and septicemia. Fulmination or extremely rapid progression of the inflammation is probably an indication for the most massive antibiotic treatment in medicine, for example 100,000,000 units of penicillin daily.

Chapter 18

Chronic pulmonary insufficiency

Typical initial orders include

1. Oxygen administration
2. Assisted ventilation
3. Bronchodilator
4. Respiratory detergent
5. Sedation
6. Corticosteroid
7. Antibiotic
8. Expectorant
9. Diuretic
10. Digitalis
11. Humidity
12. Tracheostomy
13. Diagnostic studies

CLINICAL FINDINGS

The typical patient with chronic pulmonary insufficiency requiring intensive care is a late-middle-aged or elderly man who is in borderline pulmonary decompensation at all times. His basic disease is usually pulmonary fibrosis and emphysema; then he is placed under an additional strain, usually by an acute respiratory infection or by any situation that increases metabolic demands.

He speaks in short sentences, uttering phrases between labored breaths. He is usually cyanotic and perspiring profusely and wheezing audibly. Although there will be very little movement of his barrel chest, he uses the accessory muscles of respiration for maximum respiratory effort. His expiration is prolonged and requires active effort. The fact that he is badly frightened further increases his metabolic demands. He may show signs of cerebral anoxia, as confusion or delirium; anoxia may be so severe that he becomes stuporous or unconscious.

Moderate to marked tachycardia may be present with the pulse being paradoxical, that is, disappearing during certain phases of respiratory effort because of the decreased venous return during the forceful expiration. He may be hypotensive, but the blood pressure may also fluctuate considerably according to the various phases of respiration. He is usually febrile and will frequently have dependent edema from associated right-heart failure.

PATHOGENESIS

Pulmonary emphysema accompanied by pulmonary fibrosis is the most common underlying condition. Basically emphysema is the result of partial bronchiolar obstruction so that air can be drawn into terminal groups of alveoli; then during expiration the bronchioles constrict, and air is trapped in the alveoli. Intraalveolar pressure is increased, and fragile alveolar membranes are ruptured and eventually replaced by fibrous tissue. Thus, over a long period of time a great deal of the respiratory membrane that serves to permit gas exchange between the inspired air and the blood is lost. Because of bronchiolar constriction, expiration requires active effort in contrast to the passive process typifying normal expiration. At necropsy the lungs appear hyperexpanded and heavy.

Chronic pulmonary insufficiency may also afflict patients with other conditions, such as the patient who has undergone a significant pulmonary resection for any condition, the one who has been treated for tuberculosis with pneumothorax and has failure of reexpansion, or the asthmatic individual with associated edema of the bronchial mucosa leading to obstruction of the air passages. It can also occur in the patient with pulmonary sarcoidosis or chronic fungus infection.

Treatment of these patients is quite frustrating because no single endeavor seems to be of great help. Extreme care must be exercised, with special attention given to details of numerous pharmacologic and physiologic approaches to the problem in the hope that the combined effort may return the patient to his former state of at least nearly adequate pulmonary compensation.

TREATMENT

1. *Oxygen administration* is one of the more important factors in treating this patient since he is usually suffering from extreme anoxia (page 97). Normally the primary stimulus to respiration is elevated arterial level of carbon dioxide; however, the patient has usually sustained chronic carbon dioxide retention so long that oxygen deprivation may serve as his primary stimulus to respiration. For this reason, oxygen must be administered with care.

The patient may be experiencing respiratory acidosis, also known as carbon dioxide narcosis, resulting from reduced arterial oxygen and elevated carbon dioxide. If the carbon dioxide level has been elevated for some time and oxygen deprivation is the driving force for respiratory effort, improvement of oxygen saturation may lessen respiratory effort and increase carbon dioxide retention, thus worsening the acidosis. This chain of undesirable events can usually be avoided if adequate assisted ventilation is used.

Signs of this critical complication of respiratory acidosis include restlessness, confusion, incoordination, and tremulousness. The patient may complain of a headache, or he may be disoriented to the point of hypomania. He is usually cyanotic and has marked tachycardia. Respiratory acidosis should be suspected when there is evidence of underlying pulmonary disease.

When he receives adequate oxygen, this patient may undergo apneic periods that last until the oxygen level falls, at which time he reflexly begins breathing again. The occurrence of these periods should be considered an absolute indication for some type of assisted ventilation because the patient badly needs the improved oxygen status and concomitant carbon dioxide reduction.

It is recommended that the use of oxygen for this type of patient be intermittent at a low liter flow, that is, from one to three liters of oxygen flowing for fifteen minutes and then none for five minutes. The *pulse* rather than the respiration may be used as an index of anoxia, tachycardia being the deciding factor.

2. *Assisted ventilation* by means of intermittent positive pressure breathing machine (IPPB) is usually ordered. This machine aids the respiratory muscles with respiration by automatically inflating the chest following minimal spontaneous respiratory effort. If no spontaneous effort occurs, the machine may be set to cycle automatically; this may be necessary if carbon dioxide narcosis or oversedation takes place. It can also be used prophylactically to prevent respiratory acidosis, for the carbon dioxide content is reduced at the same time the oxygen deficit is satisfied.

The conscious patient experiencing extreme pulmonary insufficiency will rarely tolerate the presence of the mask necessary to use this equipment. A tracheostomy may be done. If the patient is unconscious and this equipment is used, an adequate airway must be maintained.

3. A *bronchodilator* may be administered systemically, orally, or intranasally. Ephedrine and its analogues are frequently used.

4. A *respiratory detergent* or mucolytic agent may be administered by means of the IPPB to reduce the surface tension of the bronchial secretions and aid in their removal.

5. *Sedation* is required for this patient, who is usually quite anxious. Again, the effect of respiratory depression must be considered in selection of the drug to be used. If respiratory depression seems to be a significant factor and the patient is extremely restless or agitated, a *minimal* dose of an opiate may be helpful in reducing the metabolic requirement while also producing a certain amount of euphoria. A sedative-antidepressant or tranquilizer may also be used for this purpose.

6. A *corticosteroid* is usually given to lessen the inflammatory reaction and to reduce the allergic bronchospastic component that is fairly frequently present.

7. An *antibiotic* is routinely given to this patient since the precipitating incident for his deterioration is usually infection. Too, the patient's poor cough reflex makes his residual tissue an excellent site for infection. Empirically, a broad-spectrum antibiotic may be used until the culture reports are available. Culture samples are always taken *before* the initial dose of the antibiotic is given.

8. An *expectorant,* such as potassium iodide or ammonium chloride, helps to liquefy the sputum and increase its production. They are especially helpful in long-term management.

9. A *diuretic* is usually ordered, for the patient frequently has fluid retention and at least minimal right-heart failure.

10. *Digitalis* is usually given to this patient since an element of heart failure is almost always present. However, its use in this patient is usually disappointing, its effect seldom startling. The patient's tendency toward developing digitalis

intoxication is somewhat greater than that of the patient without chronic pulmonary insufficiency.

11. *Humidity control,* which helps to loosen secretions, may be accomplished by an area vaporizer using steam or a cold mist. Adequate fluid intake also aids in liquefying secretions.

12. A *tracheostomy* may be done in severe cases for several reasons. The patient's already small tidal volume would be more efficient if the 150 ml. of dead space of the larynx and nasopharynx were avoided by tracheostomy, which also affords ready access for tracheobronchial cleansing and may facilitate assisted ventilation via one of the positive pressure machines. These advantages must be weighed against the increased possibility of causing respiratory tract infection by temporarily removing part of the body's natural barriers to infection.

13. *Diagnostic studies* are undertaken soon after the patient is admitted. Since a respiratory infection usually precipitates the patient's difficulty, a *throat* or *sputum culture* is done to identify the offending organisms. Culture samples should be taken before initial administration of antibiotics.

A *chest x-ray* is taken soon after the patient's admission. Occasionally in this type of patient an emphysematous bleb may rupture into the pleural space, or pleural effusion may result from early congestive heart failure; the presence of pneumothorax or effusion might require a thoracentesis for relief of symptomatology.

An *electrocardiogram* is frequently made for several reasons. Since the patient has chest pain, the primary precipitating factor may be a cardiac condition, such as a myocardial infarction. Recurrent pulmonary infarction may be the primary etiology, and any acute episode of pulmonary insufficiency may be precipitated by another pulmonary embolus. Usually the electrocardiogram will not be etiologically helpful and will only show right ventricular strain or giant P waves typical of pulmonary hypertension.

Blood or serum *electrolytes* are determined early since electrolyte imbalance is common and may need correction. The *carbon dioxide combining power* is frequently quite increased because the chronic carbon dioxide retention has resulted in fixed base (sodium) retention which acts as a buffer for the acid carbon dioxide.

More specific information may be obtained from determination of *arterial blood pH* and *oxygen saturation* if these studies are available. A *complete blood count* frequently shows polycythemia as a compensatory mechanism in attempting to carry more oxygen to the tissues; leukocytosis is usually present because of infection.

Respiratory stimulants, such as caffeine, are occasionally used for this patient when carbon dioxide retention and increased oxygenation result in depressed respiratory activity. However, respiratory stimulants as such have little place in the long-term treatment of the patient with chronic pulmonary insufficiency.

In addition to noting changes in the patient that might occur as a result of the therapy just mentioned, nursing measures may include the following. A pillow might be placed at the back to exaggerate the normal lumbar curvature and allow for better excursion of the diaphragm. Since the patient habitually stays in the upright position to allow for better ventilation, the overbed table covered with pillows may aid his rest.

Postural drainage is helpful when tolerated and should be done about 15 to 30 minutes after bronchodilators or expectorants are given. Since most of these patients are elderly and may have arthritic difficulties as well, the knee portion of the Gatch bed may be elevated for the postural drainage. The drainage often precipitates nausea because of the odor and taste of the sputum; consequently it is best that it take place about an hour before meals and be followed by mouth care.

Breathing exercises can also help the patient to use his respiratory muscles more effectively, especially the diaphragm. Some patients find that wearing an elasticized abdominal support is helpful since the diaphragm has become flattened and less active.

If the patient is observed carefully and attention is paid to all of the therapeutic possibilities available for him, the outcome will generally be rewarding, with the patient returning to his former state of compensated chronic pulmonary insufficiency.

RELATED FILM

Recognition and management of respiratory acidosis. Color, 35 minutes, available from Smith, Kline & French Laboratories, 1500 Spring Garden St., Philadelphia, Pa.

The etiology, symptoms, and importance of early recognition are discussed.

The patient having central nervous system disease

Chapter 19

The unconscious patient

Typical initial orders include

1. Maintenance of adequate ventilation
2. Intravenous infusion
3. Frequent check of vital signs
4. Diagnostic studies

Care of the unconscious patient involves three major requirements: (1) maintenance of vital functions, (2) protection from further damage if possible, and (3) initiation of a systematic search to determine the cause of the unconsciousness. Once the reason for the unconsciousness is determined, definitive treatment of the primary condition is begun.

PATHOGENESIS

The many causes of unconsciousness may be divided into three broad groups: (1) those within the central nervous system, (2) metabolic or toxic factors that affect the central nervous system, and (3) exogenous materials that also affect the central nervous system either directly or indirectly.

The first group, *causes within the central nervous system,* might include such conditions as a brain tumor, hemorrhage, stroke, encephalitis, epilepsy, trauma to the brain or adjacent structures, abscess of the brain, meningitis, or increased intracranial pressure regardless of the cause.

The second group, *metabolic or toxic causes,* could include uremia, diabetic acidosis, spontaneous hypoglycemia, hepatitis, respiratory acidosis, anoxia regardless of the cause, hyperventilation, hypertensive encephalopathy, eclampsia, and marked changes in acid-base balance.

The third group, *exogenous materials,* includes accidental or intentional poisonings with chemicals such as barbiturates, tranquilizers, insulin, or alcohol. Other toxic materials include carbon monoxide by inhalation, snake venom, or antigens which produce an anaphylactic reaction. It is significant to note that the most common cause of deep coma of patients admitted to general hospitals in the United States is self-induced poisoning with depressant drugs.

The levels of consciousness vary on a continuum from somnolence to coma. Generally, in *somnolence* the patient is excessively drowsy and responds by mumbling or making jerking movements if addressed or touched. In *stupor* the patient responds, by grimacing and withdrawing, only to painful stimuli. In *coma* there is no reaction whatsoever to stimuli, and the patient cannot be aroused. In deep coma there is no gag or corneal reflex, and there may or may not be pupillary reaction to light.

TREATMENT

1. *Adequate ventilation* must be maintained by any measures feasible. Any or all of the following may be required: mouth-to-mouth ventilation; use of a portable resuscitator; oropharyngeal or endotracheal airway; nasopharyngeal, oropharyngeal, or endotracheal suctioning; tracheostomy; or mechanically assisted ventilation with automatic cycling machines.

The most frequent cause of additional damage to the unconscious patient is inadequate ventilation effecting anoxic damage. Important clues to anoxia are (1) obvious inadequate respiratory effort with absent or decreased chest or diaphragmatic motion and (2) cyanosis from inadequate gas exchange. Occasionally patients may be anoxic without being cyanotic (page 92).

2. An *intravenous infusion* should be started to provide ready access to the circulation in the event that emergency measures need to be taken to support circulation. Blood volume expanders or pressor agents may be needed. The intravenous infusion, which frequently contains glucose, is begun *after* blood is drawn for laboratory studies since these studies include analysis of blood glucose to detect diabetic acidosis or hypoglycemia. The physician may then order 50 ml. of 50% glucose intravenously slowly to counteract insulin shock, which is statistically common. This effort is harmless even in the presence of diabetic acidosis and is specific for insulin shock. The solution is hypertonic and should reduce cerebral edema as well as initiate diuresis, regardless of the cause of the unconsciousness.

3. *Vital signs* should be checked frequently. Salient deviations may be indices of certain disease conditions.

A *temperature elevation* is commonly found during infection, dehydration, and brain stem damage. *Hypothermia* may be noted following cold exposure and overdoses of depressing drugs such as barbiturates, opiates, and some tranquilizers.

Pulse changes are common in the unconscious patient. *Tachycardia* may indicate shock or congestive heart failure with decreased cardiac output that leads to inadequate cerebral perfusion. A rapid pulse may also indicate the hypermetabolic state, such as occurs with fever or with severe hyperthyroidism and produces exhaustion. *Bradycardia* is found with increased intracranial pressure, Adams-Stokes syncope, or simple fainting.

Respiration, with its changes in rate or pattern, may be very significant. Difficult respiration may be the first indication of airway obstruction. *Hyperpnea,* or respiration that is deeper and more rapid than normal, is present in any acute condition that interferes with respiratory gas exchange. *Kussmaul* respiration is a distinctive type of hyperpnea characterized by rapid, unlabored, deep respirations and is a common manifestation of diabetic acidosis. Rapid shallow breathing is often noted in shock.

Depressed respiration with shallow breathing and a slow rate is commonly seen during sedative or opiate overdosage, increased intracranial pressure, and respiratory acidosis.

The *pattern* of respiration is also significant. *Cheyne-Stokes* respiration is characterized by a gradual increase in both rate and depth to a maximum followed by an abrupt or a gradual waning of both rate and depth until a period of apnea is reached; the apneic period lasts from a few seconds to a few minutes. Although this pattern is sometimes seen in normal people in deep sleep, it is also seen in patients with congestive heart failure and uremia and is frequently a preterminal type of respiration. *Biot's* respiration is totally erratic in rate and depth; it is common in central nervous system disease, especially meningitis.

The *blood pressure* is noted frequently, its exact time interval dependent on the condition present. *Hypertension* may be seen in any condition that increases intracranial pressure, such as a subdural hematoma or a brain tumor. In addition, elevated blood pressure could be of etiologic significance in cerebral hemorrhage and hypertensive encephalopathy.

Hypotension will be noted in the fluid and electrolyte loss accompanying diarrhea, vomiting, or burns and will be noted during *shock* of any origin. Generally, shock is caused by one or a combination of three factors: (1) loss of circulating volume, due to blood or fluid loss attending either internal or external injuries; (2) loss of pump power, as seen in the shock of myocardial infarction; and (3) loss of peripheral (arteriolar) resistance, as seen in neurogenic shock with severe pain or bacteremic shock due to release and absorption of toxins.

4. *Diagnostic studies* are performed initially in an effort to further elucidate the cause of the unconsciousness. In addition to a *complete blood count, blood sugar, urea nitrogen, carbon dioxide combining power,* and *serum electrolytes* tests are usually performed. These would identify diabetic acidosis, insulin shock, electrolyte imbalances, or uremic acidosis as causes of unconsciousness.

A *chest x-ray* might further demonstrate inadequate oxygenation resulting from a pneumothorax or pleural effusion. *Skull x-rays* might reveal evidence of increased intracranial pressure or occult head injury.

Lumbar puncture is usually an important diagnostic procedure in the unconscious patient. It may yield information concerning intracranial lesions, hemorrhage, increased pressure, purulence in meningitis, or increased protein which is found in several cerebral lesions that might be responsible for unconsciousness.

If the spinal fluid is bloody, the duration of the hemorrhage may be determined by the color of the supernatant or top portion of centrifuged bloody spinal fluid; these color changes result from hemolysis. Presence of clear supernatant suggests acute hemorrhage; of pink supernatant, hemorrhage of several hours' duration with hemolysis and release of hemoglobin into the fluid; of yellow supernatant, hemorrhage of 12 hours' duration or more with the hemoglobin converted to bilirubin.

Observations to assist in diagnosis. Once adequate ventilation and circulation are established, attention can be paid to establishing a definitive diagnosis. The nurse can be of immense help by her initial careful observations and alertness to changes in the patient.

It may be that relatives or friends will arrive after the physician has left. By discreet questioning the nurse may be able to obtain enlightening information related to the patient's state of unconsciousness. Frequently a patient's identification papers will contain information that will lead to a correct diagnosis, such as cards carried by many diabetic or epileptic individuals. The nurse may note the presence of medications among the patient's personal effects, and occasionally additional medication may be found in the patient's clothing when he has taken an overdose of barbiturates or tranquilizers.

Physical examination of the patient may be the most productive source of information leading to a correct diagnosis. Some of the significant findings will be reviewed since they may be observed as frequently by the intensive care nurse as by the physician. Too, some may not be apparent during the initial examination by the physician, but they would be noted by the nurse in the course of her care of the patient.

Skin and mucous membranes. Examination of the skin and mucous membranes may reveal *multiple needle marks* over muscular areas, which may indicate that the patient is a diabetic or an addict; *multiple venipunctures* may further suggest the latter. *Lack of skin turgor* might indicate severe dehydration and accompanying electrolyte imbalance. Extreme *diaphoresis* could indicate hypoglycemia or shock. Generalized *edema* or anasarca usually indicates kidney disease, or it may result from anaphylactic shock, while localized edema may indicate trauma. If the injury has been made with a blunt object there may be no initial discoloration, but the swelling may be felt in the soft tissues.

Pallor can indicate internal bleeding if no external evidence of hemorrhage is apparent. *Rubor* may signify severe hypertension, alcoholism, or carbon monoxide poisoning as causes of unconsciousness. *Cyanosis* usually denotes inadequate oxygenation, while *jaundice* may indicate hepatic coma. *Hematomas* are usually evidence of external injury, while *petechiae* may be seen in the Waterhouse-Friderichsen syndrome in meningococcemia.

Uremic frost may be felt on the skin as graininess or seen as a white salty collection on the skin and resembles a thin layer of soapsuds that have been permitted to dry. It is more easily seen on darker-skinned individuals and indicates renal failure.

Head and neck. Examination of the head and neck may yield beneficial information. The patient should be examined as to whether his *eyes* react to light and whether he grimaces when light is shone into his eyes. The *pupils* may be equal or unequal in size (or more significantly, later become unequal), constricted or dilated or show no response to light. Almost all patients in metabolic coma retain their pupillary light reflexes. The *sclera* may be jaundiced.

On examination of the *nose,* one should note the character of any *drainage* as to whether it is purulent, bloody, or serosanguineous; clear drainage could indicate the presence of cerebrospinal fluid. The *odor of the breath* might aid in revealing diabetic acidosis, alcohol intoxication, gastrointestinal bleeding, or uremia.

Slight or moderate *frothiness* of the *mouth* may indicate that the patient is in the postictal state. Any *vomitus* should be saved for analysis; bright red color or a coffee ground appearance usually indicates gastrointestinal bleeding. Examination of the *ears* may reveal *drainage* which may be purulent, bloody, serosanguineous, or cerebrospinal.

Resistance to neck movement (nuchal rigidity) could indicate meningitis or cerebral hemorrhage with blood in the spinal fluid. *Crepitation* might indicate a fracture, in which case the head should be immobilized until the patient is again seen by the physician.

Chest. *Abnormal shape* of the chest may occur in a patient with a barrel chest who might be in respiratory acidosis. A *misshapen chest* may signify injury and subsequent suboxygenation. *Expansion* of the chest is observed for depth. Unilateral expansion may suggest a pneumothorax or pleural effusion with inadequate oxygenation.

Abdomen. The abdomen may be *enlarged* or, more importantly, enlarging. This could result from internal hemorrhage, paralytic ileus, or a ruptured bladder. A *painful response,* such as a grimace or abdominal guarding, to palpation of the abdomen could also indicate internal injury. *Melena* may be noted when the rectal temperature is taken.

Extremities. Examination of the extremities may reveal *focal twitchings, spasticity,* or *clonic movements* that may indicate brain damage. *Abnormal posture* might signify fracture or paralysis.

Body discharges. Body discharges should be noted. The urine may contain *acetone* which could indicate diabetic acidosis. *Grossly bloody urine* could denote severe trauma to the urinary system. The feces may be abnormal; severe diarrhea with *liquid feces* could be a sign of severe dehydration and electrolyte imbalance to the point of unconsciousness. *Melena* indicates gastrointestinal hemorrhage, while *clay-colored stools* might suggest hepatic coma or severe hepatitis.

Supportive treatment. Supportive treatment includes careful body alignment and frequent turning; a turning sheet is helpful since the patient will not be able to assist. All limbs should undergo full-range passive exercises to prevent contractures, and a foot board is needed to prevent foot drop. Adequate nutrition has to be maintained; if unconsciousness persists, a nasogastric tube may be inserted. If the patient has a gag reflex and will respond to verbal directions, his head should be raised and fluids and gruels may be placed by the buccal mucosa; one may use an Asepto syringe to which is attached a short length of tubing to lessen the danger of the patient's biting the tip of the syringe. He may need to be reminded to swallow, and suction should be immediately available. If it is necessary to use suction and the patient will not open his mouth, pressure should be applied to the temporomandibular joints on the side of each cheek. Frequent mouth care is necessary since this patient frequently breathes through his mouth.

If the patient is unconscious for a period of time, eye care will be needed (page 145). Care will also have to be given to elimination (page 153).

The nurse should always remember that the patient may hear but not be able to respond; therefore, all conversation in the patient's presence should be as if the patient were conscious.

Chapter 20

The convulsing patient

Typical initial orders include

1. Maintenance of adequate ventilation
2. Intravenous infusion
3. Sedation
4. Frequent check of vital signs
5. Diagnostic studies

INTRODUCTION

Convulsions may be manifestations of many and diverse illnesses. The primary problem is one of support of the vital functions until the cause can be found and definitive treatment instituted. Seizures occur in many illnesses including epilepsy, uremia, severe brain damage, eclampsia, tetanus, poisonings, meningitis, and encephalitis; they may also occur with diabetic acidosis or marked hypoglycemia, acute alcoholism or alcoholic withdrawal, numerous drug intoxications, or increased intracranial pressure. Convulsions may be the most obvious manifestation of heart disease that results in inadequate cerebral perfusion, as seen with advanced heart block which produces the Adams-Stokes syndrome.

The convulsing patient admitted to an intensive care unit is usually one having seizures of unknown etiology. While the known epileptic does not normally need intensive care, he may be admitted if complications or status epilepticus occurs.

PATHOGENESIS

Febrile state. Statistically the most common cause of a single seizure is the febrile state in the young child, as convulsions may accompany any illness capable of causing a high fever. Any febrile illness may cause an individual with latent epilepsy to have multiple convulsions necessitating hospital admission, but a single febrile convulsion does not necessarily indicate epilepsy in a child. Febrile convulsions in the nonepileptic adult are unusual.

Epilepsy. Epilepsy is a common cause of convulsions. Definitive diagnosis of this condition is dependent largely on the patient's history since physical signs may be particularly sparse. An intracranial lesion, such as a tumor, abscess, or hemorrhage, must be ruled out. Once the convulsive state is adequately controlled, specific diagnosis of epilepsy usually rests with the electroencephalogram, which is rarely available on an emergency basis.

Four types of epilepsy are recognized. *Petit mal* and *psychomotor* epilepsy are considered to be minor seizures and are of significance only in the social incapacity they produce; they rarely require intensive medical or nursing care.

The onset of *Jacksonian* epilepsy is usually a repetitive unilateral involuntary contraction of a specific muscle group, such as thumb flexors; muscle groups are progressively affected cephaladly than caudally until one entire side of the body is involved. In the individual patient the seizure always begins in the same area and migrates in the same pattern. Uncomplicated Jacksonian epilepsy would rarely require intensive care.

Grand mal epilepsy is characterized by generalized repetitive forceful clonic contractions of the major somatic musculature. It may or may not be preceded by an aura (a sensory experience involving any modality which the individual recognizes as heralding a convulsion). Bowel and bladder control may or may not be lost. There is loss of consciousness during the convulsion and amnesia concerning events closely related to the convulsive episode. The seizure is followed by a period of exhaustion and disorientation, and the patient falls into a heavy sleep (the postictal state). His only symptoms on awakening may be slight confusion for a short period of time and diffuse soreness from the muscular contractions; additionally he may have bitten his tongue.

One of the most feared complications is *status epilepticus* in which seizures occur at very close intervals and the patient does not regain consciousness between convulsions. Other complications involve the respiratory tract, such as asphyxia secondary to airway obstruction and aspiration pneumonia.

Hypertensive vascular disease. Hypertensive vascular disease with hypertensive encephalopathy, another fairly common cause of the convulsive state, may be referred to as malignant hypertension; the cause of the seizure is rather obvious, due to the elevated blood pressure. Reduction of the hypertension will usually promptly control the convulsive state; diagnostic studies are then performed in an attempt to determine the underlying cause of the hypertension (page 75).

Care of the convulsing patient with *eclampsia* is essentially the same as care of the hypertensive patient and also includes definitive obstetric care. Drugs must be chosen which will not have adverse effects upon the fetus (page 228).

Alcoholic withdrawal. Alcoholic withdrawal is a common cause of convulsions. Occasionally consumption of alcohol containing contaminants, such as lead and arsenic, may cause seizures. The patient's history may be of some help; in addition, the patient is usually quite psychotic during the interval between seizures.

Cerebral circulatory impairments. Convulsive disorders may occasionally be the manifestation of *insufficiency of cerebral blood flow,* as is classically seen in the patient who develops sudden high degrees of heart block with very low cardiac output; this produces the Adams-Stokes syncope which is often accompanied by a convulsion. An electrocardiogram might suggest this to be the mechanism of the seizure. If the patient is being electronically monitored, a strip of tracing recorded during an episode might be diagnostic. Treatment of the Adams-Stokes syncope is directed toward the primary cardiac condition, usually an abnormal rhythm.

A convulsion may occur in a patient who has *compromised cerebral circulation* as a manifestation of any condition that reduces cardiac output, such as *severe bleeding or shock* from any cause. A seizure may accompany simple *fainting,* which is also a result of impaired cerebral circulation. *Anoxia,* regardless of the cause, may produce convulsions.

Chemical imbalance. Seizures may accompany severe *acidosis,* as in uremia or diabetic coma. *Hypoglycemia* with deep insulin shock commonly results in convulsions. It is interesting to note that at one time insulin shock convulsive therapy was an accepted form of psychiatric treatment. Organic hypoglycemia, such as occurs with an insulin-producing pancreatic islet tumor, may produce a convulsive state resembling status epilepticus.

Drug overdosage. Overdosage with drugs that stimulate the central nervous system, such as dextroamphetamine (Dexedrine), may result in seizures. Many of these drugs are used therapeutically in the treatment of depression and with other compounds in an effort to control obesity. Abuse of these drugs is not uncommon.

TREATMENT

1. *Maintenance of adequate ventilation* is the most important immediate and continuous measure. Convulsing patients will frequently have moderate amounts of secretions or vomitus or both, and the convulsive unconscious state increases the likelihood of aspiration. Aspiration and asphyxia are the usual modes of death of the convulsing patient; therefore, a patent airway should be maintained at all times. Pharyngeal and, if necessary, endotracheal suctioning are used without hesitation because the patient having frequent convulsions has ineffective respiratory exchange during the convulsing period. The patient is turned to his side to allow secretions to drain from his mouth if it is carefully noted that the airway will remain patent in this position. Oxygen may be administered to assist in the control of hypoxia (page 97).

2. An *intravenous infusion* is usually initiated for ready access to the venous circulation for administration of titrations of barbiturates or other medications. To determine the blood sugar level, the blood sugar is drawn before any fluids are administered.

If the patient who is convulsing shows signs of hypoglycemia or is known to be diabetic, 50 ml. of 50% glucose may be administered intravenously *after* an initial blood sugar is drawn. Immediate recovery is diagnostic of hypoglycemia, whether organic or functional. This might occur in a diabetic who has missed meals or confused his insulin dosage, or it might be produced by an insulin-producing tumor.

3. *Sedation* is the usual treatment for the convulsive state of unknown etiology. Barbiturates are usually used, and phenomenal amounts may be needed over a relatively short period of time for control of seizures. This is especially true of uremic convulsions. The dosage is governed by whatever amount is required

to control the seizures; we have given as much as 4 gm. of sodium amytal to control convulsions during a 24-hour period. Under other circumstances this might well prove to be a lethal dose.

The rapid-acting barbiturates with medium duration are frequently administered intravenously for control of the acute convulsive situation. Amobarbital (Amytal) is a favored drug of this type. A syringe loaded with 0.5 gm. in 10 ml. of diluent is usually kept at the bedside (properly labeled) and given as necessary for control of convulsions. For long-term control of the patient's seizures, the long-acting phenobarbital is frequently used in a maintenance dose of from 50 to 200 mg. daily in divided doses. The short-acting barbiturates, such as sodium thiopental (Pentothal), are too rapidly excreted to be useful in the convulsive patient.

Diphenylhydantoin (Dilantin) is also available for parenteral administration. Each ampule contains 100 mg. which can be appropriately diluted for either intramuscular or intravenous injection. The dosage is usually limited to 0.5 gm. in 24 hours. This is a relatively safe drug although it has a slightly hypotensive and sedative effect: it causes less respiratory depression than the barbiturates.

4. *Vital signs* should be checked frequently. An accurate observation of the blood pressure, pulse, respiration, and temperature is most important in this patient since the findings may foretell impending problems and may occasionally be of etiologic importance. For example, a gradually decreasing pulse and respiratory rate and increasing blood pressure with widening pulse pressure in the convulsing patient are indicative of increasing intracranial pressure. This might be seen in a patient with a head injury, cerebral hemorrhage, brain tumor, or abscess.

Observations of a marked change in pulse rate and rhythm might suggest that the difficulty is primarily cardiac, with heart block and Adams-Stokes syndrome. The same situation may be the result of poor cardiac output from extremely rapid rates, as in ventricular tachycardia. A short period of cardiac standstill is more common with the onset of the rapid abnormal rhythms than with their conversion to normal sinus rhythm. This period of standstill or extremely rapid rates may be associated with a convulsion.

As previously mentioned, an elevated temperature may produce the convulsive state in some patients. A febrile convulsion does not necessarily indicate central nervous system disease. Many of these patients subsequently have entirely normal neurologic evaluations including electroencephalograms. Treatment for the febrile convulsion includes the use of antipyretics.

5. *Diagnostic studies* initially include studies of blood sugar, carbon dioxide combining power, blood urea nitrogen, and electrolytes.

The *blood sugar* might reveal the convulsion to be caused by the hypoglycemic state in the treated diabetic individual; seizures are occasionally seen with spontaneous hypoglycemia. Extreme hyperglycemia might also cause a convulsion.

The acidosis of uremia is a fairly common cause of convulsions and would be rapidly detected by determination of *BUN, carbon dioxide combining power,* and *electrolyte studies.* A more definitive treatment than sedation would then be instituted which would be directed at correction of electrolyte abnormalities, especially acidosis, and improvement of urinary function. This may be as simple as using an indwelling catheter in a man with a high degree of chronic prostatic obstruction and chronic kidney disease, or as complicated as having to employ peritoneal dialysis or hemodialysis to assist renal function.

An early *lumbar puncture* will frequently reveal subarachnoid hemorrhage as the cause of the convulsive state. The finding of purulent fluid will pinpoint the meningitides; further bacteriologic and chemical study of the fluid may indicate the specific diagnostic difficulty. A lumbar puncture with a finding of grossly normal fluid under increased pressure may suggest an expanding intracranial lesion, an impression that would be strengthened by chemical determinations of increased protein content of the fluid. Occasionally in the patient with subarachnoid hemorrhage or other conditions causing increased intracranial pressure, cautious removal of small amounts of spinal fluid may reduce the intracranial pressure enough to alleviate the convulsive state.

When a patient known to have epilepsy is admitted in status epilepticus, an attempt should be made to determine its cause. It may have been precipitated by omission of medications or some other condition, such as a febrile illness. Treatment includes the measures previously mentioned. In addition, inhalation anesthesia may be necessary to control the convulsions and ensure adequate ventilation; hypertonic glucose or mannitol may also be given to cause diuresis and, hopefully, reduce any increased intracranial pressure that might be present. Because of the large amounts of drugs necessary for this patient, complete apparatus for circulatory and respiratory support should be immediately available.

TYPES OF MOVEMENTS

There are various types of movements during a convulsion. *Tonic movements,* produced by simultaneous contraction of the flexor and extensor muscles, result in rigidity. Opposing muscle groups alternately contract and relax during *clonic movements.* One should determine whether the movements are generalized from the onset or whether they are focal and then spread; if the latter is the case, one should note which groups of muscles are then affected. The character of the movements and the duration are also important. A brain lesion may be the cause, and the parts of the body affected by convulsive movements may aid the physician in locating the lesion.

Observations. During a convulsion there are many observations that need to be made by nursing personnel. One should note the activity immediately before the seizure; whether the patient cries out; a change in the patient's color, respiration, and pulse. Diaphoresis should be reported, as should urinary or fecal incontinence.

One should observe the eyes for deviation up, down, or to the side. Changes in the pupils may occur, such as constriction or dilation, or there may be no change; and any inequality of movement or pupillary change is especially significant. Clenching of teeth, tongue biting, chewing movements, or any frothiness of the mouth should be noted.

The nurse should notice in the postictal state the period of time before the patient can be aroused and whether his sensorium can be characterized as somnolent, confused, or clear. Any complaints he may have, such as a headache, and any notable decreases in muscle power should be reported. He should be asked whether he can recall what he was doing immediately before the seizure and whether he had an aura.

During a convulsion one should protect the patient from injury but not attempt to restrain him. If the jaw is relaxed, a padded tongue blade or anything soft, such as a folded towel, placed between the teeth will prevent his chewing his tongue. However, if the jaws are clenched, one should *not* attempt to open them, for more injury could then be done to the gums and tissues of the mouth. If the patient is chewing, an attempt should be made to place a soft object between the teeth during the relaxing phase of the chewing process. Constricting clothing should be loosened.

Between convulsions, a padded tongue blade should be nearby but in a drawer for psychological reasons for the patient and his family. Since convulsions are a frightening experience to both the patient and his family, reassurance is an important part of the nurse's role in the management of the patient in this condition.

RELATED FILM

Modern concepts of epilepsy. Color, 24 minutes, available from Ayerst Laboratories, 685 Third Avenue, New York, N. Y.

This excellent film aids in better understanding of epilepsy, its diagnosis, and treatment.

Chapter 21

Head injuries

Typical initial orders include

1. Maintain adequate ventilation
2. Continuous intravenous infusion
3. Check vital signs frequently
4. Note state of consciousness
5. Observe weaknesses or involuntary movements
6. Note state and reactivity of pupils
7. Check hourly urine output
8. Antibiotics
9. Adrenal steroids

INTRODUCTION

The symptoms of patients suspected of having or known to have sustained a head injury are so variable that no typical picture of the clinical state is possible. A patient who has no apparent injury but who knows that he received a blow on the head of unknown severity with or without a period of unconsciousness or confusion may be sent to an intensive care unit for observation. On the other hand, nursing care may be needed for an unconscious or convulsing patient, or the patient may have gone from the emergency room to the operating room for decompression and then be brought for intensive care after the craniotomy.

Several factors combine to make care of the patient sustaining a head injury one of attention to minute detail. The skull is a rigid structure that serves to protect the extremely sensitive central nervous system tissue from being injured easily. However, this same lack of expansivity of the cranium also serves to make small volume changes in content responsible for rather sizable changes in intracranial pressure. This in turn produces rather marked changes in the patient's clinical condition. The same is true of intracranial hemorrhage, occurring either acutely or chronically with hematoma formation.

TYPES OF HEAD INJURIES

Head injuries may be classified as open or closed. An *open injury* that penetrates the skull produces obvious injury to central nervous system tissue, either the meninges or brain tissue. Additionally, evident contamination requires immediate neurosurgical intervention, with debridement and control of hemorrhage and edema. Tetanus toxoid or antitoxin is usually given.

Closed injuries may be of varying degrees of severity. A fracture of the skull may cause no depression of the fragments and no apparent injury to underlying soft tissue. A fracture may compress underlying central nervous system tissue, requiring surgical decompression as a neurologic procedure.

There may also be apparent soft tissue injury without fractures; this is further classified as concussion and contusion. *Concussion* occurs from a sudden blow and is characterized by momentary loss of consciousness but no demonstrable immediate damage, and it produces varying degrees of edema in the injured tissue. Symptoms may result from the edema displacing adjacent tissues and compressing them. A patient may have symptoms resulting from edema of the brain on the side opposite the blow due to the brain's being thrown against the cranial vault. A concussion does not necessarily imply a contusion of the brain.

A *contusion* with hematoma formation and possible laceration may be managed medically or it may require surgical intervention. Soft tissue injury may involve laceration of the dura or the brain substance itself, or it may interrupt a significantly large blood vessel so that open intervention for control of hemorrhage will be required.

TREATMENT

The observation and nursing care of patients having head injuries is similar, although the type of damage may differ. In each case, extremely close examination is required.

1. *Adequate ventilation* must be maintained. Many physicians think that a great deal more permanent damage results from anoxia than from the head injury per se. The methods of supporting respiration are discussed beginning on page 92.

Tracheostomy may be necessary under the following circumstances: (1) if secretions are copious in an unconscious or semiconscious patient, (2) if the head injury is complicated by a cervical spine injury so that the head cannot be hyperextended, or (3) if there is marked injury to the soft tissues of the neck that might compress the trachea.

Suctioning equipment should be immediately available. Until the extent of damage is ascertained, it is safer to suction through the mouth than the nose because of the proximity of the cerebrum and nasopharynx. The occurrence of vomiting in a patient whose level of consciousness is depressed may necessitate lavage of the stomach to prevent aspiration of gastric contents.

This patient should also be observed for the onset of respiratory acidosis which occurs with impairment of pulmonary ventilation (page 188). The acidosis can progress to decrease or abolish tendon reflexes and then produce coma. If not corrected, death will ensue. Oxygen administration and assisted ventilation are specific treatment.

2. *Continuous intravenous infusion* is maintained for access to the circulatory system since the patient may be treated for shock with vasopressor agents or for increased intracranial pressure with mannitol or urea, or he may receive intravenous feedings. The composition of the fluid depends on the needs of the

patient. Fluid therapy is generally thought to be adequate when the patient excretes approximately 1,000 ml. of urine daily.

Extremely careful records of fluid intake and output are mandatory regarding the patient with a head injury. Abnormalities of fluid balance (both water intoxication, page 184, and dehydration, page 183) are capable of altering states of consciousness and producing other central nervous system manifestations that may be indistinguishable from those attending progressive cerebral injury.

Soon after cerebral injury there is retention (positive balance) of water and, to a lesser extent, sodium. This positive balance phase usually lasts from 24 to 72 hours, during which time fluid therapy should not be greater than the patient's daily needs even though the urinary output is decreased. At this stage therapy with too much fluid invites water intoxication with its signs in the central nervous system.

After shock is controlled, fluid is usually limited to between 1,200 and 1,500 ml. per day for the first few days. Since there is adequate salt reserve, the fluid is largely (approximately two thirds) 5% dextrose in water. If doubt exists as to the status of body fluid, a blood volume determination may be helpful.

After the first few days, urinary output usually increases and fluid therapy may be liberalized.

If mannitol or urea is used in an attempt to reduce cerebral edema, the great increase in urine output must be considered, and steps may need to be taken to prevent significant hypovolemia.

3. *Vital signs* should be checked frequently, for much information may be obtained through observing them. While this axiom may not hold true in all cases, most disorders of vital function suggest injury to the brain stem area.

Temperature changes may indicate injury to the central nervous system in areas of temperature regulation (hypothalamus or brain stem) or edemic compression of these areas interfering with temperature regulation. The temperature may be depressed significantly. Hyperthermia may develop from petechial hemorrhages or trauma to the areas previously mentioned, or it may be indicative of infection or dehydration. Extreme elevations of from 106° to 108° F. frequently occur before death.

The *pulse rate* may be slow and full initially, sometimes being as low as from 40 to 50, and may then reach more normal levels as the patient improves. The onset of bradycardia following a period of tachycardia or normal pulse rate is almost pathognomonic of increasing intracranial pressure, especially if it occurs with rising systolic blood pressure and a widening pulse pressure. If intracranial pressure is not relieved surgically, the pulse rate may become extremely high (from 120 to 180); this usually occurs just before the patient's death. Tachycardia may also suggest anoxia, shock, or occult blood loss.

Changes in *respiration* are rather common with head injuries. Biot's respiration, which is totally arrhythmic in both rate and depth, occurs fairly frequently with increasing intracranial pressure as well as with central nervous system infection. Cheyne-Stokes respiration, especially when it has not been present previously, also suggests central nervous system difficulty and frequently occurs just before death of the patient.

Blood pressure should be checked frequently. As previously stated, a gradually rising systolic pressure with a widening pulse pressure is strongly suggestive of increasing intracranial pressure, especially if associated with bradycardia and slow, deep respirations. A drop in blood pressure may suggest associated injury with occult bleeding in another area of the body.

4. *State of consciousness* should be noted rather frequently initially, even though this involves waking a patient during his regular sleeping hours. This can be assessed by determining the patient's orientation toward time, place, and person; his performance of very simple arithmetic; or his ability to follow simple directions. Depression of consciousness may be first evident as confusion or increased restlessness and may progress to delirium, stupor with response only to painful stimulation, and then finally coma. Generally, the duration and depth of unconsciousness indicate the degree of trauma. It is most important that the physician be informed of deepening levels of unconsciousness. Increased restlessness may indicate increased intracranial pressure; however, it may be symptomatic of a full bladder if there is no retention catheter.

It should be remembered that heavy sedation or analgesia is avoided, since these drugs may depress vital signs or obscure clinical changes. Morphine is *never* given because it constricts pupils, deepens coma, and depresses respiration.

5. *Weaknesses or involuntary movements* should be observed. Weakness, paresthesia, or paralysis might be manifested by facial asymmetry, incoordination of eye movements, ocular divergence, inability to perform voluntary motor movements, or the patient's complaint that a part of his body feels "dead." A change in strength or motion of limbs may be indicative of intracranial hemorrhage.

The occurrence of involuntary movements should be reported. Their onset, nature (twitchings, tonic or clonic movements), duration and the frequency of convulsive movements may indicate the location of the injury in the central nervous system. Incontinence of a previously continent patient should be reported.

The integrity of the cranial nerves of a conscious cooperative patient can be superficially tested in a very short period of time with little special equipment.

The *olfactory* or *first* cranial nerve, which is not commonly involved in head injuries, is tested by shielding the patient's eyes and then asking him to identify items such as coffee, alcohol, or peppermint by their odor. One nostril is checked at a time. If there is such involvement, the patient may also complain that he does not taste.

The *optic* or *second* cranial nerve, which is commonly injured, is responsible for vision. It is tested by asking the patient if he can see certain objects placed before him and also by noting the presence of the blink reflex when a hand is suddenly brought toward his eyes. It is further checked by observing constriction of the pupils when a light is flashed before them.

Motion of the eyeballs is controlled by the *oculomotor* or *third,* the *trochlear* or *fourth,* and the *abducens* or *sixth* cranial nerves. The third and sixth nerves are frequently involved in head injuries, while the fourth is not commonly injured. These are usually checked together by asking the patient if he sees double at any position in the visual field with the eyes deviated to the right, left, up, or down. Oculomotor damage is further suggested by dilated pupils and ptosis of the eyelid.

The *trigeminal* or *fifth* cranial nerve, which is not commonly injured, supplies the motor nerve for biting and chewing. Three divisions also provide sensation to the area above the eye, to the upper lip, lower lip, and chin. It is tested by asking the patient to chew, noting contraction of the temporal muscles bilaterally. Sensation can be checked by testing awareness of touch above the eye and on the upper lip, the lower lip, and the chin.

The *facial* or *seventh* cranial nerve, which is quite commonly injured, supplies the muscles of facial expression. It is tested by requesting that the patient close his eyes tightly; an affected eye remains open. The angle of the mouth on the affected side droops, and there is noticeable asymmetry when the patient is asked to wrinkle the brow and to smile.

The *acoustic* or *eighth* cranial nerve, which is rather commonly injured, is tested by checking the hearing ability; deafness will be present in the affected ear. This can be further checked by placing a tuning fork on the middle of the forehead. Sound will be heard in the unaffected ear but will not be perceived by the involved ear. The vestibular branch of the acoustic nerve is concerned with balance, and disorders involving it classically produce vertigo.

The *glossopharyngeal* or *ninth* nerve, which is rarely injured, supplies sensation to the posterior portion of the tongue and to the soft palate. When it is affected there is absence of the gag reflex when the soft palate is stroked with a cotton applicator. There is also loss of taste on the posterior one third of the tongue.

The *vagus* or *tenth* cranial nerve supplies fibers for a great deal of autonomic (parasympathetic) function; this automatic function is not readily tested. It also supplies motor nerves to the soft palate which, if affected, will sag, and the uvula will deviate to the normal side. The patient may experience hoarseness from vocal cord weakness.

The *spinal accessory* or *eleventh* cranial nerve is rarely injured by head injuries but may be involved in injuries or lacerations to the neck. It is checked by noting an asymmetric response of the patient to the request to shrug his shoulders or stretch his arms forward. Involvement of this nerve may also affect the ability to turn the head.

The *hypoglossal* or *twelfth* cranial nerve provides motor function to the tongue and is rarely injured. When involved, the protruded tongue deviates toward the affected side.

6. *Pupils should be checked* for size, equality, and reaction to light at regular intervals. Inequality of the pupils, either present on initial observation or, more importantly, observed as a progressive change, strongly suggests both that localization of the injury, as with hematoma formation, is increasing and that the increasing pressure is on the side of the dilated fixed pupil. Pupils that are bilaterally fixed in the constricted state and subsequently become bilaterally fixed in the dilated state are characteristic of midbrain damage. The presence of dilated fixed pupils bilaterally suggests that irreparable injury to the central

nervous system has taken place, or it may indicate epidural or subdural hemorrhage. If conscious, a patient may complain of double vision or progressively failing vision due to papilledema.

With the increased use of contact lenses, one should ascertain whether the patient is wearing them. If so, they should be removed, since prolonged use may cause corneal ulceration. If the eyes of the unconscious patient do not close, patches may be placed over them to prevent corneal drying and ulceration.

7. *Urinary output* of the patient who is semiconscious or comatose should be checked hourly initially to aid in ascertaining the adequacy of the circulatory system (page 17).

8. *Antibiotics* are usually given if there has been a break in the skin, or they may be given prophylactically to prevent urinary or respiratory system infections.

9. *Adrenal steroids* are sometimes given in large doses in the treatment of shock; some physicians believe that these drugs also tend to lessen cerebral edema.

Additional observations. Other observations are also necessary. *Vomiting* should be noted as to frequency, amount, contents, and whether it was projectile (a sign of increased intracranial pressure) or preceded by nausea. If the patient is conscious he should be warned that if he vomits he should attempt to avoid straining, which increases intracranial pressure.

Nuchal rigidity, involuntary stiffness of the neck muscles, may occur following hemorrhage into the subarachnoid space, or it may be an early sign of irritation to the meninges due to infection. Extreme caution should be taken if nuchal rigidity is present, since it may also result from associated cervical spine injuries. The head should probably be immobilized until the latter diagnosis is ruled out.

It should be remembered that the patient suspected of having or actually having head injury may also have other injuries that may not have been noticed initially because of the more obvious difficulty; thus, careful scrutiny of the entire patient is necessary.

Any seepage of fluid from the nose or ears should be brought to the physician's attention; it may be clear, serosanguineous, or frankly bloody. Seepage of spinal fluid would indicate a tear in the meninges. Drainage from the ears may be due to traumatic rupture of the tympanic membrane. If the fluid is draining freely a compress should be placed lightly for absorbency. No attempt should be made to control the drainage by occlusion with a tamponade; since the fluid is draining into a contaminated area, occlusion would greatly increase the possibility of contamination of the cranial vault.

Oral intake of fluid is determined by the patient's condition and level of consciousness. If the patient is unconscious for a lengthy period, fluids may be given through a nasogastric tube after peristalsis has returned, usually within approximately 48 hours.

Activity of the patient with a head injury is generally restricted initially until the extent of damage is determined. If it is not contraindicated, he is turned every two hours to lessen the chance of pulmonary complications. He may be turned by so-called log rolling, his head and trunk being kept in the same relative position.

The patient is usually placed in semi-Fowler's position, his head elevated about 30° to 45° unless he is in shock, in which case the supine position is usually recommended. It is thought that the slightly elevated position reduces cerebral edema and venous congestion by improving drainage from the brain, thus also aiding in relieving increased intracranial pressure. The Trendelenburg position is not advisable since it tends to produce cerebral venous stasis and increases intracranial pressure. Too, the pressure of the abdominal contents against the diaphragm tends to produce respiratory embarrassment.

In addition to close observation of the patient, additional diagnostic procedures may be done. Roentgenograms of the skull are mandatory, and a spinal tap may be done. Special diagnostic procedures might include arteriography.

Specific medical treatment is directed toward attempting to reduce cerebral edema, thereby reducing increased intracranial pressure in the patient who shows gradual deterioration. Two potent osmotic diuretics, mannitol and urea, are frequently used for this purpose (page 272).

Other complications. Other complications may mimic an expanding intracranial hematoma. Cerebral fat embolism occasionally occurs, usually from 24 to 72 hours after the injury, especially if there has been fracture of a long bone. Early symptoms include restlessness, loss of sphincter control, disorientation, tonic and clonic seizures, aphasia, and hemiplegia. Fat droplets may be found in the sputum, spinal fluid, and urine. Petechiae may be noted on the chest, axillary folds, the sclera, and under the eyelids. The respiratory system may be affected by an increased rate, cough, cyanosis, stertorous breathing, and rales. Tachycardia and hypotension may occur. Treatment consists of use of anticoagulants beginning with heparin; dextran has also been recommended. Early fixation of fractures probably reduces the likelihood of this complication.

Rarely diagnosed, thrombosis of the carotid or vertebral artery may occur as a result of concomitant vessel injury at the time of the head injury. The time of onset of symptoms and the severity will depend on the presence of arteriosclerosis, extent of the thrombosis, adequacy of collateral circulation through the circle of Willis, severity of associated head injury, and the degree of vasospasm. Thrombosis is specifically diagnosed by means of arteriography, and its treatment is surgical.

Other specific treatment involves neurosurgical procedures. The need for early but not emergency surgery is indicated by a depression the size of a ping pong ball, persistent or recurrent rhinorrhea, a fracture depressed more than one-half the thickness of the skull, indriven fragments of bone, or a spicule of bone lodged in a major sinus.

Emergency surgery is contemplated if any of the following conditions are present: unilateral dilation of the pupils, decrease in the level of consciousness, hemiplegia or hemiparesis, hemianesthesia, deterioration of vital signs, particularly decreasing pulse rate with increasing blood pressure and widening pulse pressure.

Neurosurgical treatment includes multiple trephining to provide an area for the expansion of cerebral edema or a craniotomy with evacuation of hematoma and other neurosurgical procedures. The postoperative nursing care of the neurosurgical patient is very similar to the initial management of the patient having a head injury.

RELATED FILM

Acute head injury. Color, 28 minutes, available from Baxter Laboratories, Morton Grove, Ill. This very good film depicts the more common types of head injuries.

Chapter 22

Stroke

Typical initial orders include

1. Maintenance of adequate ventilation
2. Frequent check of vital signs
3. Drug treatment
4. Laboratory studies
5. Diet as tolerated
6. Exercises

CLINICAL FINDINGS

The patient with a stroke will have initial symptoms that vary in severity. He may be confused or semiconscious or in a deep coma. Typically, one side of his body exhibits paresis or paralysis that may be flaccid or spastic. Flaccid paralysis is more common and can be recognized by lack of muscle tone with the affected leg and foot turning outward. If the patient is able to open his eyes, the eyelid on the affected side may droop and that side of his face may sag or appear puffy. If he is able to speak, he sounds thick-tongued and his speech is usually slurred.

PATHOGENESIS

Stroke is a nonspecific term used to refer to the onset of major interference with function of the central nervous system. In its classic form stroke is associated with interference either with motor function or with cerebration; however, the term may be liberally used to refer to more or less sudden loss of any cerebral function due to interference with vascular supply. Three typical stroke syndromes are presented: (1) thrombotic, (2) embolic, and (3) hemorrhagic.

Thrombotic stroke. Thrombotic stroke classically occurs in the individual who has had fleeting signs of cerebral insufficiency, such as momentary loss of vision, facial weaknesses, or peripheral muscular weaknesses. These episodes have occurred over a period of time and have usually been ignored by the patient because of the short duration and his apparent total recovery. However, if the patient is capable of giving a history, he can usually relate this information, or relatives may be aware of these episodes.

These are symptoms representative of a state of borderline compensated cerebral circulation. When some event results in further impairment of circulation, such as hypotension from any cause or the natural progression of atherosclerosis, thrombosis causing ischemia of a portion of the cerebral cortex develops. Classically the patient awakens with this disorder. The incident precipitating thrombosis was the decreased cardiac output and hypotension associated with physiologic sleep, for this slight change decreased the blood flow. The symptoms will depend on the portion of the brain involved, but they are usually those of hemiparesis or incomplete hemiplegia. If the cerebral insufficiency involves the dominant hemisphere, associated aphasia is likely. The thrombotic stroke may also be precipitated by any event that reduces cardiac output or peripheral blood flow, such as marked hemorrhage or a myocardial infarction.

When first seen, the patient is usually conscious but has a more or less definite unilateral involvement that may vary from slight weakness to total paralysis. On initial examination of the patient it is impossible to know his eventual outcome; therefore, the facility in which the patient with a thrombotic stroke is treated should proceed through the full gamut of all possible supportive measures because it is impossible to ascertain from initial examination which patient will experience greater difficulty and which will improve spontaneously. Some patients recover rather promptly as soon as cardiac output and cerebral blood flow are improved, while other patients' thrombosis may be progressive, with proximal propagation of the area of insufficiency and progressive symptoms. Because of the drastic effect on these patients of reduced blood flow, only minimal or preferably no sedation is desirable.

The diagnostic features of the thrombotic stroke include a gradual onset associated with the precipitating factor, premonitory signs, and usually the absence of headache or pain.

Embolic stroke. Embolic stroke may follow myocardial infarction or subacute bacterial endocarditis, for mural thrombi or valvular vegetations may be discharged into the systemic circulation and enter carotid or intracranial vessels.

Embolic stroke usually differs from thrombotic stroke in that the former is sudden in onset, reaches a maximum deficit promptly, and usually stabilizes after having caused considerably less cerebral damage than the initial involvement seemed to suggest. The key to the diagnosis of the embolic stroke is discovery of a potential source of embolism, as the fibrillating heart, the murmurs of valvular heart disease, or the silent myocardial infarction. It is estimated that approximately 10% of patients with strokes have a coronary occlusion simultaneously, perhaps precipitating the stroke by decreasing cardiac output or by embolism.

The embolic stroke is likely to be confused with the hemorrhagic stroke because of the sudden onset of difficulty, usually without premonitory signs.

Hemorrhagic stroke. The hemorrhagic stroke is likely to occur in the patient with severe hypertension; and, conversely, the patient with severe hypertensive encephalopathy may present with the stroke syndrome in the absence of frank cerebral infarction or cerebral hemorrhage. The hemorrhagic stroke may also occur in an individual when there is rupture of a presumably congenital aneurysm in the circle of Willis producing subarachnoid hemorrhage; occurrence of a hemorrhagic stroke in a young individual is usually the result of such a malformation.

Hemorrhagic stroke usually differs from the thrombotic and embolic strokes by having a sudden onset, usually accompanied by a severe headache, although the abruptness is not an absolute essential. The severity of headache, evidence of meningeal irritation, and early instability of vital signs with elevated blood pressure are hallmarks of the hemorrhagic stroke.

Hemorrhagic stroke is more likely to be confused with acute meningitis than is a thrombotic or embolic stroke because of the associated signs of meningeal irritation; these include nuchal rigidity, severe headache, tachycardia, and evidence of increased intracranial pressure; fever may also be present.

TREATMENT

1. *Adequate ventilation* must be maintained. Since the patient may be comatose or semiconscious, special attention must be given to maintenance of a patent airway. As excessive salivation frequently occurs, he may be turned on his side to allow drainage to prevent aspiration. Suctioning equipment should be readily available. It may be necessary to assist ventilation in some manner (page 92). If respiratory effort is inadequate, respiratory stimulants such as caffeine may be given.

2. *Vital signs* should be checked frequently so that changes indicating increasing difficulty can be noted. An elevated *temperature* may indicate dehydration or infection; this patient is prone to develop pneumonia and infections of the urinary tract. Depressed temperature may indicate progressive deterioration.

While checking the rate and rhythm of the *pulse,* one should watch especially for other signs of congestive heart failure if tachycardia develops (page 21).

An increased *respiratory rate* may also indicate the onset of congestive heart failure. Biot's and Cheyne-Stokes respiration are both common with brain damage.

The *blood pressure* is commonly elevated during hemorrhagic stroke. Progressive hypotension may indicate vascular collapse and the necessity for vasopressors.

3. *Drug treatment* may include the use of antihypertensive drugs for the patient with a hemorrhagic stroke, or of anticoagulants for a patient with an embolic or thrombotic stroke.

The therapeutic value of anticoagulants for the patient with a thrombotic stroke is an unanswered question, but many physicians believe that prompt use of anticoagulants may minimize the area of damage by preventing its extension. Because a stroke usually occurs in a patient with an already compromised vascular tree, he is particularly prone to developing other complications of a vascular nature, such as stasis thrombophlebitis and pulmonary embolism. This may be considered another indication for use of anticoagulants.

On the other hand, by using anticoagulants the incidence of hemorrhagic complications may be greater, and one will also occasionally inadvertently prescribe anticoagulants for a patient with occult bleeding whose precipitating episode was one of hemorrhage. For this reason it is important to smell the patient's breath; the patient with gastrointestinal bleeding may have the breath odor typical of digested blood before the bleeding is manifested by vomitus or melena.

There is fairly general agreement that the embolic stroke patient should be treated with anticoagulants, at least during the acute phase, in order to perhaps reduce the amount of cerebral necrosis as well as prevent the recurrence of embolism from the original site.

4. *Laboratory studies* include analysis of the spinal fluid and complete blood count, studies of blood urea nitrogen and blood sugar, chest x-ray, and electrocardiogram.

The *lumbar puncture* is a positive diagnostic study only for the stroke caused by hemorrhage. The presence of bloody spinal fluid is diagnostic, although the intracerebral hemorrhage may not be determined in this manner. A lumbar puncture yielding normal cerebrospinal fluid under normal pressure tends to rule out other possible causes of the difficulty such as subarachnoid hemorrhage, meningitis, or an expanding intracranial lesion that can sometimes mimic the stroke syndromes.

Additional treatment of the hemorrhagic stroke may involve serial lumbar punctures with cautious removal of spinal fluid in amounts necessary to reduce the increased intracranial pressure to a safe level. One will occasionally be rewarded by the almost instantaneous improvement of an apparently moribund patient with a hemorrhagic stroke by the simple expedient of the slow removal of approximately 10 ml. of cerebrospinal fluid.

The occurrence of a hemorrhagic stroke in a young individual demands cerebral arteriography once the condition has stabilized so that lesions of the cerebral circulation may be identified. These may be amenable to surgical correction.

An abnormal *complete blood count* with decreased hematocrit and hemoglobin would reveal the presence of occult bleeding, while a *blood urea nitrogen* gives an indication of renal status. An *abnormal blood sugar* may produce symptoms similar to a stroke if there is marked elevation or depression. The *chest x-ray* might reveal cardiac hypertrophy and pleural effusion with congestive heart failure. An *electrocardiogram* is also done to detect any abnormalities.

5. The *diet* that will be tolerated is largely dependent upon the patient's state of consciousness. Intravenous fluids may be needed for a few days if the patient is unconscious or semiconscious. Fluid balance must be carefully maintained because this patient is particularly prone to get increased damage from hypovolemia. On the other hand, hypervolemia is also hazardous; since his circulation is sometimes poor, he is usually more likely to be in borderline congestive failure, and a fluid overload can precipitate pulmonary edema.

Administration of fluids should be started by mouth as soon as the patient is able to accept them without aspirating or choking. Thicker fluids or gruels, such as ice cream or strained oatmeal, are easier for him to manage than liquids of less viscosity, such as fruit juices. When the patient is being fed, the food should be placed in the unaffected side of his mouth; it may also be necessary that his head be tilted slightly to this side so that he can handle the food more easily. As soon as he is able, the patient should start feeding himself to encourage him to become independent.

6. Passive and active *exercises* should be initiated as soon as feasible. While

there is some concern over the early institution of passive exercises, it is thought that they should be begun after the first 24 to 48 hours on each patient who is not in shock or who has no other evidence of remaining critically ill. Since most of these patients have stabilized during the period of initial observation and muscle stiffness begins fairly soon after periods of immobilization, it is recommended that full-range passive exercises be begun for all limbs as soon as feasible. Since ankylosis can occur when a normal joint is simply immobilized, it is most important that these exercises be done frequently and regularly (for example, each exercise done five to ten times during each of two or three periods daily). In this manner the joints remain mobile until there is maximum return of function. Ankylosis of the joints adds an additional disability to that of the stroke.

Many patients become disabled from inactivity rather than from the stroke; they assume they will not be able to use an extremity since they had a stroke, and they never try to use it. In addition to preventing contractures and improving circulation by increasing blood flow, these exercises give *hope* to both the patient and his family. They can get this feeling when the nursing and physiotherapy staff tell them that the exercises are done so that the patient will walk sooner. The public still has to be educated to the fact that a patient who has had a stroke is not necessarily an invalid for the rest of his life. It is true that strokes do sometimes severely cripple a person for the remainder of his life, but it is also a fact that a great number of patients can be returned to almost their previous state of health if an effort is made in this direction.

After eight years' experience at the Baldwin County Stroke Clinic, Milledgeville, Ga., we are impressed by the fact that many patients are able to do much more than they or their families thought possible *if the patient will try,* with his family giving him moral support and the needed physical aid. The patient is encouraged to do as much for himself as his capacity permits. For this reason it is recommended that exercises be started as soon as the patient's condition stabilizes (within from 24 to 48 hours) and ambulation be begun by approximately 72 hours. The patient should be gotten out of bed before he and his family have time to consider him an invalid.

An excellent guide for nursing personnel to use in teaching the patient and his family the passive and active exercises is the booklet "Strike Back at Stroke," which can be secured from the American Heart Association or the Government Printing Office, Washington, D. C.

Since many family members are fearful of performing the exercises incorrectly, a helpful explanation is that the exercises are those actions which each person can do normally. For example, each person can normally flex and extend his lower arm, so this is all anyone can be expected to do in the way of motion in this joint.

First one should demonstrate full range of motion in each joint, and then the family member should return the demonstration. Next, the nurse should perform full range of motion exercises on the patient's unaffected side and then on his affected limbs. Next, the family member performs the exercises on the patient. This aids in showing the family member the degree of disability the patient may have to overcome. The patient should be encouraged to move the affected extremities in any way he can.

The nurse should instruct the family member to produce the full range of motion in each joint of each limb as nearly as possible. If there is spastic paralysis, he should be instructed to go *to* the point of tightness and just a little farther in order to stretch the muscles. Patient and family can be encouraged by the knowledge that some patients continue to get return of function one or two years following a stroke.

The remainder of the treatment is supportive. In positioning the patient in bed, it is preferable that he lie flat much of the time so that he does not experience flexion contracture of the hip. It is best to have no pillow under the head since flexion contracture of the neck can occur. If the patient prefers a pillow, it should be tucked under his shoulders. The hand is positioned with the fingers outstretched to favor the extensors.

Since flexor muscles are generally stronger than extensors, the patient should be positioned so that the joints are in neutral position or so that the extensors are favored. The gastrocnemius is an exception, for this powerful extensor of the foot needs to be overcome by a footboard, which aids in preventing footdrop and helps the return of the proprioceptive ability as the patient presses against it. A two- to three-inch block placed between mattress and board allows heel room and lessens the possibility of formation of decubiti on the heels. A trochanter roll under the outer aspects of the thighs will help to prevent outward rotation of the leg.

This patient requires good skin care since he is usually older and has more fragile skin. Many of these patients have urinary incontinence initially. A retention catheter is to be avoided if possible since it increases chance of infection and lessens opportunity for retraining the patient. Incontinence is embarrassing to the conscious patient; he should be reassured that his control usually returns with a short passage of time, and he can be aided in its reestablishment by offering the urinal or bedpan every one or two hours. There may be bowel incontinence, but fecal impaction, the more frequent disturbance, may be prevented by small enemas.

One should approach this patient from his unaffected side since visual disturbances are more common on the affected side. In addition, occasionally a patient will completely ignore the existence of the disabled side.

Emotional lability is very common and most distressing to the family and to the patient if he is aware of it. The nurse should reassure the family that this is a symptom of the illness and tends to be temporary. Since many patients are aware of occurrences in their presence even though they cannot respond, one should *always* remember to be careful of what is said in the patient's presence.

One should watch for changes in the patient's level of consciousness and his increasing abilities. As he becomes more alert, he should do more for himself, and more activity should be expected of him.

In conclusion, one must respect and understand this patient and emphasize his capabilities rather than his deficiencies. He should be given the reassurance he needs and the motivation toward developing as much independence as possible.

RELATED FILMS

Cerebral vascular disease: the challenge of diagnosis (EM 246A). Color, 30 minutes.

Cerebral vascular disease: the challenge of management (EM 246). Black and white, 38 minutes.

Second chance (EM 242). Black and white, 28 minutes.

Each of these films is available from state heart association.

Chapter 23

Meningitis

Typical initial orders include

1. Maintenance of adequate ventilation
2. Intravenous infusion
3. Antibiotics
4. Control of convulsions
5. Frequent check of vital signs
6. Diagnostic studies
7. Fluid intake and output record

CLINICAL FINDINGS

The typical patient having meningitis is admitted to the hospital in a serious or critical condition characterized by fever, backache, and an excruciating headache. He may have an altered state of consciousness varying from mild confusion to stupor or unconsciousness, and he may be convulsing. If conscious, he may complain of diplopia or photophobia or both.

His medical history usually indicates that he was in reasonably good health until shortly before admission, at which time coryza or an upper respiratory tract infection may have been noted which seemed to become progressively worse.

Upon physical examination the individual appears lethargic and is usually flushed from a high fever. There is nuchal rigidity, with pain on movement of the neck. Nausea and vomiting, common with increased intracranial pressure, may be present. The pulse rate is usually elevated, and respiration is usually slow and irregular; moderate elevation of the blood pressure is common. Muscular twitchings may be present due to meningeal irritation.

PATHOGENESIS

The skull and spinal canal are lined by the three-layered meninges which protect the brain and spinal cord. The tough outer layer is the dura mater. The two inner layers are adherent to the surface of the brain and spinal cord and to each other; together they are known as the pia-arachnoid. Spinal fluid fills the space between the dura and pia-arachnoid and acts as additional insulation.

Inflammation of these membranes, called meningitis, can be of viral, bacterial, or occasionally chemical etiology. The chemically induced type is usually the result of medication and is ordinarily limited to a local reaction involving primarily the arachnoid membrane (chemical arachnitis).

155

The most common types of meningitis are bacterial and viral. More than 90% of all cases of bacterial meningitis are caused by meningococcus, pneumococcus, or *Haemophilus influenzae* organisms. *H. influenzae* is the organism most commonly causing the disease in children, especially attacking the debilitated infant. The meningococcus is usually the etiologic agent in the middle-aged individual, while the pneumococcus commonly attacks the elderly.

Meningoencephalitis or aseptic meningitis is generally presumed to be of viral etiology and may occasionally occur as a complication of almost any of the epidemic viral diseases. Meningitis occurs more often during the fall and winter months when upper respiratory infections are common; the enteroviruses are more common in summer and fall.

Certain conditions seem to predispose individuals to specific types of meningitis. The patient with a skull fracture may suffer direct contamination of the meninges from organisms in the sinuses and respiratory tract. Purulent involvement of the sinuses or ears may spread directly to the meninges; this is more frequent with pneumococcic organisms. The severely debilitated alcoholic is especially susceptible to meningitis caused by the *Klebsiella pneumoniae* or Friedländer's bacillus.

TREATMENT

1. *Maintenance of adequate ventilation* is imperative in this patient because frequently he is stuporous or comatose and is quite prone to airway obstruction. He is also subject to aspiration, especially if he has convulsions.

2. *Intravenous infusions* are ordered if it is necessary to continuously infuse an antibiotic during the early critical period. Intravenous fluids are also required to maintain hydration if the patient is comatose or unconscious.

3. The choice of *antibiotics* depends somewhat on identification of the causative organisms. Many physicians believe that a suspicion of meningococcus warrants the use of a soluble sulfonamide since many of the antibiotics cross the spinal fluid barrier rather poorly; however, control series have revealed that antibiotic therapy alone is quite satisfactory.

Penicillin in doses of several million units daily parenterally or ampicillin 2 gm. daily are usually the drugs of choice in meningococcic meningitis. Different antibiotics may be used when other causative organisms are suspected. Antibiotic combinations in large doses by the parenteral route of administration are frequently used.

4. *Control of convulsions* is necessary if they occur (page 136).

5. *Vital signs* should be checked frequently for they may foretell complications. A falling blood pressure accompanied by a rising temperature may indicate septicemic complications and associated adrenocortical insufficiency (the Waterhouse-Friderichsen syndrome). The occurrence of this complication demands specific and immediate treatment (page 157).

A rising blood pressure with widened pulse pressure accompanied by decreasing pulse and respiratory rates may indicate increased intracranial pressure.

6. *Diagnostic studies* include a *lumbar puncture* that is performed soon after the patient's admission; this is the only definitive method of diagnosis. The char-

acter of the spinal fluid and the cellular content will enable one to rapidly differentiate the purulent or bacterial meningitides from aseptic or viral meningoencephalitis. The spinal fluid typical of the former disease is cloudy, while it is usually clear or only slightly turbid with the latter. The spinal fluid pressure may be elevated with either type although it is usually higher with purulent meningitis.

The cellular exudate of the purulent spinal fluid generally contains cell counts greater than 3,000 per cubic millimeter, 90% or more being polymorphonuclear leukocytes. The spinal fluid in aseptic meningitis typically has fewer than 3,000 cells per cubic millimeter, 70% or more of which will be mononuclear cells.

The causative organism of the bacterial meningitis may be presumptively identified from direct stain or a smear of the spinal fluid. Tentative identification of the meningococcus, pneumococcus, *H. influenzae,* or Friedländer's bacillus may suggest the choice of an antibiotic until results of the culture are obtained.

Blood studies include a complete blood count and culture. The complete blood count in bacterial meningitis is usually characterized by a pronounced elevation of the leukocytes with a predominance of polymorphonuclear cells in the differential count. The leukocyte count of the patient with aseptic meningitis may vary considerably from leukopenia to quite high counts; however the predominant cell is usually a mononuclear cell. The presence of atypical mononuclear cells in the peripheral smear may suggest the difficulty to be viremia. Elevated hematocrit and hemoglobin may suggest accompanying hypovolemia.

Blood cultures are obtained for possible confirmation of the causative organism; bacterial meningitis is frequently bacteremic and may occasionally be septicemic.

7. Fluid *intake and output* are followed closely; it is fairly easy for this patient to become dehydrated due to the high fever and inadequate fluid intake if he is comatose or semiconscious.

General supportive care includes careful attention to fluid and electrolyte balance, general hygiene, and skin care. Any diet that can be tolerated is allowed, and increased fluid consumption is emphasized. It may be necessary to apply alcohol sponges to lower the patient's elevated temperature. The room must be kept quiet and somewhat darkened since the patient is extremely sensitive to extraneous stimuli. He needs to be turned frequently; so-called log rolling may cause the least amount of pain in his neck.

This patient is usually isolated, and personnel should be especially careful regarding discharges from the nose and mouth. If the patient is disoriented, side rails may be necessary. Reassurance of his family is important since the patient appears critically ill; yet most patients have a fairly good prognosis.

COMPLICATIONS

Complications of meningitis are sometimes seen for which urgent treatment is needed. The most common life-threatening complication of meningococcic meningitis is the *Waterhouse-Friderichsen syndrome,* presumably caused by adrenal hemorrhage and adrenal insufficiency. This is heralded by a marked drop in blood pressure and is almost always preceded by the appearance of petechiae followed by ecchymoses. For this reason the nurse's observation of petechial hemorrhages in the course of general hygiene and skin care is exceedingly important, and the information should be relayed to the physician *immediately*.

Treatment of the profound shock of the Waterhouse-Friderichsen syndrome involves the parenteral administration of adrenocortical hormones, such as hydrocortisone or dexamethasone. The use of pressor agents, such as metaraminol or levarterenol, is rarely effective in these cases without the concomitant use of the adrenal steroids (page 261).

Other later complications are *pneumonia* due to aspiration or *septic embolism*. A central nervous system complication very commonly seen with pneumococcus, *H. influenzae,* or Friedländer's meningitis is *brain abscess*. In this situation, the patient seems to gradually improve until there is a rather marked change usually characterized by localized signs suggesting development of a focal lesion; the symptoms include signs of cranial nerve involvement, localized twitchings, and increasing intracranial pressure.

Hydrocephalus is also an occasional complication of meningitis, especially pneumococcic meningitis, because the exudate produced is very tenacious and occludes the free egress of spinal fluid from the ventricular cavities to the arachnoid space. The development of a brain abscess or hydrocephalus or both produces a much higher mortality than meningitis alone and will usually require neurosurgical intervention.

The patient with aseptic meningitis or meningoencephalitis which complicates an epidemic viral disease usually recovers completely, having required only careful supportive treatment. No specific therapy is known.

RELATED FILM

Bacterial meningitis. Color, 25 minutes, available from Ayerst Laboratories through Ideal Pictures Offices. 685 Third Avenue, New York, N.Y.

This is a very good film on this subject; however, it neglects mention of steroid therapy for the Waterhouse-Friderichsen syndrome.

The patient having gastrointestinal disease

Chapter 24

Bleeding of upper gastrointestinal tract

Typical initial orders include

1. Intravenous infusion
2. Blood typing and cross matching; transfusion
3. Frequent check of vital signs
4. Gastric suctioning
5. Drug therapy
6. Milk and antacid administration every hour
7. Surgical (medical) consultation
8. Diagnostic studies
9. Record of urinary output
10. Notation of all vomitus and stools

CLINICAL FINDINGS

The appearance of the patient presenting with upper gastrointestinal tract bleeding varies considerably, depending on the amount and rapidity of blood loss. Usually the patient seeks treatment after having vomited blood or having had black, tarry bowel movements. The vomitus may be bright red or of coffee-ground appearance due to partial digestion of the blood. The patient whose bleeding is rapid in onset is more likely to have faintness, pallor, tachycardia with a thready pulse, sweatiness, thirst, and other signs of acute blood loss; whereas the patient with gradual, slow bleeding may experience only weakness and faintness. The latter patient may be aware of having had black bowel movements but unaware that this usually signifies blood loss.

Digested blood has a specific odor that may be noted on the patient's breath even before the onset of melena or the first expulsion of vomitus. This odor is qualitatively the same as that of melena but is usually fainter.

PATHOGENESIS

The patient who vomits blood is usually bleeding from a source above the ligament of Treitz; reverse peristalsis is seldom sufficient to cause hematemesis if the bleeding point is below this area. Statistically the patient with upper gastrointestinal tract bleeding is likely to have ulcer disease; however, other bleeding conditions of the upper gastrointestinal tract can occur, such as gastric carcinoma or esophageal varices.

161

Bleeding occurs in ulcer disease when a blood vessel is eroded. The amount of bleeding depends on several facts, such as the size and type of the vessel and the elasticity of the vessel wall. Tarry stools occur more frequently with duodenal ulcer, while hematemesis is more common with a gastric ulcer; however, both may be present in either condition.

When the patient is first seen, the severity and rapidity of the blood loss may not be determined immediately, but the presence of shock or hypotension with tachycardia usually signifies a moderate blood loss (in excess of one to two pints).

Knowing several facts of the patient's medical history may assist one in determining the probable source of bleeding and the definitive treatment. The chronic alcoholic patient is likely to be bleeding from esophageal varices, while the patient with prior ulcer symptoms is frequently bleeding from an ulcer.

The decision for surgical treatment of the patient with upper gastrointestinal tract bleeding is a matter of judgment; however, several factors must be considered. The patient with repetitive bleeding, or the individual who has had one or more previous bleeding episodes, is more likely to require surgery as soon as the condition stabilizes than the patient with his first episode of bleeding. The age of the patient must be considered. Because of arteriosclerosis of blood vessel walls, the older patient is more likely to continue to bleed than the younger patient. He is also less likely to tolerate repeated bleeding episodes or prolonged bleeding because of secondary damage, notably that caused by hypovolemia to organs whose circulation is already compromised by atherosclerosis. Both cerebral thrombosis and coronary thrombosis are occasionally precipitated by a bleeding episode.

The amount and rapidity of bleeding deserve consideration. Physicians have various rules of thumb concerning the decision to proceed with surgery for presumed ulcer in the presence of continued bleeding. One might be the requirement of from three to five pints of blood given daily for two consecutive days to maintain blood volume and cardiac output. Another might be a total transfusion requirement of six pints given within three days; however, these are only rules of thumb, and their use must be tempered by judgment. One might be more inclined to operate sooner on a patient with a rare blood type if there were difficulty in obtaining blood to maintain blood volume. If at all possible, the patient should not be subjected to anesthesia until adequate circulation is established and maintained. Here again, a judgment must be made as to whether to operate on a patient in shock when blood cannot be replaced rapidly enough to improve the shock situation. The patient with a gastric ulcer is somewhat more likely to require surgery when bleeding occurs than the patient with a duodenal ulcer.

Care of the patient is so designed that early in the course of management the severity of blood loss is assessed, a sufficient amount of blood is replaced to counteract shock, and a definite type of treatment is planned.

TREATMENT

1. An *intravenous infusion* is begun immediately by means of a large caliber needle. The venipuncture may be kept patent with 5% glucose in water or plasma

volume–expanders such as plasma or dextran until whole blood can be typed and cross matched.

2. Blood is *typed and cross matched* immediately after the patient is admitted, and initial transfusion treatment is based on the presence of hypotension and tachycardia, as well as the results of the blood count and blood volume.

3. *Vital signs* are checked frequently until they become stable, and thereafter at close intervals. Apprehension accompanied by thirst, an elevated pulse and respiration, and a decreasing blood pressure may indicate additional bleeding. If ice water lavage is done, any abnormal cardiac rhythms should be carefully noted.

4. *Continuous gastric suctioning* may be ordered to keep the stomach empty and remove irritating gastric secretions. Suctioning may be alternated with iced physiologic saline lavage, for the coldness seems to decrease bleeding tendencies. However, this fluid must usually be suctioned right away since the coldness causes blood to clot in the stomach and in the tube.

For inserting a Levin tube, the tube is first lubricated well with a water-soluble lubricant. After the procedure has been explained to the patient and he is placed in an upright position if possible, the tube is inserted with gentle pressure into one of his nostrils. A slight twisting motion usually suffices to deflect the tube downward when it reaches the posterior pharyngeal wall. If he is conscious and cooperative, the patient is asked to swallow and the tube is slowly advanced until it reaches the stomach. The patient may be allowed to take small sips of water to make swallowing easier. (A straw should be used so that the glass will not be in the way.)

If there is difficulty in passing the tube, flexion of the neck with the chin toward the chest helps in smoothing the curve of the posterior pharyngeal wall and makes the tube's entering the trachea less likely; the flexion also makes it easier for the patient to swallow.

If the patient is unconscious, the tube should be advanced between respirations to lessen the likelihood of its entrance into the larynx.

A nasogastric tube is very uncomfortable for a patient, and he may complain of sore throat, hoarseness, or earache. Because of increased mucus formation in his nose, he requires paper tissues nearby to wipe his nose; cream may be applied to keep the nasal tissues soft and prevent encrustation. The sore throat may be aided by gargling with warm saline solution, or the physician may permit the use of throat lozenges or a local anesthetic spray. If the patient breathes through his mouth, which is a common occurrence, cream may be applied to his lips, and frequent mouth care is beneficial. Some physicians allow the patient small amounts of cracked ice or chewing gum for overcoming the dryness.

Irrigation of the tube is usually ordered at regular intervals, using 30 ml. of isotonic sodium chloride solution. It is important to keep accurate records of the amounts of fluid used for irrigation so these can be subtracted from the total amount of gastric suction drainage to ascertain the true amount of drainage.

If there is no drainage, several checks can be made to ascertain the reason. The tubing is milked toward the machine to dislodge any obstruction, and then functioning of the machine is checked. After the Levin tube is clamped, the tubing to the machine is disconnected at the glass connection. The distal end of this tubing is placed in a glass of water; if water can be suctioned from this container, one can assume that the machine is working properly.

If the machine is found to be functioning properly, one should irrigate the Levin tube with normal saline solution and then attempt to aspirate it. If it does not return, the physician should be notified, for distention can cause serious difficulty for the patient.

The amount and character of the drainage should be noted. It is especially important that the physician be advised of any newly occurring bright red bloody drainage.

There should be no kinks in the tubing and no pins placed in it. If it is necessary that the tube be kept in place, a small piece of adhesive tape can be fastened around the tube and then pinned in place.

A sump tube is similar to a regular Levin tube except that it has an extra lumen to the stomach which allows a small amount of air to enter the distal end of the tube. Because this continuous stream of air bubbles facilitates suction, this smaller tube is not clamped. Occasionally drainage will return through this lumen. If this separate tubing is placed higher than the drainage tube, the fluid will seek the lower level.

At the time of gastric surgery, some physicians insert the tube for gastric decompression into the stomach by gastrostomy rather than through the nose since it is more comfortable to the patient and presents less danger of causing respiratory complications. Irrigation of the tubing and care of the suctioning apparatus is the same as mentioned previously.

5. *Drug therapy* may be necessary. *Sedation* is required because this patient is usually quite excited and frightened. If nausea and vomiting are prominent symptoms, sedation is perhaps best achieved with injectable *antiemetics,* such as prochlorperazine (Compazine), although simple barbiturate sedation parenterally is quite effective. If the patient is allowed fluids by mouth, mild barbiturate sedation orally may be effective. This is usually combined with an *anticholinergic,* such as methantheline (Banthine) or atropine, to reduce motility and secretion of hydrochloric acid.

6. *Milk and antacids* during alternate hours may be ordered. The protein in milk and the alkali aid in neutralizing the hydrochloric acid. A nonabsorbable alkali is commonly used to prevent electrolyte imbalance.

7. Prompt *consultation* is requested. If this patient is admitted to a medical service he deserves immediate surgical consultation so that the surgeon will be familiar with him before the decision for surgery must be made. Likewise, if he is admitted as a surgical patient, immediate medical consultation is needed for detection of coexisting disease and ideas relative to time and condition for surgery.

8. *Diagnostic studies* are done as soon as possible for the purpose of establishing a definite diagnosis. These include a complete blood count, blood volume, prothrombin time, sulfobromophthalein test, gastrointestinal series, and electrocardiogram.

Complete blood count and *blood volume* are done to indicate blood loss. A *prothrombin time determination* is performed for two reasons: many patients are currently undergoing long-term therapy with anticoagulants. That one is dealing with such a patient may not be immediately made known in the excitement of the episode of gastrointestinal bleeding in a strange patient; also, a prolonged prothrombin time may be indicative of liver disease.

A normal *sulfobromophthalein* (Bromsulphalein, BSP) *test* is considered by most to be adequate in ruling out esophageal varices as a source of bleeding. However, elevated retention of the dye does not necessarily mean that the bleeding is from varices, for there is a higher incidence of peptic ulcer in the patient having cirrhosis than in the population at large.

As soon as the patient's blood pressure and clinical condition stabilize, a gentle *upper gastrointestinal series* is performed. In this situation the radiology personnel should be made aware of the patient's acute bleeding situation so that the patient may be handled with care. This applies to their transporting him to the radiology department and their readiness to perform the examination expeditiously. The early G.I. series is of immense value to the physician in deciding definitive treatment and determining prognosis.

An *electrocardiogram* is made soon after admission; this is especially important if a period of significant hypotension has been present or if the patient is old. The hypotensive episode may have been sustained long enough to produce myocardial damage in the presence of arteriosclerotic coronary narrowing. The presence of a superimposed acute myocardial infarction would make conservative medical management the treatment of choice unless surgery were mandatory.

9. *Urinary output* is recorded as an indication of the degree of shock (page 17).

10. Color, frequency, amount, and consistency of *vomitus and stools* should be noted. An accurate record of intake and output should be maintained.

ESOPHAGEAL VARICES

In any consideration of upper gastrointestinal tract bleeding, one must discuss the management of the patient with bleeding esophageal varices. These varices are quite likely to bleed repeatedly because of the nature of the condition and the uncooperativeness of the patient, who is usually a chronic alcoholic. In addition, such a patient is a poor surgical risk and usually has considerable associated disease. For these reasons management of these patients is at best unsatisfactory.

The normal venous drainage of the intraperitoneal structures is into the portal vein and through the liver. A hardened and distorted liver offers resistance to this blood flow, producing portal hypertension. A small plexus of veins around the lower end of the esophagus (esophageal plexus) and around the anus may drain into either the systemic or the portal venous system. With portal hypertension, considerable blood may be shunted from the portal into the systemic circulation through these collateral channels and may thus produce distention and hypertrophy. These hypertrophied vessels in the esophageal plexus are called *esophageal varices*. The hypertrophied anorectal plexus forms hemorrhoids. Thus, the patient bleeding from esophageal varices is likely to have hemorrhoids, the portal hypertension being a contributory cause of both.

Treatment. Generally the first therapeutic approach to the patient suspected of bleeding from esophageal varices is identical to that for the patient with a bleeding ulcer. However, when bleeding persists, use of the Sengstaken-Blakemore tube may be necessary as a temporary measure to gain time for definite treatment and to prevent further blood loss. The tube has three lumens, one of which leads to an esophageal balloon, another to a gastric balloon, and the third to distal openings which allow suctioning from the stomach.

The tube is usually inserted through the mouth because it cannot be accommodated by most nares because of its large size. Since this patient usually has a diseased liver and since many sedatives are detoxified in the liver, an antihistaminic may be preferred for its drowsy side effects. The technique for insertion is one of asking the patient to swallow as the tube is simultaneously gently pushed until it enters the stomach, as determined by the aspirate from the free tip. The tube is then inserted a little farther, and the gastric balloon is inflated with from 100 to 150 ml. of air. Once this balloon is inflated, the tube is slowly withdrawn until the gastric balloon fits snugly against the cardia of the stomach. This should be indicated by cessation of blood returning through the gastric tube and also by epigastric discomfort produced by the tension of the balloon against the cardia of the stomach. This procedure may be sufficient to control bleeding if the varices are distal to the cardia.

If blood continues to be withdrawn from the tubing, the esophageal balloon is distended, thus producing tension on the varices in the esophagus above the cardia. Since the patient cannot swallow saliva, paper tissues should be available, and suctioning may be needed to prevent aspiration. Frequent mouth care is necessary.

If bleeding continues after both balloons have been inflated, the stomach balloon is further inflated with from 300 to 400 ml. of air and a two-pound weight is suspended from the end of the tube to produce traction, thereby increasing pressure against the cardia. Ice water and alcohol may be used to inflate the balloon.

With the Sengstaken-Blakemore tube in place, the patient's condition may stabilize, and he may be ready for surgery. However, since this patient is usually a cirrhotic who tolerates the breakdown products of intestinal bleeding very poorly, it may be desirable to wait several hours. During this period, the intestinal tract may be sterilized to prevent accumulation of some of the breakdown products of the blood. For this reason, these patients may be given cathartics by this tube periodically as well as nonabsorbable antibiotics to sterilize the gastrointestinal tract. Vitamin K may also be given.

Since esophageal varices are usually caused by portal hypertension due to obstruction to blood flow at some point in the portal venous system, surgery is directed toward relieving this obstruction, and the approach is that of a portal-caval anastomosis or spleno-renal anastomosis for the alleviation of portal hypertension. If the obstruction is intrahepatic, the portal vein is anastomosed to the inferior vena cava, thus bypassing the liver (portacaval shunt). When the portal vein is obstructed a splenectomy may be done; then the splenic vein is anastomosed to the left renal vein (a spleno-renal shunt), thus relieving pressure on the portal vein since approximately 30% of its blood comes from the splenic vein.

The surgical approach to bleeding from the upper gastrointestinal tract may be either definitive or palliative, whether the bleeding is from a peptic ulcer, esophageal varices, or malignant disease. The condition of the patient may be such that definitive procedures would not be tolerated whereas simple ligation of the bleeding point might be efficacious. Again, this would be a matter of judgment, both preoperatively and in the operating theatre.

RELATED FILM

Human gastric function. Color, 18 minutes, available from Smith, Kline and French Laboratories, 1500 Spring Garden St., Philadelphia, Pa.
This interesting film demonstrates the effect of stress on gastric function.

Chapter 25

Gastrointestinal surgery

Although the average patient recovering from abdominal surgery does not require intensive care, there are those who do, such as (1) the poor risk patient who requires emergency abdominal surgery and who has other complicating factors, (2) the patient who has undergone unusually extensive or meticulous abdominal surgery, or (3) the patient who develops anesthetic or postoperative complications regardless of the specific surgical procedure.

COMPLICATIONS

The intensive nursing care for these patients is directed toward careful attention to details of treatment, such as nasogastric suctioning, fluid balance, and medications. However, the primary need is for close observation to detect the occurrence of complications. These can generally be considered as follows: (1) anesthetic complications, (2) shock that may result from hemorrhage or bacteremia in contaminated cases, (3) infection or developing peritonitis, (4) obstruction that may occur in the gastrointestinal or genitourinary tract, (5) electrolyte imbalance, (6) circulatory complications that may be either thrombotic or ischemic, or abnormalities of blood volume, and (7) jaundice.

Anesthetic complications. Anesthetic complications occasionally occur, usually as atelectasis or aspiration pneumonia. *Atelectasis* occurs when a branch of the bronchial tree is plugged by inspissated mucus; the air distal to this plug is absorbed into the circulation, resulting in collapse of the area. Subsequent infection of this atelectatic area may result in pneumonia. The development of inspissated secretions leading to atelectasis may sometimes be prevented by intermittent positive pressure breathing. Mucolytic enzymes or respiratory detergents may be added to the water or saline solution used to humidify the inspired air. Another preventive measure is adequate hydration in the postoperative state.

Pneumonia may also result directly from aspiration, or infection may be introduced by the endotracheal tube with direct contamination of the respiratory tract. These complications are usually directly proportional to the duration of anesthesia. They can be prevented to a great extent by meticulous attention to endotracheal suctioning during surgery and careful attention to deep breathing, coughing, frequent turning, and suctioning in the postoperative state.

The onset of these respiratory complications may be heralded by an increased respiratory rate, chest pain, fever, tachycardia, audible rales, or rhonchi. In extreme cases consolidation or mediastinal shifting and cyanosis may occur. Treatment is the same as is described for pneumonia (page 118).

Shock. Shock in the postoperative patient is most commonly due to *occult bleeding;* however, it can result from *bacteremia*. If it results from occult bleeding, serial hemoglobin, hematocrit, and blood volume determinations should help to elucidate the problem. Adequate blood volume replacement may be the only treatment needed, or if continued bleeding is suspected, reexploration may be indicated. *Bacteremic shock* is especially likely if the causative organism is a gram-negative bacillus. It may produce a severe shock state with hypotension, decreased urinary output, and death. Evidence of peritonitis might be present, such as fever and tachycardia, in which case the abdomen may become increasingly tender, painful, or rigid. Patients with either peritonitis or intraperitoneal bleeding may show signs of intrathoracic pathology because of irritation of the diaphragm, and they may have pain referred to the suspender area of the shoulder. Hiccups may also be a fairly common sign of diaphragmatic peritoneal irritation.

Strenuous treatment is required, including administration of appropriate antibiotics, vasopressor drugs and adrenocorticosteroids. The adequacy of urinary output can be used as an index of effective treatment of the shock.

Infectious complications. Infectious complications, likely to result from abdominal incisions into gangrenous or contaminated fields, include *septicemia and bacteremia,* as previously mentioned, plus *peritonitis* and *localized abdominal abscesses.*

A *subphrenic abscess,* or pus beneath the diaphragm, is one of the more difficult diagnoses to establish. Diaphragmatic irritability may be suggested by pain referred to the shoulder, increasing pulse rate, fever, respiratory guarding with painful, grunting respirations. This diagnosis can usually be confirmed by a fluoroscopic examination of the chest that shows the diaphragm on the involved side being markedly splinted and moving very little. Such abscess usually requires surgical drainage.

Obstruction. Obstruction in the gastrointestinal tract may occur as a complication of intra-abdominal surgery. Almost all patients who have undergone abdominal surgery will have a period of paralytic ileus during which peristalsis is absent, and some of the signs of obstruction may be present. However, mechanical obstruction may occasionally result from circulatory interference, formation of adhesions, or intestinal tortion. Uncommonly, ureteral injury or obstruction may occur following abdominal, and especially pelvic, surgery.

Electrolyte imbalance. Electrolyte imbalance is prone to occur in these surgical patients for several reasons. They usually lose blood and tissue fluid incident to surgery. Most are receiving limited oral intake or may have continuous nasogastric suctioning for intestinal decompression; this makes them particularly susceptible to electrolyte complications, especially hypokalemia. They may also develop water intoxication with its relative hyponatremia, hypochloremia, and hypokalemia. This syndrome is described on page 184.

Circulatory complications. Circulatory complications, either *thromboembolic* or *ischemic,* may occur following abdominal surgery but are much more likely after pelvic surgery. Nevertheless, they may be seen after any surgery and are usually proportional in frequency to the duration and magnitude of the surgery.

There are numerous reasons for the likelihood of developing pelvic and peripheral phlebitis following abdominal surgery. Increased coagulability of the patient's blood after surgery is a natural homeostatic mechanism. There is minor trauma to venous circulation during performance of the surgery, sluggish circulation in the postoperative period when there is little exercise of the legs, and compression of venous tributaries by edema incident to surgical trauma. Thrombophlebitis and subsequent pulmonary embolism are two of the more serious complications of abdominal surgery (see page 29).

Direct ischemic complications are rare and result from inadvertent interference with arterial blood supply that leaves behind a nonviable tissue mass, such as a duodenal stump. Indirect ischemic complications usually result from periods of hypotension produced by surgery and anesthesia in patients who have arteriosclerotic disease. In view of the excessive coagulability of the blood following surgical trauma, even short periods of hypotension may be sufficient to precipitate coronary, cerebral, or peripheral arterial insufficiency and damage.

Abnormalities of blood volume may result in either hypovolemia or hypervolemia. Inadequate fluid replacement during the early operative and postoperative periods brings about symptoms of *dehydration* (page 183). The hemoglobin and hematocrit are usually elevated in this situation if there is no concomitant blood loss.

A somewhat more common complication is overreplacement of fluid and blood, producing *hypervolemia*. There will be visible distention of the venous system, especially noticeable in the jugular veins. The pulse is elevated, and the patient is hyperpneic and may actually have pulmonary edema resulting from the excessive fluid volume. If the overreplaced fluid is blood, the patient may appear somewhat flushed. This situation can be managed by fluid restriction and diuresis; occasionally phlebotomy may be necessary. Here again, the nurse's role is one of observation in order to assist in early detection.

Jaundice. Jaundice occurring in the postoperative period suggests either *hemolysis* or *obstruction* to the biliary outflow tract.

Jaundice from hemolysis, becoming evident immediately postoperatively, is usually seen as a result of transfusions with incompatible blood. The anesthetized patient is particularly prone to experiencing hemolytic blood reactions because the presence of anesthesia is likely to mask many of the early signs that would suggest incompatibility of transfusions and prompt discontinuance in the conscious patient. Therefore, the anesthetized patient is more likely to receive a larger amount of incompatible blood than is the conscious patient. There are also situations in which it is necessary that blood be given under pressure; this significantly decreases the survival time of the transfused red cells although no incompatibility may be present.

Hemolysis may occasionally take place following prostatic or bladder surgery when distilled water leaks into the circulation, producing intravascular hemolysis. Water is hypo-osmotic and will pass into the normo-osmotic red cell in an effort to achieve osmotic balance between the intracellular and extracellular fluids; the red cell is thereby distended to the point of rupture, destruction and hemolysis. This was a frequent occurrence years ago following urologic procedures that required bladder distention; however, urologists now use an iso-osmotic solution for bladder distention.

This complication may also arise from the erroneous use of rather large volumes of distilled water as the vehicle for intravenous medications or occasionally from inadvertent use of distilled water intravenously.

The presence of hemolysis is usually confirmed by a marked increase in urinary urobilinogen and a mild or negligible increase in urinary bile.

Jaundice occurring during the immediate postoperative period may be due to complicating pancreatitis, but it occurs more commonly as a complication of biliary tract surgery. It is occasionally seen in gastric surgery from associated edema of the structures around the biliary outflow tract and is occasionally due to inadvertent injury to the common bile duct during surgery.

The most common cause of obstructive jaundice is a stone in the common duct. It may be overlooked at the time of operation, or it may drop down to an obstructing position immediately after the surgery. This complication occasionally happens to the patients of the best of surgeons in spite of all efforts to demonstrate patency of the biliary tract at the time of surgery by use of cholangiograms and scrupulous examination.

Obstruction may also occur following gallbladder surgery due to associated edema of the common bile duct. Surgeons leave a T tube in the common bile duct in order to remove biliary drainage, which is toxic to the tissues, from the operative site. This tube must **never be clamped** unless ordered by the surgeon.

Obstructive jaundice is usually differentiated from *hemolytic jaundice* by the absence of urinary urobilinogen and the presence of large amounts of bile in the urine. It can be distinguished from hepatitis on the basis of several additional laboratory studies. Obstructive jaundice typically produces a marked elevation of alkaline phosphatase, whereas this test is usually normal during hepatitis. Classically hepatitis produces an elevation of cephalin flocculation and thymol turbidity, which remain normal or are only very slightly elevated in the presence of obstructive jaundice.

The nurse's role in these observations is that of recognizing early a yellow tint of the skin and sclera and the presence of unusually dark urine, as well as noting grayish-colored stools due to the absence of bile in the intestinal tract.

In addition to these general considerations, certain complications that are more likely to be associated with specific abdominal procedures will be considered briefly.

Colectomy is especially noted for causing peritoneal soilage, peritonitis, and sepsis with the gram-negative organisms because of the large amount of generally contaminated tissue dealt with, the richness of its blood supply, and the size of the serous surfaces. The patient is also predisposed to electrolyte difficulties because of continued nasogastric suctioning, loss of fluid through an associated ileostomy or cecostomy, and loss of tissue fluid from the fairly large area of tissue involved. The patient having a resection of a relatively small amount of small bowel is not likely to have difficulty unless the area is contaminated, as by gangrenous bowel. In this situation he is susceptible to bacteremia, shock, and fluid and electrolyte imbalance with hypovolemia.

The patient having undergone a *gastrectomy* is particularly prone to bleeding because of the rich blood supply of the stomach mucosa; the production of serous fluid may also deplete the body's stores of plasma proteins. Following surgery the gastric secretions obtained by nasogastric suctioning are normally reddish-tinged for approximately eight hours. Any continued reddish coloration of the secretions after that time should be reported to the surgeon.

Leakage of the duodenal stump is the complication following gastric surgery most feared by surgeons. It is most likely to occur about the fifth postoperative day, when the tissues are more likely to slough where ligatures have been placed. The leakage will result in sudden deterioration of the patient, with hypotension, fever, tachycardia, marked abdominal pain and rigidity, leukocytosis, and rapid decline. The treatment may be surgical or the same as is described on page 120 for bacteremic shock.

Following gastrectomy, the patient is also fairly susceptible to pancreatitis because of mechanical trauma from the anatomic proximity of the stomach and pancreas. This will usually result in the classic signs of pancreatitis with or without associated biliary tract obstruction (symptoms, page 173). The patient recovering from biliary tract surgery is also particularly prone to pancreatitis. When the field of surgery is contaminated, there is also more likelihood of development of a subphrenic abscess.

Chapter 26

Acute pancreatitis

Typical initial orders include

1. Analgesic and anticholinergic drugs
2. Intravenous infusion
3. Continuous gastric suctioning
4. Frequent check of vital signs
5. Antibiotic
6. Diagnostic studies

CLINICAL FINDINGS

The typical patient having acute pancreatitis goes to a medical facility after being awakened by sudden agonizing epigastric pain that radiates to his back. Usually this pain is at its peak intensity at the time of onset. This patient is usually older than 40 and frequently reports that he consumed a heavy meal on the evening prior to admission.

The patient is extremely restless and seeks a more comfortable position; he is also very anxious and may be confused. He may be in shock *out of proportion* to the rest of the clinical findings. This is signified by hypotension which may be mild or profound, weakness, diaphoresis, and tachycardia. He is frequently febrile, usually dyspneic due to diaphragmatic irritability, and may be cyanotic. There may be nausea and profuse vomiting.

The physical signs include an exquisitely tender epigastrium, sometimes with rigidity suggesting a perforated hollow viscus. The patient may be slightly jaundiced and moderately distended. Left lower chest pathology may be suggested because of the proximity of the pancreas to the diaphragm.

PATHOGENESIS

The exact etiology of acute pancreatitis is not known, although a number of predisposing factors are recognized. Many of the patients have a history of gall bladder or other biliary tract disease. This may have been caused by stones or strictures from repeated inflammation which, in turn, may occasionally produce partial obstruction. Many of these patients also have a history of chronic alcoholism.

Pathologically, an occasional case may be explained by inflammation of the sphincter of Oddi. There may be a common channel from the biliary tract and the pancreatic duct with possible reflux of bile into the pancreatic acini which produces scattered hemorrhage, edema, and necrosis of pancreatic tissue. This necrotic tissue can lead to intra-abdominal hemorrhage and abscess formation.

Acute pancreatitis may occasionally be caused by infectious organisms that may come from the bloodstream, as in mumps or scarlet fever, or from the duodenum such as staphylococcic food poisoning; or they may arise in the biliary tract.

Pancreatitis may be caused by trauma such as that experienced during abdominal surgery or from an external blow. Drugs, such as adrenocorticosteroids and thiazides, have been implicated in occasional cases. In addition it may be related to metabolic factors such as hyperlipemia or hyperparathyroidism. However, pancreatitis may occur in the absence of any of these factors, the patient's only significant history being that of dietary indiscretion, especially of overindulging in a meal high in fat a few hours preceding the onset.

TREATMENT

The treatment of acute pancreatitis is primarily medical. An occasional patient will require surgical exploration acutely when the possibility of a perforated hollow viscus cannot be excluded, or subacutely for the drainage of a pancreatic pseudocyst. However, usually the patient is treated medically, the treatment depending on the severity of the condition. Surgery is avoided if at all possible because the patient is very intolerant of any additional stress; furthermore, some anesthetic agents are detoxified or excreted by the liver whose function may also be impaired.

1. *Analgesia* necessitates the use of a potent narcotic because pain relief is difficult to obtain. Prior to the initial dose of analgesia the serum amylase must be drawn since the opiates increase the tone in the sphincter of Oddi; this can result in false-high amylase readings. Dihydromorphinone (Dilaudid) and meperidine (Demerol) seem less likely to produce sphincter spasm than morphine. Due to the severe and recurring pain there is an ever-present danger of drug addiction.

An *anticholinergic* such as atropine is usually administered systemically to lessen vagal stimulation of pancreatic secretions and decrease tone in the sphincter of Oddi. Nitroglycerine may also be used parenterally occasionally to assist in relaxing biliary tract spasm.

2. An *intravenous infusion* of 1,000 ml. of 5% dextrose in water with 15 to 25 units of regular insulin may be begun slowly. This allows access to the circulation and also initiates replacement of fluid lost. The regular insulin is administered with the glucose so the latter can be utilized by the body since the pancreatic disease may alter insulin production. Furthermore, hyperglycemia is avoided when possible since it will stimulate the pancreas.

The patient will require careful fluid maintenance, both for blood volume and electrolytes, because the pattern of loss is not consistent. Since he may lose tremendous quantities of fluid into the peritoneal cavity or by vomiting, he will require at least from 3 to 4 liters of parenteral fluids every 24 hours to prevent dehydration. Loss of blood may require replacement with the appropriate component, such as plasma, albumen, or whole blood.

3. *Nasogastric suctioning* is instituted in a severe case. A large-caliber Levin tube is used to decrease the incidence of occlusion of the tube; extreme care is exercised to be sure the tube remains open. Emptying of the acid gastric contents into the duodenum stimulates the pancreas to produce more enzymes. Therefore, continuous evacuation of the stomach allows resting of the gland as much as is physiologically possible.

4. *Vital signs* are checked frequently since this patient must be observed closely for the development of hypovolemia and shock. The findings characterizing hypovolemia are listed on page 183. The treatment is fluid replacement with electrolytes as required.

The signs of shock include a decreasing blood pressure; tachycardia with a weak, thready pulse; increased respiration; cool, clammy skin; and decreasing urinary output although the urine is not necessarily concentrated (treatment, page 19).

The patient may be electrocardiographically monitored since the electrolyte imbalance may produce changes in the electrocardiogram. Changes in both form (peaked T waves with hyperkalemia, long Q-T interval with hypokalemia) and rhythm may be seen.

5. A broad-spectrum *antibiotic* is usually given since necrotic tissue is a good culture medium.

6. *Diagnostic studies* executed are serial determinations of serum amylase, electrolytes, blood volume, bilirubin, and blood counts. Additional laboratory studies include survey films of the abdomen, roentgenogram of the chest, and electrocardiogram.

The *amylase* is a measure of a digestive enzyme ordinarily released from the pancreas into the duodenum to assist in the digestion of carbohydrates. A small amount is normally present in the blood, but large amounts are released by the diseased tissue when there is acute pancreatic injury. A level greater than 400 units is considered diagnostic.

As was mentioned previously, the serum amylase should be collected before administration of the initial dose of analgesia; otherwise, a false-high reading can result. If the level is several hundred units this would not be a factor, but it would need to be considered in the borderline elevation. The amylase must be determined early in the course of the disease since the elevation is commonly transient, usually returning to normal by the third day. The serum lipase and urinary amylase may also be helpful, and they remain elevated longer.

Almost any conceivable pattern of *electrolyte* abnormality may be seen. The serum *calcium*, which is determined serially, is a useful test for prognostication in pancreatitis. Release of the digestive enzymes into the peritoneal cavity results in a large weeping of fluid. The alkaline digestive juices act on the peritoneal fat with the serum calcium drawn from the blood to form soft soaps so that needle aspiration of the peritoneum may yield frankly soapy aspirate. Hypocalcemia may occasionally be present to the point of tetany on the second or third day; as such, this is a bad prognostic sign. Treatment for this condition is mentioned on page 268.

Potassium level must be followed carefully. Hyperkalemia and acidosis may be present from excess tissue destruction; hypokalemia may occur from vomiting and nasogastric suctioning (symptoms, pages 185 to 187).

A *complete blood count* usually shows leukocytosis, with an increase in the number of neutrophiles. The hemoglobin and hematocrit may be variable. They may be elevated from hemoconcentration with fluid loss, normal with both fluid and volume loss so that hemodilution is not possible, or low if hemorrhage is a marked feature. A *blood volume* would help to elucidate this problem. There may be considerable blood loss into the peritoneal cavity either in addition to or caused by associated hemolysis. The *bilirubin* may be elevated as a result of associated biliary tract obstruction, cholangitis, or hemolysis.

Survey films of the abdomen in either the upright or the left lateral decubitus position should be done for the following two reasons: (1) The differential diagnosis includes the possibility of a perforated hollow viscus, which is best detected with the left lateral decubitus or a ten-minute upright abdominal film that may show the presence of air under the diaphragm. (2) The presence of pancreatic calcification may suggest that the present episode is recurrent.

A *roentgenogram of the chest* may show elevation of the diaphragm with collection of infradiaphragmatic fluid, or it may occasionally reveal a basilar pneumonia which on rare occasions will mimic pancreatitis with most of the symptomatology being in the upper abdomen. It may also reveal areas of atelectasis, especially in the left base, or there may be signs of pleural effusion. All of these findings may result from contiguous inflammation because of the proximity of the pancreas to the diaphragm.

The *electrocardiogram* should help in differentiating the occasional patient with a myocardial infarction who experiences primarily epigastric pain. However, pancreatitis may produce electrocardiographic changes of a nonspecific nature due to irritation of the diaphragm or electrolyte abnormalities, especially calcium and potassium. These nonspecific changes should not prevent a correct diagnosis of pancreatitis.

Blood glucose levels are checked frequently since these patients may develop acute diabetes. Failure to metabolize glucose leads to incomplete fat metabolism with its resultant ketosis; therefore, including enough regular insulin to utilize the glucose administered in intravenous fluids is desirable.

Since no specific treatment is available, medical and nursing management of the patient having acute pancreatitis is entirely supportive by the following measures:

1. Symptoms are relieved.
2. Antibiotics are given to prevent secondary infection.
3. The organ is physiologically rested (gastric suctioning and insulin administration).
4. Abnormal physiologic events (hypovolemia and electrolyte abnormalities) are detected early and treated specifically.

The patient having renal disease

Chapter 27

Basic anatomy and physiology of the kidney

Since the kidney is one of the most important organs for maintaining homeostasis of the body, a brief outline of its basic anatomy and physiology is presented.

THE NEPHRON

The functional unit of the kidney is the *nephron*. It is composed of a *glomerulus* or capillary tuft, *Bowman's capsule,* and a long *tubule* that empties into the *renal pelvis*. There are approximately one million nephrons in each kidney (Fig. 27-1).

TASK OF THE KIDNEY

The kidney has the primary task of regulating the composition and volume of the blood. It does this by (1) removing toxic metabolic wastes from the blood and (2) regulating the amount of nontoxic substances, such as water and electrolytes, in the blood. It accomplishes this task by *filtration, selective reabsorption,* and *secretion*.

Filtration. The glomerular capillary tuft is quite unique to body vasculature. It differs from ordinary capillaries by having an arteriole leading to *(afferent arteriole)* and away from *(efferent arteriole)* the glomerulus so that the hydrostatic pressure within the capillaries can be very finely controlled. Glomerular hydrostatic pressure is regulated by relative dilatation or constriction of the afferent and efferent arterioles, as well as by systemic blood pressure.

Glomerular filtrate is produced primarily by hydrostatic pressure. This glomerular filtrate is quite similar in concentration and composition to cell and protein-free plasma, for it is composed of water, electrolytes, and nutrients. Blood cells, platelets, and plasma proteins normally remain in the arterioles.

Each *glomerulus* sheds its filtrate into a small funnel-shaped microscopic structure called a *Bowman's capsule*. The filtrate is then conducted from the capsule into the *proximal convoluted tubule, the loop of Henle,* the *distal convoluted tubule,* and finally into the *collecting tubule*.

Selective reabsorption. The *efferent arteriole* leading from the glomerular capillary tuft again divides into a *secondary capillary network* that surrounds divisions of the renal tubules. This is the site of selective reabsorption, for certain

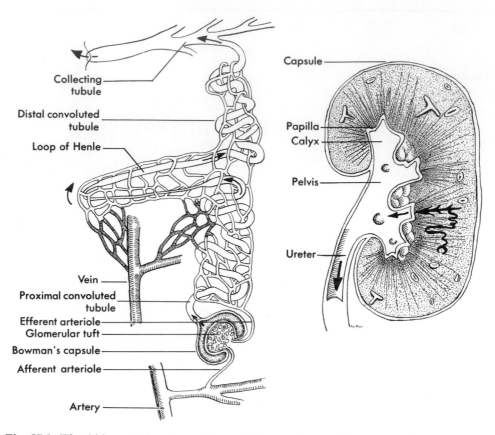

Fig. 27-1. The kidneys. The glomerulus and Bowman's capsule are actually microscopic structures; however, the nephron (glomerulus, Bowman's capsule, and tubules) is represented in the kidney macroscopically for orientation only.

desirable solutes, such as glucose and electrolytes, as well as water, are normally reabsorbed into the capillaries. This results in concentration of the glomerular filtrate.

Secretion. Secretion takes place when certain substances, such as creatinine and some drugs, are secreted from the secondary capillary network into the convoluted tubules. Approximately 150,000 ml. of glomerular filtrate progress daily through the glomeruli and convoluted tubules. Approximately 99% of this filtrate is reabsorbed into the circulation. The remaining 1%, or 1,500 ml., is excreted as urine, which is composed of water, metabolic waste materials, and those solutes which occur in excess and are no longer needed by the body or which exceed the capability of the system to reabsorb.

The *collecting tubules* merge, and urine empties through the *papillae* into the *calyces* of the kidney and then into the *renal pelvis*. It then progresses through the *ureter* to the *bladder,* where it is excreted from the body through the *urethra.*

Chapter 28

Fluid and electrolyte problems

Normal ranges

pH—7.35 to 7.45

CO_2—22 to 30 mEq./liter—45 to 70 vol.%

Sodium (Na)—135 to 145 mEq./liter

Potassium (K)—3.5 to 5.0 mEq./liter

Calcium (Ca)—4.5 to 6.0 mEq./liter—
    9 to 11 mg.%

Chlorides (Cl)—100 to 110 mEq./liter

INTRODUCTION

One can most easily understand problems of fluid and electrolyte balance by considering them as either deficits or excesses of individual electrolyte components. Since electrolytes and water are interrelated and a single electrolyte abnormality is seldom seen, the syndromes are usually considered in terms of the dominant electrolyte abnormality. An awareness of the situations in which the anomalies are likely to occur and the symptoms of their presence will aid in their recognition. It should be remembered that an electrolyte deficit may be produced either by increased intake of water, excessive loss of electrolytes, or a combination of these factors. The reverse is also true: an excess amount of an electrolyte may occur with decreased intake of water, excessive loss of water, excessive intake or retention of an electrolyte, or a combination of these factors.

Basic understanding of fluid and electrolyte abnormalities depends on some realization of their normal physiology and balance. The term *electrolyte* is used to refer to chemicals which, when dissolved, are capable of conducting an electric current. This capability is the result of dissociation of the compound into electrically charged particles called *ions*. Positively charged particles are called *cations;* negatively charged particles are called *anions*. Any solution should contain an equivalent number of positively and negatively charged ions. Clinically, the term *electrolyte* may refer to such a compound or any individual ion.

Some compounds dissociate almost completely. For example, sodium chloride (NaCl) dissociates into sodium (Na+) and chloride (Cl−) almost completely when dissolved in water. Other compounds, such as proteins, dissociate very little and, as such, are weak electrolytes.

The commonly encountered cations within body fluids are *sodium, potassium, calcium,* and *magnesium*. The commonly encountered *anions* are *chlorides, carbonic acid, sulfates,* and *phosphates*. Because positively and negatively charged particles are attracted to each other, any cation may chemically unite with an equivalent amount of any anion.

181

The chemical strength or chemical reactivity of a compound depends on the extent to which it dissociates into charged particles. The term *milliequivalent* (mEq.) is used to represent a unit of chemical activity of a compound. With reference to body fluids, this is expressed in milliequivalents per liter (mEq./liter). In chemical activity, a milliequivalent of one ion is equal to a milliequivalent of any other ion.

BODY FLUID

Body fluid is divided into two major compartments: *intracellular* fluid, which is located *within* the cells and *extracellular* fluid, which is located *outside* the cells of the body. The two fluids are separated by the cell membrane.

When a state of balance exists, the total osmotic concentration within the cell and in the extracellular fluid is equal. In the process of osmosis, fluid moves from an area of lesser concentration to an area of greater concentration. Therefore, if the concentration within the cell is excessive, water is drawn into the cell from the extracellular fluid. Conversely, if the concentration in the extracellular fluid is excessive, water is drawn from the cell to dilute the extracellular fluid.

Potassium (K+) is the dominant cation in the intracellular fluid, and *sodium* (Na+) is the dominant cation in the extracellular fluid. This is the major electrolyte difference between the two fluid compartments.

The *extracellular fluid* is subdivided into two types: the *intravascular fluid* (fluid within the blood vessels) and the *interstitial fluid* (fluid between the body cells). The chemical composition of the intravascular fluid and interstitial fluid is very similar, with the major difference being in protein content. Likewise, they are in equilibrium.

Water and small molecular solutes, such as oxygen, carbon dioxide, sodium, potassium, chlorides, and nutrients are forced through the capillary walls into the interstitial space by the hydrostatic pressure within the vascular tree. As this water and these small molecular solutes leave the intravascular system, the plasma protein, which is much less diffusible, becomes more concentrated in the intravascular fluid. Thus, osmotic pressure is increased in the intravascular space which in turn causes fluid to be brought back into the intravascular space to relieve the hyperosmolarity of this fluid. Therefore, the hydrostatic pressure within the vascular tree is held in equilibrium by the osmotic pressure. Generally, electrolyte concentrations diffuse freely from the vascular to the interstitial space.

Ultimate control of the body fluid and electrolytes depends on the individual's fluid intake and output. A cardinal rule is that *intake must equal output* for the fluids, electrolytes, and acid-base balance to remain in equilibrium.

With reference to the body, sources of *water intake* are these three: liquids consumed, water contained in food, and water formed by food metabolism.

Water loss is much more complex. It involves moisture lost through the skin as perspiration and through the expired air (insensible water loss), and water excreted through the intestinal and urinary tracts. By its ability to excrete concentrated or dilute urine, the normal kidney is able to maintain water balance within very narrow limits in spite of great variation in intake.

ACID-BASE BALANCE

There must be proper *acid-base balance* in the body; this is maintained by controlling the concentration of hydrogen ($H+$) ions, which is indicated by pH. A solution that has a pH of 7 has a balance of $H+$ and $OH-$ ions and is neutral (water). An *acid* solution contains more $H+$ ions, and the pH is decreased; a base or *alkaline* solution contains fewer $H+$ ions, and the pH is increased. The body fluid is slightly alkaline, for the normal pH range for the body is from 7.35 to 7.45.

To maintain this acid-base balance, the body has a *system of buffers,* which are substances that act as chemical sponges in the body. The balance is also regulated by two other paired organs: the *kidneys* and the *lungs.*

The buffer systems can give off $H+$ ions or absorb $H+$ ions as necessary, thereby dissociating in such a manner as to form either weak acids or weak bases. If excessive acid is present, the buffer dissociates to form a weak base to neutralize this acid. If excessive base is present, the buffer dissociates to form a weak acid to counteract this base.

The major buffer systems are the carbonic acid–bicarbonate system, the plasma protein system, and the hemoglobin system. The operation of the buffer systems is similar and, strictly speaking, is a temporary measure.

Regulators. In normal situations the *kidneys* serve as the prime regulator of electrolyte content; they maintain a relatively narrow tolerance of the various electrolytes despite wide variations in intake.

A secondary function of the *lungs* is control of electrolyte balance. The moisture lost during respiration is obligatory (fluid is lost through expiration, regardless of the fluid intake) and varies according to respiratory volume and temperature. However, some electrolyte adjustments are possible through the ability of the lungs to expire carbon dioxide, which when dissolved in water is an acid, in certain conditions of excessive acid production. This adjustment is made by increasing or decreasing respirations, by which mechanism the lungs have an important function in the maintenance of pH. They also assist in the maintenance of pH by oxygen exchange and its effect on the hemoglobin buffer system.

FLUID ABNORMALITIES

Hypovolemia. Hypovolemia, or extracellular fluid volume deficit, usually represents a deficiency of both water and electrolytes. Hypovolemia is frequently referred to as dehydration which, strictly defined, refers to water loss. In common clinical usage these terms are interchanged.

Predisposing factors. Predisposing factors include decreased fluid intake, diuresis, fever, diaphoresis, vomiting or diarrhea or both, intestinal intubation, or intestinal obstruction. During intestinal obstruction, a great deal of fluid is ineffective for use by the body since it remains within the distended loops of the intestinal tract. Hypovolemia may also be caused by drainage from skin lesions, fistulas, wounds, or burns.

Clinical findings. Clinical findings include dry skin with poor turgor, dry mucous membranes (which one can ascertain by feeling the junction of the gums and buccal mucosa), coated tongue, sunken soft eyeballs, listlessness, and acute weight loss. The pulse is generally elevated, the blood pressure is depressed, and the voice is husky. There may be oliguria or anuria. Hypovolemia causes a longer venous filling time of peripheral veins. (When the hand is elevated, hand veins should empty within from three to five seconds and then refill in the same length of time when the hand is lowered.)

Laboratory studies. Laboratory studies reveal an increase in hemoglobin and hematocrit values because of hemoconcentration. There is a depression of blood volume since intravascular and extracellular water are freely exchangeable, and both are lost in hypovolemia. The urine is concentrated and has a high specific gravity.

Hypervolemia. Hypervolemia, or extracellular fluid volume excess, usually represents elevated levels of both electrolytes and water in approximately physiologic proportions.

Predisposing factors. Predisposing factors may have been intravenous infusions given too rapidly or in excessive amounts, especially isotonic saline solution. There may have been excessive salt ingestion or prolonged administration of the adrenocorticosteroids. The patient may have predisposing heart or kidney disease, such as congestive heart failure or the nephrotic syndrome.

Clinical findings. Clinical findings include edema which pits on compression; this may progress to anasarca or pulmonary edema. There is also acute weight gain, coarse facies due to edema, puffy eyelids, and venous engorgement that may be seen in the distended jugular veins while the patient is in the semisitting position. Hypervolemia may cause shortness of breath, coughing, moist rales, and excessive sputum production. Urinary output is usually diminished.

Laboratory studies. Laboratory studies usually reveal normal electrolytes with depression of hemoglobin and hematocrit from hemodilution, and blood volume is elevated. The urine usually has a low specific gravity.

ELECTROLYTE ABNORMALITIES

Hyponatremia. Hyponatremia, or sodium deficit, may occur with or without hypovolemia. When it occurs without hypovolemia, it is responsible for most of the symptoms of the syndrome of *water intoxication.*

Predisposing factors. Predisposing factors are heat exhaustion and diaphoresis with excessive water consumption without concomitant salt replacement. It may follow repeated water enemas or potent diuresis; and it may occur with nasogastric suctioning when water is being consumed, for the water facilitates the removal of gastric juices. Iatrogenically, it is produced when infusion of electrolyte-poor fluid, as 5% dextrose in water, is excessive. Hyponatremia is found in patients who have adrenal insufficiency since they are unable to conserve sodium, and it also occurs following inhalation of water when a patient almost drowns in fresh water (as opposed to salt water).

Clinical findings. Clinical findings include evidence of central nervous system irritation, such as headache, confusion, anxiety, or delirium. The patient may complain of cramping abdominal pain or other muscular irritability with twitching that may culminate in convulsions. There may be hypotension and tachycardia if hypovolemia accompanies hyponatremia. Additionally, there is loss of skin turgor, and the eyeballs are sunken and soft.

Laboratory studies. Laboratory studies reveal a low plasma sodium, usually less than 130 mEq./liter with a low chloride less than 98 mEq./liter. The specific gravity of the urine is also low.

Hypernatremia. Hypernatremia, or sodium excess, is seen in special conditions.

Predisposing factors. Predisposing factors include situations in which extra sodium (and usually chloride) is taken into the body without enough water to dilute the solute to osmolarity. If water is available, water is retained to balance the electrolytes thus producing an excess of extracellular fluid or hypervolemia. The classic example of this syndrome is consumption of sea water when no other water is available; it also occurs in the patient who inhales or swallows sea water during near-drowning. Inadvertent infusion of hypertonic saline solution will effect the same state.

Excessive adrenal secretion of aldosterone is the only physiologic predisposing factor. This may be primary aldosteronism or secondary to congestive heart failure or cirrhosis.

Clinical findings. Clinical findings include agitation that may progress to convulsions, dry mucous membranes, marked thirst, flushed facies, hypertension, and tachycardia.

Laboratory studies. Laboratory studies reveal an elevation of plasma sodium, usually greater than 150 mEq./liter. Serum chloride is also elevated, usually greater than 110 mEq./liter, and the urine specific gravity is elevated. If the condition is prolonged, the blood urea nitrogen level becomes elevated.

Hypokalemia. Hypokalemia, or potassium deficit, is one of the more common electrolyte abnormalities seen in clinical practice. In recent years recognition of this deficiency has become much more frequent.

Predisposing factors. The most common predisposing factor is administration of potent diuretics, especially the thiazides. Nonetheless, this deficit may also accompany excessive loss of intestinal juices through diarrhea, vomiting, intestinal fistulas, or intestinal intubation.

Hypokalemia is also common during the recovery phase of diabetic acidosis since the administered insulin tends to drive the extracellular potassium into the intracellular space. Because this occurs at the same time that osmotic diuresis is taking place, there is a deficiency of potassium in the extracellular fluid.

Clinical findings. Clinical findings are progressive weakness, which can culminate in flaccid paralysis, due to lack of nerve impulses to the muscles; diminution of reflexes; apathy; anorexia; vomiting; and intestinal ileus. The patient's voice is very weak, respirations may be shallow, pulse may be weak, and there may be progressive hypotension. The electrocardiogram may reveal abnormal rhythms and a prolonged Q-T interval with low voltage T waves.

Hyperkalemia. Hyperkalemia, or potassium excess in extracellular fluid, seldom occurs except in the presence of chronic kidney disease.

Predisposing factors. Predisposing factors include severe burns, severe trauma, and adrenal insufficiency. In burns and trauma the situation is produced by the release of the intracellular potassium into the extracellular fluid by the disruption of the integrity of the cell membranes.

Clinical findings. Clinical findings include muscle irritability, nausea, and abdominal cramps or mild diarrhea or both. There may be weakness progressing to flaccid paralysis, and respiratory difficulty may also be present. The patient may remain alert while these symptoms are present.

Laboratory studies. Laboratory studies indicate a serum potassium level elevated to greater than 5.5 mEq./liters, usually confirmed by an elevated urea nitrogen level or other evidence of chronic renal disease.

The electrocardiogram may show a high peaked T wave and fairly frequent extrasystoles. With increasing hyperkalemia, the extrasystoles frequently progress to more ominous arrhythmias. Hyperkalemic death is usually due to ventricular fibrillation.

Hypocalcemia. Hypocalcemia, or calcium deficiency in extracellular fluid, occurs fairly frequently.

Predisposing factors. The most common predisposing factor is probably the hyperventilation syndrome that produces respiratory alkalosis. This binds the calcium to the serum protein (a buffer system) so that it is functionally rather than absolutely decreased.

Administration of large amounts of citrated blood binds serum calcium to the citrate in the blood; this is probably the most common cause of significant hypocalcemia likely to be seen in the intensive care situation. For this reason calcium gluconate is usually administered when multiple transfusions are given; however, when the patient is bleeding rapidly, this order may be neglected.

Calcium deficit may also take place during acute pancreatitis in which the release of pancreatic enzymes into the tissue results in fatty necrosis, and the serum calcium is bound to the partially digested fats as soaps. Chronic diarrhea or malabsorption syndromes, such as sprue, may also result in faulty calcium absorption and chronic deficiency.

Hypocalcemia may occur with massive infection of subcutaneous tissue or following removal of or injury to the parathyroid glands. Its advent may be intentional in the treatment of parathyroid adenoma or inadvertent during a thyroidectomy.

Clinical findings. Clinical findings include tingling of the fingers, toes, ears and nose that may progress to carpopedal spasm and tetany. Abdominal and muscle cramping may also be present. If persistent and increasing, hypocalcemia may terminate in convulsions or cardiac arrhythmias or both.

Laboratory studies. Laboratory studies reveal serum calcium to be depressed to less than 4.5 mEq./liter. Sulkowitch's urine test shows no precipitation. Nonspecific electrocardiographic abnormalities may also be noted.

Hypercalcemia. Hypercalcemia, or calcium excess in extracellular fluid, occasionally occurs; however, it rarely produces acute symptoms requiring intensive care.

Predisposing factor. The primary predisposing factor is hyperparathyroidism. A secondary cause is metastatic disease of the bone resulting in bony destruction and liberation of excessive calcium into the extracellular spaces.

Clinical findings. Clinical findings are usually referable to the gastrointestinal tract and include diarrhea, constipation, nausea, and indigestion. There may be kidney stones, pathologic fractures, or multiple bone cysts.

Laboratory studies. Laboratory studies reveal a serum calcium level elevated to greater than 6.0 mEq./liter and considerable loss of calcium in the urine as revealed by heavy precipitation in Sulkowitch's test. Specific roentgenographic findings on examination of the bones may aid in diagnosis.

ACID-BASE IMBALANCES

Acid-base imbalances are generally classified according to their cause. The etiology may be either *metabolic,* due to defective metabolism, or *respiratory,* due to abnormalities in respiration. These classifications can be subdivided into *metabolic acidosis, metabolic alkalosis, respiratory acidosis,* and *respiratory alkalosis.*

Metabolic acidosis. In metabolic acidosis, there is an increase in acid resulting from a deficit in the base or bicarbonate.

Predisposing factors. A primary predisposing factor is diabetes. Diabetic acidosis is the result of a relative deficiency of bicarbonate because of retention of acetoacetic acid, acetone, and other acids when fats are partially metabolized. Metabolic acidosis may also occur in severe diarrhea.

Clinical findings. Clinical findings include deep, rapid, unlabored breathing (Kussmaul respiration). This hyperpnea is a compensating mechanism, for the lower pH with its increased hydrogen ion concentration stimulates the respiratory center. Therefore, the respirations are increased in an attempt to lower the plasma acid content by increased expiration of carbon dioxide.

Other symptoms include headache and drowsiness that can progress to unconsciousness; abdominal pain is common, and fluid deficit usually accompanies this condition.

Laboratory studies. Laboratory studies reveal a carbon dioxide combining power less than 22 mEq./liter and plasma pH less than 7.35. The urine pH is below 6, and acetonuria is present. In diabetic acidosis, glycosuria occurs, and the specific gravity of the urine is elevated.

Chronic metabolic acidosis is seen in the retention of sulfates and phosphates (acids) in chronic renal disease, almost regardless of the type of renal disorder. Probably the lowest bicarbonate levels encountered in clinical practice are present in the patient who has chronic kidney disease. Marked elevation of the urea nitrogen tends to confirm the level of the carbon dioxide–combining power that is so low that it is first thought to represent a laboratory error. As the acidosis develops over a long period of time (months or years), the patient's body has an opportunity to compensate. An occasional patient may seem to be in fair general condition with a carbon dioxide–combining power of less than 10 mEq./liter and urea nitrogen greater than 100. Potassium elevation is a common accompaniment because of failure of the kidney to excrete potassium.

Metabolic alkalosis. Metabolic alkalosis occurs when there is an increase in the base (usually bicarbonate) due to a deficiency in acid. This can occur when chloride-rich solutions are lost, resulting in a relative increase in bicarbonate. Metabolic alkalosis is usually associated with and potentiates potassium deficiency, and the dominant symptoms are those of potassium deficit.

Predisposing factors. Predisposing factors such as intestinal intubation and persistent or excessive vomiting produce loss of hydrochloric acid. Metabolic alkalosis can also be caused by excessive ingestion of alkalis.

Clinical findings. Clinical findings include symptoms resembling those characteristic of potassium deficiency (page 185). There is also slow respiration and headache.

Laboratory studies. Laboratory studies indicate a high pH and elevated carbon dioxide–combining power.

Respiratory acidosis. Respiratory acidosis occurs when there is an increase in carbonic acid; this is caused by *hypoventilation*.

Predisposing factors. Predisposing factors are any conditions that depress respiration and therefore result in retention of carbon dioxide by the lungs and, consequently, the presence of excessive carbonic acid in body fluids. Two major classifications are *drug intoxications* such as overdosage of barbiturates, opiates, or tranquilizers and *respiratory conditions* including chronic pulmonary insufficiency, asthma, emphysema, pneumonia, or pneumothorax.

Clinical findings. Clinical findings include slow, inefficient respirations, some degree of cyanosis, restlessness, headache, incoordination, tremors, and confusion that may progress to mania. Papilledema and decreased reflexes may also be present.

Laboratory studies. Laboratory studies reveal plasma pH less than 7.35. The plasma carbon dioxide content is actually elevated if the condition has developed slowly, for the sodium bicarbonate may have been retained in an attempt to compensate for the elevated carbonic acid (due to retained carbon dioxide).

Respiratory alkalosis. Respiratory alkalosis, or carbonic acid deficiency, is caused by hyperventilation. The loss of carbon dioxide causes a depletion of carbonic acid in the extracellular fluid.

Predisposing factors. Predisposing factors include fever or extreme emotional stress, as in the hyperventilation syndrome.

Clinical findings. Clinical findings include hyperpnea and symptoms of calcium deficiency (page 186). These symptoms probably result from the effect of alkalosis on the available calcium. The symptoms can rather promptly abate after the patient is given an injection of calcium gluconate.

Laboratory findings. Laboratory findings include a plasma carbon dioxide level less than 22 mEq./liter and a plasma pH greater than 7.45.

RELATED FILM

Parenteral fluid therapy (Introduction to Water and Electrolytes). Color, 15 minutes, available from Baxter Laboratories, Morton Grove, Ill. 60053.

This is an excellent film to aid in teaching electrolyte therapy.

Chapter 29

Azotemia and peritoneal dialysis

The terms *azotemia* and *uremia* are generally used interchangeably and refer to retention of the end products of protein metabolism.

Azotemia may be classified as (1) prerenal, or due to factors other than diseased kidneys; (2) postrenal, or caused by obstruction to the discharge of urine without initial damage to the kidneys; or (3) resulting from renal disease and further classified as acute renal failure or chronic renal failure.

PRERENAL AZOTEMIA

Prerenal azotemia, which is usually acute, is present in any condition that causes inadequate kidney perfusion. This might occur with *prolonged hypotension from any cause* or *protracted hypovolemia* as might occur with acute gastroenteritis with little fluid retention. It may result from *severe crush injuries* that effect an extremely heavy overload of waste materials to be removed from the body, *inadequate renal perfusion* as in congestive heart failure, or *impeded blood supply* to the kidney as might happen in renal artery thrombosis.

Clinical findings. The clinical findings are those of the underlying condition and usually include preceding hypotension. The patient's state of consciousness is depressed, and he usually has a rapid pulse and respiration. Symptoms of abnormal fluid state, either hypovolemia or hypervolemia, are common. Urine is usually scanty and concentrated and may contain albumen. The blood urea nitrogen and creatinine are elevated.

Treatment. Treatment involves management of the underlying condition, such as assuring adequate renal perfusion and replacing volume deficits as required. For example, if the volume deficit is predominantly blood, as in gastrointestinal bleeding, blood would be the fluid needed, while fluid and electrolytes would be necessary following gastroenteritis. If the deficient fluid is primarily serum, as in burns, serum proteins, plasma, or plasma expanders may be helpful. If the major difficulty is inadequate perfusion, as with congestive heart failure, primary treatment is directed toward this problem. Prior to therapy, serum electrolytes, complete blood count, and blood volume determinations should be done to serve as a guide for fluid and electrolyte therapy.

POSTRENAL AZOTEMIA

Postrenal azotemia results from obstruction to the discharge of urine although there has been no initial damage to the kidneys. Treatment of this condition

189

rarely requires admission of the patient to an intensive care unit, but patients who have this syndrome may be admitted to a unit for other reasons.

Postrenal azotemia may be caused by *ureteral strictures* that perhaps result from a calculus, tumor, infection, or external pressure that partially occludes the ureters. The severity of the condition usually depends on whether one or both kidneys are affected. This condition may also result from *urethral strictures,* the most common cause being *prostatic hypertrophy.*

This type of azotemia is rarely produced acutely because sudden obstruction to the urinary tract usually produces symptoms that demand relief before it has been present long enough to produce significant azotemia. On the other hand, chronic obstruction to the urinary tract is capable of producing significant azotemia. Because of constant urinary retention characteristic of prostatic hypertrophy, the hydrostatic pressure within the bladder increases. This greater pressure is transmitted retrograde through the ureters to the renal pelves, and thence to the parenchyma of the kidneys, causing damage. Because this decreases production of urine, nitrogenous waste materials are not filtered from the body; therefore azotemia results.

Clinical findings. The clinical findings in the patient with postrenal azotemia resulting from severe prostatic hypertrophy reveal that he is frequently confused and may have had recent mental deterioration. He usually complains of anorexia and gives a history of difficulty in urination, either in starting the stream or having a small stream of urine. The bladder does not empty completely, so residual urine is constantly present even though he urinates frequently. The odor of urine that may emanate from him may actually be the smell of azotemia. This is produced by the excretion of nitrogenous material through the breath and pores of the skin, or it may result from repeated minor soiling from urinary dribbling.

This patient has usually been existing on a marginal amount of renal function for some time. His acute deterioration may be precipitated by almost any event that increases his metabolic rate, such as fluid imbalance resulting from a gastrointestinal illness, or by an increase in the degree of urinary tract obstruction. A major cause of difficulty is a urinary tract infection, since stagnant urine is a good culture medium for bacterial growth.

Laboratory studies. Laboratory studies commonly reveal an *elevated blood urea nitrogen* that may be as high as 75 or more. Since his diet has usually been marginal for some time, he is basically *anemic* and *hypoproteinemic;* however, since hemoconcentration is usually present due to hypovolemia, the true anemia may not be indicated by the hemoglobin and hematocrit until there is adequate hydration. A blood volume determination will aid in determining the degree of *hypovolemia.*

Almost any pattern of electrolyte abnormality may be seen in this patient due to the variations of intake, tissue breakdown, infection, and so forth. Generally, the pattern is hypovolemia with retention of protein breakdown products that are basically acid (sulfates and phosphates). This retention depresses base bicarbonate and the carbon dioxide–combining power, indicating *metabolic acidosis. Hyperkalemia* is usually present because of the inability of the kidneys to excrete potassium.

Treatment. Treatment for this patient consists of adequate urinary drainage, usually by means of an indwelling catheter, and adequate hydration by the intravenous or oral route of administration. Associated illnesses, such as infection of the urinary or respiratory tract or congestive heart failure, are appropriately treated. Definitive treatment for this patient is a prostatectomy when his general condition has improved. Nursing care following this surgery is discussed on page 202.

ACUTE RENAL FAILURE

The patient with acute renal failure (also known as acute tubular necrosis, lower nephron nephrosis, or acute renal suppression) has a recent history of oliguria followed by anuria. Its onset frequently follows some acute event that is well known, such as a transfusion reaction or any of the conditions mentioned among the clinical findings with prerenal azotemia. This condition may also follow the ingestion of poisons, such as cyanide, arsenic, or lead. It is occasionally seen without its cause being known, as in the patient with acute glomerulonephritis.

The pattern of acute renal failure is conveniently divided into three phases: (1) the oliguric, (2) the anuric, and (3) the polyuric or recovery phase. Manifestations and treatment vary with each phase.

Oliguric phase. The oliguric phase begins shortly after injury and is characterized by gradually decreasing urinary output. During this phase, the urine may show definite abnormalities, such as casts, albuminuria, and hemoglobinuria.

Treatment. Treatment is directed toward minimizing damage by such measures as alkalinization in transfusion reactions to increase the solubility of the free hemoglobin. This is done by administration of sodium bicarbonate, either intravenously or orally. At this stage the injury is frequently compounded by fluid overload in an erroneous attempt to "wash out" the toxic products. This is acceptable only if water balance can be maintained in a negative state by persistent mannitol diuresis.

Anuric phase. The oliguric phase may merge into the anuric phase during which there is total absence of urine production. If injury is less severe, the oliguric phase may pass directly into the recovery or polyuric phase.

Because the anuric patient's major disability is his inability to produce urine, nitrogenous waste materials and sulfates are retained. He will frequently be in metabolic acidosis since he cannot rid his body of acid tissue-breakdown products. He is also on very treacherous ground because of his inability to rid his body of excessive fluid. Frequently on arrival in the intensive care unit, this patient will have been overhydrated to the point of obvious edema. Excess fluid in an amount equivalent to from 5% to 10% of body weight is required for visible edema. If the patient is seen from the onset or oliguric phase, this dangerous state of overhydration may be avoided by limiting fluid intake.

Treatment. The major therapeutic endeavor during acute renal failure is to maintain vital functions and keep the chemical status within reasonable limits in order to give the kidneys an opportunity to recover their function. Fortunately, in most situations in which acute renal failure is produced, recovery is possible, and the anuric phase lasts only a few days. Among the several measures taken in an attempt to maintain homeostasis in this altered state are the following: (1) limited fluid intake, (2) high carbohydrate and moderate fat intake with as little protein ingestion as possible, and (3) correction of electrolyte imbalances.

1. *Limited fluid intake* is very important for this patient. Fluid may be limited to a volume equaling insensible fluid loss, or that fluid usually lost through the pores of the skin and respiration (usually from 500 to 1,000 ml. daily), plus a volume equal to the urine output of the preceding day. If the patient is in an overhydrated state, the amount of fluid allowed may be limited to the volume of the urine output of the preceding day.

Fluids allowed are those low in protein, potassium, and sodium. Ginger ale is generally permitted. Lemonade whose sweetening agent is white sugar increases the caloric intake but provides a low intake of potassium since only a small amount of lemon juice is needed. It is also noted that cranberry sauce and juice are low in both potassium and sodium. These acid liquids might help to diminish the nausea that frequently accompanies a diet high in fat content.

2. *High carbohydrate, moderate fat,* and *minimal protein ingestion* is attempted to keep the level of nitrogenous wastes and acid protein-breakdown products as low as possible. In addition, protein digestion or metabolism usually results in release of rather large amounts of potassium, which is quite toxic to the anuric or oliguric patient.

To provide from 1,500 to 2,000 calories, the patient is given fairly large amounts of carbohydrates and as much fat as he can tolerate. Although fat is high in calories, the fact that it can be nauseating has to be taken into consideration. This patient may be given sweetened butterballs made with unsalted margarine or butter if he is able to eat. A slice or two of toast spread with unsalted margarine and sprinkled heavily with white sugar (and lightly with cinnamon) gives a little variety. The patient is also encouraged to suck hard candy. If he is unable to eat or needs supplemental calories, these may be provided by 10% to 20% glucose by slow infusion with the volume determined as previously mentioned.

3. *Correction of electrolyte imbalance* is vitally important because this imbalance is the primary cause of death in this patient. The major imbalance is hyperkalemia with its associated abnormal cardiac rhythms, and for this reason close attention is paid to potassium metabolism, especially in the oliguric and anuric phases. Since there is a certain amount of tissue catabolism incident to living, there is considerable intracellular potassium liberated into the extracellular fluid and blood. This shift in potassium causes a rise in serum potassium and the accompanying manifestations of hyperpotassemia (see page 185).

Significant relative hyperpotassemia may at times be reflected in the electrocardiogram prior to marked elevation of serum levels. Consequently, continuous electrocardiographic monitoring may be desirable during some phases of acute renal failure. The *electrocardiographic signs* of hyperkalemia are tall, peaked T waves and evidence of cardiac irritability as manifested by frequent extrasystoles, sometimes multifocal, or other ectopic rhythms.

Temporary treatment. Temporary treatment for hyperpotassemia may include the administration of 50 ml. of 50% glucose intravenously with 50 units of regular insulin. This produces a shift of potassium into the intracellular space and may be quite dramatic in its effect on cardiac arrhythmias. Unfortunately this treatment is quite temporary, lasting only a few hours; therefore, more definite treatment must be instituted.

Other procedures to reduce hyperpotassemia include the use of intestinal intubation with continuous suctioning since gastric secretions are high in potassium, or the use of potassium-binding resins such as polystyrene sodium sulfonate (Kayexalate). Resins are insoluble powders that have an affinity for a certain electrolyte, binding it to the resin molecule. In this case a potassium-binding resin is used. This resin, which may be given by Levin tube (although it can be taken orally), binds the available potassium in the gastrointestinal tract, after which the potassium passes out of the body with the feces. This effect must be augmented by inducing diarrhea by simultaneous strong laxation, a measure necessary to increase fluid output with the feces and to counteract the constipating effect of the resins. The resins may also be administered by retention enema; they act by absorbing potassium from the interstitial space in the lower colon. In addition to the therapy just described, peritoneal dialysis (page 195) or hemodialysis may be done.

Polyuric phase. During the polyuric or recovery phase of acute renal failure, there is usually a rather marked diuresis. However, because renal function is not uniformly improved, there may be rather marked wasting of various electrolytes, especially sodium, potassium, and base bicarbonate, either altogether or one independent of the other.

Treatment. Careful attention must be given to the type of replacement fluid used. Again, the volume of fluid replacement can be fairly well controlled if one refers to the volume of the previous day's urinary output. Frequent determinations of electrolyte levels should be made.

Other therapeutic measures include antibiotics and sedation or tranquilization or both. Selection of all medicines must be made on the basis of their mode of excretion. Since many drugs are excreted through the kidneys, dangerous levels will accumulate if the routine doses are administered to the oliguric or anuric patient.

The patient with azotemia, either acute or chronic, is prone to gastrointestinal bleeding because of both interference with coagulation and the tendency toward ulcer formation. The bleeding places a severe load on the azotemic patient because of the very high content of potassium and nitrogenous waste products present in digested blood. This can be partially negated by evacuation of the gastrointestinal tract by intubation and gastrointestinal sterilization, as with the neomycins, in order to reduce the effect of intestinal bacteria, which cause increased breakdown of protein products.

Chronic renal failure. The patient with chronic renal failure is encountered in the intensive care unit because of other conditions that may precipitate decompensated renal insufficiency, or he may be admitted for an exacerbation of his primary renal disease. The major reason for admission may be gastrointestinal hemorrhage, which is rather common in this patient.

Numerous *etiologic factors* predispose one to chronic renal insufficiency, such as chronic glomerulonephritis, chronic pyelonephritis, renal nephrosclerosis complicating hypertensive vascular disease, the Kimmelstiel-Wilson syndrome complicating diabetes, or congenital polycystic kidneys. Additional causes may be long-standing obstruction of the lower urinary tract leading to parenchymal destruction, or the damage may be caused by crystals of uric acid or calcium or by certain drugs used, such as the sulfonamides.

Usually the patient with chronic renal failure is not anuric or even oliguric. Nevertheless, because of the decreased renal function, he has a chronic metabolic acidosis, with accumulation of sulfates and phosphates, and retention of nitrogenous waste products. In spite of this abnormal renal function, the patient's body has usually adjusted to compensate for these anomalies.

Many of these patients have a compensatory hypertension, and any situation decreasing cardiac output and renal blood flow may tip the balance toward decompensated renal insufficiency. This is occasionally seen following overzealous treatment of the patient with chronic hypertension. Decreased renal blood flow may also follow diuretic therapy with the more potent products now available that are quite likely to produce electrolyte abnormalities or exaggerate those present.

Treatment. The objective of the treatment of this patient is to restore him to his previous precarious balance. This treatment involves close attention to fluid intake and output, careful electrolyte replacement, antibiotic therapy for treatment of chronic pyelonephritis, and restoration of blood volume if the patient is hypovolemic. In addition, the gastrointestinal tract may be evacuated and occasionally sterilized by drug therapy (page 193).

Complications. Primary complications are metabolic acidosis and hyperkalemia. The *acidosis* may be treated by administration of base bicarbonate such as sodium lactate or sodium bicarbonate. Because it is frequently desirable to use a small volume of replacement fluid, these solutes may be administered as hyperosmotic solutions and given rather slowly.

The *hyperkalemia* may be treated by removing excessive potassium from the body through the use of ion exchange resins (page 193) or peritoneal dialysis (page 195). Both of these procedures are being used more frequently for the patient with chronic renal failure.

During the acute exacerbation, the patient must be watched carefully, especially for hyperkalemia. Electrocardiographic monitoring may be desirable; frequent determinations of the electrolytes need to be made.

RELATED NURSING CARE FOR THE PATIENT WITH AZOTEMIA

Since the azotemic patient is likely to have deficits and excesses of electrolytes, the nurse must know the signs of imbalances. One can look for signs of overhydration and dehydration by noting the turgor of the skin and presence of edema. Since most of these patients may be resting in bed, presacral edema particularly should be noted.

Urine and stools and any vomitus are checked for evidence of bleeding. The first indication of hematuria is smoky urine.

Careful record of fluid intake and output is made because the physician will partially base his treatment on figures reported by the nursing personnel. All intake (oral and intravenous) and all output (urine, vomitus, watery diarrhea) must be recorded and note made of excessive perspiration.

To measure water taken in by his sucking cracked ice, the patient is given a container of cracked ice and an equal amount is put in a similar container; then the water is measured after the ice melts.

If sodium is restricted, one should be sure that salt substitutes do not contain potassium.

Any change in the patient's sensorium is noted and reported. The patient must turn and breathe deeply at frequent intervals to lessen the possibility of respiratory tract infections. Frequent mouth care is necessary.

PERITONEAL DIALYSIS

Peritoneal dialysis offers the average well-equipped general hospital many of the advantages of hemodialysis without the tremendous expense in both equipment and personnel involved in the latter.

Rationale for use of peritoneal dialysis. The peritoneal cavity contains a surface area of approximately 20 or 25 square feet of semipermeable membrane called the peritoneum. The peritoneum separates the peritoneal cavity from the interstitial fluid (which is, in turn, in equilibrium with the intravascular fluid).

Small molecules diffuse from an area of greater concentration to one of lesser concentration across a semipermeable membrane with only the concentration difference affecting the speed of transfer.

Generally speaking, molecules with a molecular weight less than 25,000 (smaller than the albumen molecule) are fairly freely diffusible. Any solution introduced into the peritoneal cavity will rather rapidly achieve equilibrium with the tissue and vascular fluid level of all small molecules. If this fluid is replaced frequently, short periods of time being allowed for equilibration, very large quantities of low molecular weight solutes can be removed from the body. By one's varying the osmolarity of the fluid introduced, a fluid volume lesser than, or greater than, that introduced can be recovered; fluid may actually be added to or removed from the body in this manner. Among the diffusible molecules are the body electrolytes, such as sodium, calcium, potassium, and chloride as well as urea, creatinine, acetoacetic acid, glucose, sulfates, phosphates, and many of the medicinal chemicals used therapeutically.

The major laboratories producing intravenous fluids and electrolyte solutions also produce various combination dialysate fluids. These fluids are basically electrolytically equivalent to ideal blood, with the exception of the materials that are desired to be changed; for example, in treating hyperkalemia, a dialysate containing no potassium would be used.

Technique. The technique of peritoneal dialysis, straightforward and uncomplicated, involves performing a paracentesis and introducing a catheter into the peritoneal cavity. This catheter is fixed in place, used for the introduction of fluid for a period of time, and then used for withdrawal of the same fluid after time is allowed for equilibration (Fig. 29-1).

Fig. 29-1. Peritoneal dialysis. Fluid in 2 liter exchanges is introduced into the peritoneal cavity through a catheter. In the cavity the fluid equilibrates with body fluid solute content and is then withdrawn through the same catheter.

In an adult the dialysis is ordinarily performed by the rapid introduction of 2 liters of solution over a period of from 10 to 15 minutes; then a period of from 15 to 60 minutes is allowed for the solution to equilibrate with body fluid. The solution is then drained by gravity siphon into a bedside container. The volume of each dialysis and withdrawal is carefully recorded. The exact procedure varies slightly with the different types of sets provided by various laboratories. In dealing with children or smaller adults, one may reduce the volume per unit.

During the dialysis procedure the patient is observed frequently for any changes in blood pressure, pulse, and respiration that might indicate excessive retention of fluid with resulting hypervolemia (page 184) or excessive loss of fluid producing hypovolemia (page 183).

Ordinarily the peritoneal dialysis is continued for as long as necessary to achieve the desired removal of waste products, electrolytes, or intoxicants. The customary course is considered to be from 24 to 48 hours, performed at the rate of approximately one dialysis (of 2 liters) per hour.

The greater portion of equilibration of dialysate with body fluid occurs during the first few minutes after introduction. In acute phases the equilibration period may be shortened so that more exchanges can be done in the same length of time; for example, a maximum withdrawal of barbiturates in as short a period of time as possible is helpful in barbiturate intoxication.

Customarily, a small amount of heparin is added to the infusion to reduce the likelihood of catheter obstruction because of fibrin clots. Initially, a small amount of an antibiotic was considered advisable, but this is not generally used now.

Patients requiring peritoneal dialysis. There are three groups of patients who may need peritoneal dialysis. The first is the group experiencing *acute renal failure*. In this situation the kidney tubule has considerable regenerative powers if the patient can be kept alive for a few days (rarely longer than three weeks). Potassium retention and acidosis are the factors most likely to result in the patient's death. Potassium can be removed quite effectively from the body by dialysis. The same situation is present following massive burns or crush injuries.

A second group of patients who may need peritoneal dialysis are those with *chronic renal failure* (page 193). They have barely adequate renal function and may be aided in ridding the body of excessive nitrogenous wastes by dialysis. The third group is patients with *poisonings* by dialyzable compounds such as barbiturates, salicylates, alcohol, carbon tetrachloride, amphetamines, bromides, and numerous other intoxicants. Occasionally when intoxication is suspected and the exact poisoning is not known, dialysis may be attempted while awaiting laboratory studies to determine the exact nature of the poisoning.

Among relatively few absolute *contraindications* to the use of peritoneal dialysis are peritonitis and recent abdominal surgery.

Precautions. Several precautions must be taken when peritoneal dialysis is done. The peritoneal catheter must be inserted deep into the abdominal cavity. A careful record of cumulative fluid balance must be kept, usually on a specific record sheet. Prolonged dialysis may result in significant loss of protein since some of the lower molecular weight proteins are diffusible. There is also a slight weeping of protein from the peritoneal surface secondary to mechanical irritation.

When one uses hypertonic solutions, removal of body fluid may be quite rapid and thus may produce undesirable hypovolemia and hypotension except in patients with massive edema. Because dialysis may also bring about paralytic ileus, especially if prolonged in a patient already critically ill, the patient may occasionally require nasogastric suctioning, thereby introducing another factor in fluid balance.

Attention should be paid to the temperature of the fluid. Rather large volumes of fluid are used over a short period of time, and these equilibrate with body temperature as well as body chemistry; therefore, it is important that the fluid be warmed to body temperature before it is used. Cool fluids may produce significant hypothermia, while excessively warm fluids can produce fever.

Complications. Complications of dialysis include perforation of the bowel. Such perforation can be made less likely by the use of a twisting motion to augment its cutting action when the trochar is inserted. Cardiac arrhythmias may develop during rapid changes in potassium. If the patient has normal potassium levels, 4 mEq. of potassium should be added to each liter of dialysis solution.

Abdominal pain is rarely a problem; however, it may be relieved by addition of a small amount of a local anesthetic to the fluids. Bleeding is seldom troublesome, but if it is persistent or excessive, the procedure should be interrupted and additional diagnostic steps taken to confirm or exclude intra-abdominal hemorrhage.

The most common complications are drainage difficulties that result from occlusion of the catheter tip by the omentum and by fluid pooling in the peritoneal cavity. Various maneuvers to change the patient's position may improve the drainage as may gentle pressure applied to the abdomen with both hands. Rarely, it may be necessary to replace the catheter because of fibrin occlusion; but with the small amounts of heparin included in the infusion, this is seldom a problem.

Three general groups of dialysates are available. These all contain 150 mEq. of sodium per liter, 4 mEq. of calcium per liter, 1.5 mEq. of magnesium, 100 mEq. of chloride, and 44 or 45 mEq. of lactate or acetate. The solution containing 1.5% dextrose is used to remove abnormal solutes from the general circulation, while the 7% solution is hyperosmotic and is used for removing excessive fluids. The 4.2% dextrose dialysate solution also results in a less marked loss of fluid, but enough fluids should be removed to result in a negative fluid balance for the body. Sorbitol is also used to substitute for dextrose and would be preferable for the diabetic patient.

Related nursing care. In addition to the measures already mentioned, one must be sure that the patient's bladder is empty prior to the paracentesis. The abdominal wall may be shaved over a small area where the catheter will be inserted. The patient may be weighed before and after dialysis.

The bedpan is offered and back care is given at the end of each period of dialysis. Dialysate fluid should be labeled appropriately when medication is added.

Fluid intake and output should be meticulously recorded. This includes intake and output both through the usual routes and through the dialysis procedure.

RELATED FILM

Practical aspects of peritoneal dialysis. Color, 23 minutes, available from Film Service Department, Abbott Laboratories, North Chicago, Ill. 60064.

This is an excellent film on this subject.

Chapter 30

Surgery of the urinary tract

The nursing care of the patient who has undergone urologic surgery differs only slightly from the care given patients having general surgery. They may require intensive nursing care during the postoperative phase for essentially the same reasons as patients having abdominal surgery with a few possible exceptions.

Surgery of the upper urinary tract

Typical initial orders following surgery might include

1. Sips of water and cracked ice for 48 hours and intravenous fluids for adequate hydration
2. Frequent check of vital signs
3. Analgesia
4. Antibiotics
5. Blood studies within 24 hours
6. Prophylactic postoperative care
7. Record of fluid intake and output with close observation of urinary drainage

Patients who have undergone either nephrectomy or other upper urinary tract surgery require deep general anesthesia with laryngeal intubation and controlled respiration. The surgery involves a retroperitoneal area, and tension is placed upon peritoneal structures.

POSTOPERATIVE CARE

1. *Sips of water and cracked ice* are usually given during the first 48 hours since these patients have had general anesthesia and may experience attendant nausea; paralytic ileus may also be present because of retroperitoneal irritation. Nasogastric suctioning may be necessary if peristalsis does not return within 48 hours; medications to stimulate peristaltic action, such as neostigmine salts (Prostigmin), may be given. Care of the patient undergoing nasogastric suctioning is described on page 163.

If bowel sounds are present at the end of 48 hours, the patient may have surgical liquids. If there are no signs of distention 72 hours postoperatively, he may then progress to a soft diet.

After he has recovered from surgery and if there are no contraindications, the patient should be encouraged to take from 2,000 to 3,000 ml. of fluid daily spaced over a 24-hour period. This prevents waste products from passing through the urinary system in a concentrated form that predisposes him to calculi, and it also helps keep the urinary system irrigated; adequate spacing prevents overhydration.

2. One should *check vital signs* frequently, especially observing indications of complications, either hemorrhagic, respiratory, or cardiac, all of which are heralded by changes in the vital signs, such as tachycardia, hypotension, and increased respiration. The skin may also become pale and clammy. Hemorrhage may occur following renal surgery and is more likely when the highly vascular parenchyma of the kidney is incised.

Since most of these patients have a drain from the operative site, the nurse should especially note the posterior portion of the dressing since secretions would drain toward the lumbar area.

The patient requiring kidney surgery frequently has a degree of hypertension that may be a compensatory mechanism initiated by the damaged kidneys. The nurse should be aware of the preoperative blood pressure since the patient may actually be experiencing hypotension when his blood pressure is within normal range according to the usual criteria.

3. *Analgesia* is given as necessary. The patient may complain of muscular aches on the contralateral side resulting from the hyperextended side position used in surgery. If this is particularly troublesome, muscle relaxants may be ordered for a few days.

4. *Antibiotics* are usually given to reduce the danger of infection.

5. *Blood studies* including a complete blood count, blood volume, and electrolytes are frequently done 24 hours postoperatively because of impaired renal function, poor fluid intake, and possible bleeding. Abnormalities of body fluid may be fairly frequent and require specific treatment. Page 184 begins a discussion of electrolytes.

6. *Prophylactic postoperative care* includes the patient's turning, breathing deeply, and coughing every two hours and walking as soon as possible. Since the upper pole of the kidney is directly below the diaphragm, the patient may find it painful to breathe deeply and cough. The patient should execute these activities about 30 minutes after he has been given analgesia to lessen the discomfort. Splinting the incision manually or with pillows will also help during this procedure and will lessen the discomfort when the exercise is done without prior analgesia.

Intermittent positive pressure breathing may be ordered to prevent atelectasis, especially if the patient is debilitated.

The patient should begin to walk as soon as possible to lessen the likelihood of thromboembolic complications. If he has a history of these complications, his legs may be wrapped with ace bandages before surgery and then rewrapped two or three times daily after surgery. Active exercises of the legs are also done.

If there is moderate drainage, the physician usually orders the dressings to be changed as necessary. Montgomery straps will reduce skin irritation caused by frequent changes of adhesive tape. Copious drainage from the wound, of which the physician should be notified immediately, may indicate obstruction to urinary flow that could produce dire results.

7. *Fluid intake and output* are recorded with care since the patient may have borderline renal function. Nasogastric suctioning can severely alter his water and electrolyte status.

The importance of *adequate observation of the urinary drainage* cannot be overemphasized. The catheter of a patient who has just returned from surgery should be checked each time the vital signs are checked. If there is frank bleeding, the surgeon should be notified immediately. If the patient is restless or convalescing, one should check the catheter frequently to be sure it is not occluded, because obstruction to urinary flow can cause complications. It is also checked often if the patient has hematuria.

The character of the drainage should be noted at frequent intervals. A urinary catheter may be inserted in the bladder or the patient may urinate spontaneously. The urine is usually dark red or pink immediately following surgery but should not be bright red or viscid or contain clots. If these findings are noted, the surgeon should be called immediately.

When surgery is done for removal of calculi and a drain is in place, there may be large amounts of light red urine on the dressings for several days. The surgeon should be notified immediately if this drainage becomes bright red.

The color of the urinary drainage should be noted as it appears in both the glass connecting tubing and the collecting bag. Early bleeding may be detected in this way; the changes in the appearance of the urine in the glass connector as it gradually becomes more bloody may be noted within a short period of time. The bleeding may be so slight that it might not be noticed in the glass connector, but the darker reddish color would be seen in the collecting bag in this case.

When the patient's urine is emptied at the end of each eight-hour nursing shift, the nurse should total and record the amount and then describe it if it appears unusual. Reddish or smoky hues may indicate bleeding, cloudiness usually indicates albuminuria, and thick consistency ordinarily indicates infection.

Unless specifically ordered, a catheter should never be clamped. Clamping causes distention and pressure which, if not relieved in a short while, produce pain and predispose the patient to paralytic ileus. In addition, increased pressure produced in the kidneys can lead to renal damage, and infection may be precipitated by urinary stasis.

One must never clamp a catheter draining a kidney. Since the capacity of the normal adult renal pelvis is only from 4 to 8 ml., the catheter must *never* be clamped, and care should be taken that it does not become plugged or partially occluded. If a catheter in an incision is accidentally removed, the surgeon should be notified immediately; prompt reinsertion is imperative since these openings diminish in size rapidly.

If there appears to be inadequate drainage in the collecting bag from a urethral catheter, the bag is checked and then inspected upward to ascertain the reason. Occasionally the clamp becomes loose and allows urine to leak from the bag; the nurse should check with the other personnel to find out if this has happened. A clot obstructing the flow to the bag can be dislodged by milking the catheter and tubing *toward* the bag.

A catheter may be occluded due to the weight of the patient's leg. For this reason it is preferable that the tubing be brought over the anterior portion of the patient's thigh. If the patient's obesity interferes with gravity flow, the catheter may be run underneath the leg with a *smooth* trough (so as not to interfere with venous return) made with towels on either side of the catheter. Any time the patient lies on his side, one must make certain that drainage tubes are patent; this is especially true with nephrostomy and ureterostomy catheters.

Surgery of the lower urinary tract

Typical initial postoperative orders following a *transurethral resection* might include

1. Cracked ice and sips of water and surgical liquids if tolerated	5. Analgesia
	6. Antibiotics
3. Continuous bladder irrigation	7. Blood studies
4. Record of fluid intake and output	8. Prophylactic postoperative care

The elderly male requiring prostate surgery comprises a significant portion of urologic practice. Because of advancing age, the patient frequently also has numerous other conditions that may require medical supervision in addition to the urologic surgery, for example, coexisting heart disease, diabetes, or pulmonary insufficiency. With improved techniques and careful supervision, this type of elderly man, usually considered a poor anesthetic risk, seems to tolerate these procedures quite well if they are accomplished within a reasonable period of time. Much of this improved outlook is attributed to the fact that most prostatic surgery is now done under spinal anesthesia so that the patient does not have the added risk of general anesthesia. Since he is given less sedation and requires little analgesia, he is considerably less likely to develop respiratory complications.

POSTOPERATIVE CARE

1. *Cracked ice and sips of water* are allowed immediately after surgery. If there is no nausea, the patient can usually take surgical liquids the night of surgery and then progress to a full diet the following day. This early tolerance of food is probably the result of his not having had general anesthesia or an incision into the peritoneal cavity.

2. *Vital signs* are checked frequently for reasons mentioned on page 200. In addition, special attention is paid to the temperature of this patient, for he may develop hypothermia. He is usually elderly, his temperature-regulating mechanism may be somewhat impaired, and the anesthesia and analgesia also have depressing effects on this mechanism. Additionally, moderate quantities of irrigating solutions are introduced within his body through the catheter. Since these solutions equilibrate with body temperature, the patient may actually lose considerable body heat through the drainage of irrigating solutions from his bladder.

These patients must be watched closely immediately after surgery for many will bleed freely from the prostatic bed. The surgeon may produce slight traction on the catheter to control venous ooze. The next most frequent period for secondary bleeding is within two or three weeks when the eschar begins to slough.

3. *Continuous bladder irrigation* is usually ordered. Sterile normal saline solution is used as the irrigating fluid in preference to distilled water to prevent the likelihood of water intoxication by absorption of water into the vascular bed.

A large two-way catheter is inserted into the bladder and held in place with a large retaining balloon. The drip is regulated to a continuous flow in order to prevent any obstruction of the catheter by clots. It is thought that the continuous irrigation is much superior to the previous method of periodic irrigation whereby infection was often introduced.

4. *Fluid intake and output* records are extremely important and must be kept with care because of the additional fluid involved in irrigation. One must remember to determine the amount of fluid used for the bladder irrigation and then subtract this amount from the total urinary drainage to ascertain the true drainage.

5. *Analgesia* in minimal doses may be needed. Since many of the elderly become disoriented when given opiates, an antihistaminic, such as diphenhydramine (Benadryl), may be ordered for pain, nausea, and restlessness. Opium and belladonna rectal suppositories may be used if there is severe bladder spasm due to the presence of the catheter.

6. *Antibiotics* are usually given to prevent infection since prostatic surgery is considered contaminated.

7. *Blood studies,* including a complete blood count, electrolyte study, and perhaps a blood volume determination, are frequently checked 24 hours postoperatively because the patient may lose considerable blood diluted with urine and it may be difficult to determine the amount of blood loss. Electrolyte studies are usually performed since there has been notable exchange of fluid during the course of the procedures and the patient is intolerant of electrolyte imbalances, which are treated as necessary. He is especially prone to water intoxication or low-sodium syndrome (see page 184).

CARE AFTER OPEN PROSTATIC SURGERY

When open prostatic surgery is performed, the nursing care is similar to that of transurethral resection surgery with a few exceptions. Since there is more danger of paralytic ileus, giving cracked ice is usually continued for from 36 to 48 hours, and intravenous fluids are necessary to maintain the patient's hydration. A suprapubic catheter and an indwelling urethral catheter may be used for continuous irrigation, with physiologic saline solution flowing into the bladder through the urethral catheter and leaving through the suprapubic catheter; the latter catheter is usually removed within 24 hours.

Since the patient is likely to hemorrhage, a hematocrit and possibly a blood volume are done 12 hours after surgery and are repeated 24 hours after surgery.

If distention is a problem, a rectal tube may be helpful. A good carminative enema is a mixture of four ounces of milk and four ounces of molasses.

Nursing care of the patient having bladder surgery is not significantly different from the care just described.

Injuries to the lower urinary tract

The patient suffering injuries to the lower urinary tract, usually in conjunction with multiple injuries, may be seen frequently in the intensive care situation.

Some of the lower urinary tract injuries, especially intraperitoneal rupture of the distended bladder, are insidious in their symptomatology and require constant awareness of their possibility. Most lower urinary tract injuries require studies of the tract with radiopaque contrast media before a definite diagnosis can be made. Only contrast material suitable for intravenous injection is used since there is always danger that these materials may enter ruptured veins.

Intraperitoneal rupture of the bladder may produce almost no early symptoms. This can result from a sudden blow to the lower abdomen over a distended bladder. Abdominal pain or other evidence of injury may be almost absent soon after the injury because sterile urine is not greatly irritating to the peritoneum initially. Frequently the patient's only early complaint is inability to urinate. The absence of early symptoms of intraperitoneal rupture of the bladder has made maintenance of a high index of suspicion mandatory. Any patient with an abdominal or pelvic injury who is unable to urinate should be considered as having a ruptured bladder until it is proven otherwise. A retrograde cystogram is diagnostic.

Extraperitoneal rupture of the bladder is common with a fractured pelvis, especially if the fracture is disrupted. This condition may also occur in the absence of a fracture but with sudden blows to the soft tissues in the pelvic cavity. The patient is unable to urinate, and the catheterized urine is usually bloody. Presence of lower abdominal pain is not a reliable indication because many patients have a great deal of pain from spasm relative to the fracture. Diagnosis again depends on retrograde cystogram.

Rupture of the membranous urethra, a fairly common injury, is suggested by blood at the external meatus and inability to urinate. Catheterization yields blood rather than urine. In this situation, the extravasation of blood and urine occurs behind the urogenital diaphragm in the area of the bladder so that ecchymoses of the perineum, scrotum, and abdominal wall are not noted. A definite diagnosis is suggested when a boggy mass is felt by means of rectal examination; the tentative diagnosis is confirmed by a retrograde urethrogram. Definitive treatment is usually retrograde surgical exploration and suturing.

TREATMENT

Since the cardinal symptom of all lower urinary tract injuries is the patient's inability to urinate, the nurse should immediately report his inability to the physician when it occurs concomitantly with trauma to the abdomen or pelvis. That the patient cannot urinate and that there is an increase in size over the bladder area may indicate leakage of blood or urine into the tissues. Scanty or bloody urine should also be immediately reported.

Inability to urinate may indicate damage to the lower urinary tract; but it may also indicate renal shutdown, obstruction by clots in either the ureters or the urethra, or laceration of one or both ureters during the injury.

The patient who has these conditions should be given treatment for shock, if it is present, and then reparative surgery as soon as his condition warrants.

During traumatic injuries the kidneys may suffer contusions or complete rupture. Since spontaneous healing can occur following contusions, surgery is withheld unless absolutely necessary. Surgery is indicated for the ruptured kidney but is never undertaken unless there is evidence that the other kidney is functioning.

Catheterization. A few additional points in nursing care need to be mentioned. When catheterizing a female patient, one should pull upward on the labia minora to stretch the tissues and expose the urinary meatus more clearly. For male catheterizations, the penis should be held perpendicular to his body to lessen the urethral curvature. If resistance is felt from the urethral sphincter as the catheter is inserted, one should pause until the sphincter relaxes and then continue with the insertion.

An indwelling catheter is inserted about an inch farther after the urine flows. The patient should not experience pain when the balloon is inflated; but if he does, the balloon should be deflated immediately and the catheter inserted farther. After the balloon is inflated, the catheter is gently tugged to check the balloon. It should also be irrigated to be sure it is patent and will drain adequately.

All indwelling catheters are anchored to the interior of the thigh so that tension on them will not cause irritation in the trigonal area. A patient who needed an indwelling catheter for a period of time taught us that a *loose*-fitting garter works nicely for this purpose. This can also be made from adhesive tape folded onto itself and made into an encircling band that will slip up the patient's thigh to anchor the catheter.

If the tubing is excessively long, it should be looped *on* the bed; if the extra tubing has a dependent loop *beside* the bed, more pressure is needed for the urine to travel upward through this loop, hence there is greater chance of partial obstruction. A portion of the tubing should be anchored to the bed in such a way that the tubing is not occluded and no pinholes are in the tubing. A short length of adhesive tape can be placed around the tubing, and this tape can be pinned to the sheet.

The genitals and the catheter at the point of insertion are bathed daily with a germicidal soap when an indwelling catheter is present. If there is increased risk of infection, as with diabetics or those suffering traumatized genitals, additional cleansing at regular intervals with benzalkonium chloride (Zephiran) or hydrogen peroxide sponges may reduce this likelihood.

Catheter irrigation may occasionally be ordered to ensure that the catheter is patent. Ordinarily irrigation should not be necessary if the patient is adequately hydrated unless there is hematuria with clot formation. The nurse must remember that the purpose of the irrigation is not to irrigate the bladder. Irrigation done under pressure will only irritate the bladder mucosa and tends to spread infection.

Irrigation is always performed under sterile conditions. Sterile normal saline solution is usually used since it is isotonic with the body fluids. *Before* the catheter is disconnected from the drainage tubing, the area of the connection is cleansed with alcohol sponges. After disconnection, the end of the tubing is kept sterile by being wrapped in a sterile compress or alcohol or benzalkonium sponges. Before reconnection, the ends of the catheter and glass or plastic connector are always wiped to prevent the introduction of microorganisms into the drainage system and the possible risk of an ascending bladder or kidney infection. Another possible source of ascending infections is the end of the drainage tubing that is allowed to communicate with the urinary drainage.

During the irrigation, the fluid is allowed to enter and return from the bladder by gravity. If it will not enter, the catheter is milked toward the distal end in an attempt to dislodge the obstruction. If this does not prove successful, pressure is *gently* applied to the irrigating solution, for occasionally mucous threads will occlude the eyes of the catheter. If an obstruction is still encountered, the physician should be notified.

After removal of an indwelling catheter, one should note time, amount, and appearance of initially voided urine. If the patient has not urinated in eight hours he should be catheterized; however, the surgeon may order this procedure before this period of time has lapsed. After prostate surgery, the patient should urinate at least every three or four hours. The surgeon should be alerted if the urine appears cloudy since some patients develop cystitis from residual urine. It is fairly common for hematuria to persist for a few days following removal of a catheter after bladder or prostate surgery.

Section VII

The patient having endocrine disorders

Chapter 31

Diabetes

Patients with diabetes are frequently admitted to an intensive care unit. The diabetic condition may be the primary illness if the patient is in diabetic acidosis, or he may be admitted for other conditions, diabetes being a secondary condition. Additionally, nursing personnel should be aware of symptoms of acidosis, a condition that may develop in the acutely ill patient who has undiagnosed diabetes.

PATHOGENESIS

Diabetes is primarily a condition in which there is an insufficient amount of functional insulin in the bloodstream. Insulin, a hormone produced in the isle of Langerhans in the pancreas, is required for the passage of glucose through the cell membrane and enables the cell to utilize the glucose. This insulin deficit increases blood levels of glucose (*hyperglycemia*).

In the normal kidney, glucose is a part of the glomerular filtrate; the glucose is entirely reabsorbed in the tubule if blood sugar (and glomerular filtrate) levels are normal. However, the capacity of the tubule to reabsorb glucose is limited; and when the blood (and glomerular filtrate) glucose level exceeds the normal limit (usually from 150 to 200 mg./100 ml.), the excess glucose is not reabsorbed but is excreted in the urine (*glycosuria*). The blood sugar level at which glycosuria occurs is referred to as the renal threshold for sugar.

The excess blood glucose acts as an osmotic diuretic that accounts for two of the classic symptoms of diabetes: *polyuria* and *polydipsia*. This diuresis is also responsible for a part of the fluid and electrolyte imbalance. Other classic symptoms of diabetes may be explained. The inability of the body to use sugar for energy leaves a consistent energy deficit resulting in *polyphagia, weakness,* and, in more severe cases, *weight loss.*

Diabetes is probably more than one disease entity since there is little similarity between the brittle (or juvenile) diabetic and the maturity-onset diabetic, but both may be thought of as experiencing relative insulin insufficiency. This relative insulin insufficiency may be caused by (1) inability of the insulin-producing beta cells of the pancreas to respond to glucose loads, as occurs in the maturity-onset diabetic; (2) beta-cell destruction, as in the individual developing diabetes following pancreatitis; or (3) the presence of insulin antagonists, as is thought to be the case of the person with severe brittle diabetes. Most juvenile diabetics are of the brittle type; that is, their disorder is controlled with difficulty. Both juvenile and brittle diabetics are prone to acidosis and shock, and insulin requirements are likely to be greater than 40 units daily and change erratically.

Absolute insulin deficiency is seen following pancreatectomy and rarely requires more than from 30 to 40 units of insulin daily for control. This suggests the likelihood of factors other than the pancreas affecting the diabetic who requires large doses of insulin.

The patient with maturity-onset diabetes does not usually form acetone, but he may do so during periods of unusual stress. His diabetes can frequently be regulated by reducing insulin requirements through weight reduction and carbohydrate limitation or by the use of the insulin-sparing drugs, such as chlorpropamide (Diabinese). If insulin is required, the dose is usually small.

The diabetic patient is predisposed to atherosclerosis, probably resulting from the secondary effect of altered glucose metabolism on fat metabolism. With incomplete utilization of fats, blood levels of fatty acids and cholesterol are increased. This predisposition to atherosclerosis is common to both the maturity-onset diabetic and the labile diabetic. Vascular complications account for a large percentage of the complications of diabetic patients. Both types of diabetics are also more prone to infection than are nondiabetics, perhaps because the increased glucose content of body tissue makes good culture medium.

The labile diabetic almost always requires insulin for control. In addition to the infectious and vascular complications, he is more likely to develop severe difficulty than the patient with maturity-onset diabetes. These complications include acute metabolic acidosis, insulin reactions, and chronic renal failure from intercapillary nephrosclerosis.

DIABETIC ACIDOSIS

Since the diabetic is unable to use glucose (and carbohydrates) as primary sources of energy without adequate insulin, fats are utilized for this purpose. Since a certain amount of glucose is required to effect complete fat metabolism in the cells, incomplete fat utilization results. Acetone, acetoacetic acid, and similar compounds that are acid in nature are the end products of this incomplete fat metabolism. If these substances, also known as ketone bodies, are excessive, metabolic acidosis develops.

If the patient is known to have diabetes, some event altered his usual course and precipitated the acidosis. This may be a missed insulin dose, confusion in the dose, marked dietary indiscretion, infections, or gastrointestinal upsets with vomiting or diarrhea or both.

Clinical findings. The typical patient is in a state of altered consciousness and is somnolent, confused, or in frank coma. His state of consciousness is related more to the degree of metabolic acidosis than to the level of blood sugar. His face is flushed, which may result from fever or dehydration; his pulse is rapid, and his blood pressure is usually depressed to some degree. His skin and mucous membranes are quite dry, while his eyeballs are likely to be soft due to extreme dehydration. If he is conscious he may complain of abdominal pain. He has Kussmaul respiration with increased rate and depth; this is the body's attempt to blow off acid carbon dioxide to compensate for the acidosis. His breath has the sweet, fruity odor of acetone.

Treatment. The treatment of the patient with diabetic acidosis includes the following orders:

1. *Adequate ventilation* must be maintained. Since this patient is frequently confused or totally unconscious, airway patency is a major responsibility of attendant personnel. Care must be taken that the patient does not aspirate, since vomiting is common. The abdomen is frequently distended, and paralytic ileus may develop; therefore, it may be necessary to insert a Levin tube to prevent further vomiting and possible aspiration. The gastric fluid may be tobacco colored because of occult gastrointestinal bleeding.

2. *Fluid replacement, intravenously and orally,* is necessary because most of these patients are severely dehydrated since hyperglycemia causes massive diuresis. The fluid must be replaced and adequate diuresis maintained to assist in flushing the ketones from the body. A rapid infusion with 1/6 molar sodium lactate or physiologic sodium chloride solution may be given. Sodium lactate or sodium bicarbonate is used if there is marked acidosis.

Although the diabetic patient is usually considered as having almost continuous diuresis, the extremely ill patient with diabetic acidosis may become anuric due to the marked fluid deficit and electrolyte imbalances. This situation is commonly accompanied by hypovolemic shock and might require the use of plasma expanders.

When the patient is able to accept fluids by mouth, liquids high in potassium and sodium, such as orange juice, tomato juice, and salty broth, are forced. Soon thereafter food with no fat, such as saltines, cereals, and milk, is given.

3. There are many rules of thumb regarding *insulin administration,* yet none are very helpful since the amount of insulin required to reverse the picture of altered glucose metabolism may vary greatly in comparable levels of acidosis. Almost all of the rules involve giving a rather large amount of regular insulin (50 to 100 units) initially intravenously and then repeating various doses at intervals with the dosage being determined from the tests for acetonuria, glycosuria, and the level of hyperglycemia.

Many physicians begin treating the patient suffering diabetic acidosis by giving him 100 units of regular insulin intravenously and later give divided dosages as great as from 200 to 300 units of regular insulin if he has not improved. Insulin may be given hourly, proportional to the acetonuria and glycosuria. If acidosis persists and hyperglycemia is controlled, glucose in saline solution may be given; this continues the diuresis and provides glucose for metabolism.

Improvement is heralded by return of consciousness, loss of abdominal pain, loss of fruity odor of the breath, and return of appetite. During the recovery phase the patient must be watched closely because he may become hypoglycemic. *Signs of insulin shock* include sweatiness, tachycardia, weakness, tremulousness, headache, blurred vision, pallor, and confusion which can progress to coma and convulsions.

Personnel are *forewarned* by the disappearance of the urine sugar. After the patient's recovery from acidosis, insulin seems to be more effective. Frequent blood sugar determinations are helpful.

The *treatment of insulin shock* is to give sweetened orange juice. If the patient is still swallowing but the nurse is afraid to give liquids, one or two packets of granulated sugar may be emptied beside the buccal mucosa. The sugar will dissolve in the saliva and may provide enough glucose to produce return of consciousness.

If a diabetic patient becomes unconscious and the differential between shock and acidosis is uncertain, the patient may be given 10 ml. of 50% glucose intravenously while the nurse awaits further orders or laboratory results if this is permitted by the attending physician. If the patient responds promptly, shock was the problem. If he does not respond and acidosis is present, this small additional sugar load will not be harmful.

Usually after 24 hours of treatment, the sliding-scale order is reduced both in the frequency of determinations and the amount of insulin given per plus of urine sugar. Generally after from 24 to 48 hours of regular insulin administration according to sliding scale, long-acting insulin is begun.

Although regular insulin and longer-acting insulin are fairly frequently combined in the management of the diabetic patient, regular insulin should never be mixed with protamine zinc insulin. There is an excess of the protamine zinc molecule that will bind to the regular insulin so that it, too, becomes protamine zinc insulin. Other long-acting insulins may be mixed with regular insulin without changing the characteristic of either.

4. *An indwelling catheter is inserted and the urine tested.* The urine is usually checked initially every 30 minutes or every hour. As the patient improves, these tests are done less frequently.

When performing urine tests, it is most important that the specimen be *fresh*. If the patient has an indwelling catheter, one must always get the specimen *directly from the catheter* and never from the drainage bag. After the patient regains consciousness and is stable, the catheter is usually removed. In order to check fresh urine and not a specimen that has been in the bladder several hours, one should have the patient urinate 30 minutes before the test and then give him a glass of water to drink. When the nurse returns in 30 minutes she can collect the necessary specimen.

5. *Laboratory studies* typically reveal moderate or marked hyperglycemia and the carbon dioxide–combining power as moderately or markedly decreased. Glycosuria and acetonuria are common. The primary endeavor is to get the patient acetone-free, for in acetone formation lies the danger. The complete blood count is generally elevated because of hypovolemia.

Intially electrolyte studies frequently show hyperkalemia; but as the treatment with insulin and fluid progresses, potassium is rather rapidly depleted. This hypokalemia results from polyuria and from the potassium being driven into the cells by glucose and insulin. After the second and third hour of treatment, one should watch the patient for signs of hypokalemia, a condition that may be recognized clinically but whose clinical appearance is usually obscured by the diabetic acidosis. One point of difference may be recognized: The patient's respiration is deep and rapid during acidosis, while it is weak and shallow during hypokalemia. Although this breathing pattern may be similar to that during insulin shock, the other symptoms of shock would not be present.

The guide to addition of potassium to the therapeutic routine is usually based on electrocardiographic interpretations (the patient may be monitored continuously) or on frequent determinations of serum potassium levels. It should be remembered that a patient may have a potassium deficit although the laboratory report is within normal range; this can occur with hypovolemia and intracellular dehydration.

In addition to management of acidosis, a search for the precipitating cause should begin, especially for infections of the respiratory or urinary tract.

TREATMENT OF THE DIABETIC PATIENT REQUIRING SURGERY

The brittle diabetic who requires surgery presents special problems and may therefore require intensive nursing care. The individual having mild nonacetone-forming maturity-onset diabetes rarely presents a problem in the management of the acute surgical situation. The ketone-forming diabetic is typically one who requires more than 40 units of long-acting insulin daily, whose control is less than adequate, and who has a history of previous episodes of insulin shock or diabetic acidosis or both. Following the surgery, this patient will require very careful attention to prevent the occurrence of both insulin shock and acidosis in the immediate postoperative period.

In addition to the patient's usual preoperative orders, one-half his usual dose of long-acting insulin may be given on the morning of surgery, and a continuous intravenous infusion of 10% glucose in water begun. This may be regulated during the immediate preoperative, operative, and early postoperative periods to maintain slight glycosuria or hyperglycemia so as to avoid insulin shock.

During the preoperative phase, the renal threshold will usually be established. If the renal threshold is such that glycosuria occurs at a level of less than 200 mg./100 ml., the urine sugar may be used as a guide to insulin and sugar requirements.

Following surgery, in addition to the routine postoperative orders for the type of surgery performed, this patient will require special observation concerning the diabetic condition. This would include frequent urine checks or blood sugar determinations with type of fluid and amount of insulin governed by these studies.

To prevent the occurrence of insulin shock, it is usually preferable to maintain a slight glycosuria. The intravenous fluids should be continued postoperatively to keep a trace of sugar present in the urine. Fluid used is generally 5% glucose administered in water or saline solution, depending largely on the presence or absence of acetonuria.

The presence of acetone in the urine necessitates the administration of isotonic saline, sodium bicarbonate, or sodium lactate. If acetonuria is strongly positive, blood sugar and carbon dioxide-combining power determinations are indicated. If the blood sugar or urine sugar level is quite elevated, additional small increments of regular insulin may be used. Glucose in saline solution may be necessary under these conditions: positive acetonuria, negative glycosuria, depressed carbon dioxide–combining power, and normal or low blood sugar. If there is a tendency for the postoperative patient to retain sodium, the amounts of sodium bicarbonate, sodium lactate, or isotonic saline will usually be less than the amounts ordered for mild diabetic acidosis.

As soon as the patient's condition stabilizes postoperatively, the frequency of examination of the blood sugar, carbon dioxide–combining power, and urine is decreased. By the time the patient is eating his full diabetic diet, he will usually be receiving approximately half his daily dose of long-acting insulin and small increments of regular insulin as determined by urine determinations made periodically. The patient may need additional carbohydrates if there is a tendency for hypoglycemia to occur, or the dosage of insulin may be reduced. As soon as his activity and dietary intake approach normal, his dose of long-acting insulin may be carefully increased.

Alternate management. An alternate method of management has been found particularly useful when the patient's routine is not interrupted for long periods of time. Long-acting insulin is totally omitted on the day of surgery, and a slow intravenous infusion is begun which contains glucose and regular insulin in a ratio of one unit of regular insulin for each 2 gm. of glucose. In this type of management, the amount and type of fluid replacement depend entirely on the patient's fluid balance. Additional increments of insulin may be given as indicated by urine sugar studies. The onset of acetonuria and depressed carbon dioxide–combining power requires the use of sodium bicarbonate, sodium lactate, or sodium chloride for the reversal of acidosis.

Since the diabetic patient is particularly prone to experiencing infectious complications and thromboembolism, careful observation for the occurrence of these conditions is warranted.

RELATED FILM

Diabetes—what you don't know *can* hurt you. Color, 27 minutes, available from the Ames Company, Division Miles Laboratories, Inc., Elkhart, Ind. 46514.

This very good film is concerned with the diagnosis and treatment of diabetes.

Chapter **32**

Hyperthyroidism and thyroid crisis

Typical initial orders include

1. Sedation
2. Control of tachycardia
3. Antithyroid treatment
4. Corticosteroids
5. Fluid and electrolyte management
6. Vitamins
7. Diagnostic studies
8. Nonstimulating environment
9. Diet control

CLINICAL FINDINGS

The patient experiencing hyperthyroidism may require intensive care if (1) hyperthyroidism is complicated by other conditions, or (2) the patient suffering severe hyperthyroidism has delayed seeking medical attention and develops thyroid crisis or thyroid storm. The latter occasionally happens as an acute situation when, without evidence of prior thyroid disease, the patient rather suddenly becomes critically ill with severe hyperthyroidism. This usually occurs following severe emotional stress or physical trauma, such as following surgery or an accident, or some acute major illness.

The condition of the typical patient with hyperthyroidism is not difficult to diagnose. This patient is classically a young adult, frequently a female since this illness occurs from four to eight times more often in the female, especially during puberty, pregnancy, and menopause. The patient has anxious facies and complains of extreme nervousness, irritability, weight loss despite increased appetite, palpitation, breathlessness, and heat intolerance. She may also experience gastrointestinal symptoms, such as frequent bowel movements and maybe nausea and vomiting. The female may also complain of hypomenorrhea or amenorrhea. Emotional lability is apparent.

On examination the patient's skin is soft, warm, and flushed, the palms are moist, and the hair is of fine texture. There may be exophthalmos and lid retraction brought about by increased orbital contents and said to be present when sclera can be seen above the cornea when the patient looks straight forward. Another eye sign of exophthalmos is lid lag, when the eyelid moves slower than the eyeball. Pupils are frequently dilated, and the brow fails to wrinkle when the patient looks up. Exophthalmos, or proptosis, may be unilateral or bilateral and is thought to be due to sympathetic nervous system overactivity or mediated through the pituitary gland. Malignant exophthalmos

215

with destruction of orbital contents is a dreaded complication occasionally seen with hyperthyroidism but progressing independently of it. Treatment is generally unsatisfactory and includes efforts to suppress pituitary function with radiation and large doses of adrenal steroids. Surgical decompression is sometimes undertaken.

A goiter is usually palpable; a thrill or bruit or both may be felt or heard over the gland due to increased vascularity. The very fine tremors present can be seen best when the eyelids are gently closed and the tongue or fingers are extended; placing a sheet of paper on the extended hands may help to demonstrate the tremors.

The speech is generally rapid, and there may be hoarseness from local pressure on the recurrent laryngeal nerves over the gland. The patient may also experience difficulty in swallowing due to the increased size of the gland. She is generally hyperkinetic, the deep tendon reflexes are hyperactive, and there may be pretibial myxedema of the lower extremities.

The pounding pulse is rapid, and various abnormal rhythms may be present. The blood pressure may be moderately elevated with a wide pulse pressure, and the respiration is generally rapid.

Severe hyperthyroidism in the elderly may lack many of the typical features seen in the young adult.

PATHOGENESIS

Little is known about the remote etiology of hyperthyroidism. Normal thyroid function is influenced by the central nervous system through the hypothalamus and pituitary gland by release of thyroid-stimulating hormone (TSH). Production of adequate thyroid hormone in turn suppresses pituitary TSH release (a so-called feedback mechanism). Hyperthyroidism is presumed to result from failure of this control. An excessive amount of thyroid hormone is rarely released in association with inflammatory changes of the thyroid gland.

All of the manifestations of hyperthyroidism are attributable to the pharmacologic effects of thyroid hormone. Almost all phases of metabolism are accelerated under its influence, and each finding is simply another manifestation of the hypermetabolic state.

Thyroid crisis. Thyroid crisis or thyroid storm was fairly common many years ago as a postoperative occurrence following surgery for goiter on an incompletely prepared hyperthyroid patient. While it is rarely seen in this situation today, thyroid crisis may come about under the aforementioned conditions. Thyroid crisis has also been recorded following insulin reactions, diabetic acidosis, tooth extractions, digitalis intoxication, pneumonia, or vigorous palpation of the thyroid gland. In these situations one suspects that the patient was mildly hyperthyroid prior to the stressful situation, although this is not always true. Thyroid crisis may also occur following the abrupt withdrawal of antithyroid drugs. The patient may or may not have a history of recent trauma or surgery, especially an operative procedure affecting the neck or upper thorax.

Symptoms. The symptoms of thyroid crisis resemble those of hyperthyroidism except that they are more exaggerated. The patient is extremely agitated and may be delirious or frankly psychotic. She is perspiring profusely and is feverish. The tremors are more marked, there is severe insomnia and hyperpnea, and tachycardia is extreme (from 150 to 200) with or without abnormal rhythms.

Thyroid crisis produces a rather high patient mortality, occasionally reported as high as 50%, the cause of death generally being exhaustion and heart failure. The critical period usually lasts about three days.

The diagnosis of extreme hyperthyroidism is rarely a problem; however, the diagnosis of thyroid crisis in the absence of known prior hyperthyroidism or goiter may frequently be overlooked since there is little to direct one's attention to the thyroid gland. This condition may mimic postoperative or post-partum psychoses.

TREATMENT

The treatment for severe hyperthyroidism and for thyroid crisis is essentially the same except that therapy for the latter is more rapid and intense.

1. *Sedation* is required in doses considered much larger than the usual dose. Reserpine has been found to be effective and may be given by injection, usually in fairly large doses (from 5 to 15 mg.) intramuscularly in divided doses over a 24-hour period. Fortunately this drug is a good sedative and aids in controlling anxiety as well as decreasing the tachycardia. In addition, it does not interfere with specific diagnostic tests or other therapeutic endeavors that may be required.

2. *Control of tachycardia* in these patients is extremely difficult, especially if failure has supervened. Tachycardia accompanied by abnormal rhythms is notorious in its resistance to digitalis therapy. Congestive heart failure, when it occurs in this patient, is also refractory to treatment. Digitalis to the point of digitalis intoxication will rarely produce much effect on the tachycardia. Quinidine or propranolol (Inderal) may be ordered to treat atrial fibrillation or other abnormal rhythms that are common.

3. *Specific antithyroid treatment* is begun; however, because there is a delay before the antithyroid drugs become effective, the necessity of sedation to control the symptoms may be prolonged. The effect of these drugs, thought to block production of thyroid hormone, is not evident until the excess hormone stored in the thyroid gland has been secreted into the bloodstream.

Methimazole (Tapazole) in as high a dosage as 100 mg. daily may be ordered. This is given in divided doses at regularly spaced intervals to maintain constant blood levels. Frequently a somewhat depressing effect on thyroid function is noted within one week at this large dose. With lower doses it may be as long as four weeks before the depressing effect becomes manifest.

Propylthiouracil may also be given in dosages as large as from 1,000 to 1,500 mg. daily. It is also given in divided dosages at evenly spaced intervals since it is excreted rapidly.

Potassium iodide or Lugol's solution is usually added to the intravenous fluids during the first few days of treatment for extreme hyperthyroidism. Its action is more rapid than that of the other antithyroid drugs, but it has a shorter sustained action. It is given in a dosage of between 20 and 60 drops daily. After the initial treatment, the iodide may be given orally if the patient is cooperative and able to take the medication by mouth. It is more palatable if given in milk or fruit juice; to prevent staining of the teeth it is diluted to at least 100 ml. and drunk through a straw.

Radioiodide sodium (I^{131}) treatment is rarely used in extreme hyperthyroidism because of the time lag of from three to six weeks before it becomes effective. However, once the severe hyperthyroidism is controlled by drug, the patient may be given fractional doses of I^{131} for long-term treatment. This is usually reserved for those patients more than 40 years old.

4. *Adrenocorticosteroids* may be used in the treatment of the severe or resistant thyrotoxic patient as a supportive measure. These drugs are necessary because the severely hyperthyroid patient undergoes extreme stress, and normal physiologic response by the adrenal gland may be inadequate. When used in this situation the parenteral preparations, such as hydrocortisone, are given initially and are followed by a gradually tapering oral dose as necessary. A usual injectable dose of hydrocortisone might be 50 mg. every six hours, while a comparable oral dose of prednisone might be from 5 to 10 mg. every six hours.

5. *Fluid and electrolyte management* of the patient is extremely important. Due to very rapid metabolism, marked diaphoresis, hyperpyrexia, and hyperventilation, large quantities of fluids are lost daily so that the patient may require an intake of from 4 to 6 liters of fluid daily. Because of this large fluid exchange, the patient is particularly prone to electrolyte imbalance, and serial electrolyte studies are necessary. The patient also seems to be somewhat susceptible to water intoxication (see page 184), which aggravates the general metabolic condition and mental aberrations.

6. *Vitamin therapy* is particularly important for the hyperthyroid patient. As the function of most vitamins, especially the B group, is to act as a catalyst in the metabolic pathways, the tremendous increase in metabolic activity requires large amounts of vitamins. Some physicians think that the heart disease and failure accompanying severe hyperthyroidism are similar to those seen in vitamin B deficiency (beriberi heart). With vitamins, as with other drugs considered in this treatment, doses are larger than those ordinarily used.

7. *Diagnostic laboratory studies* ordered for this patient might include the protein-bound iodine (PBI), T-3, I^{131} uptake, serum cholesterol, and a thyroid scan. The PBI is noticeably elevated, often on the level of 14 gamma per 100 ml. The T-3 is also generally elevated to or greater than 40%. The serum cholesterol is classically depressed, and figures less than 150 mg. per 100 ml. are not uncommon. The cholesterol level, once established, is probably the simplest method used by the laboratory to follow the patient with hyperthyroidism.

The I^{131} uptake is noticeably increased, usually greater than 50%. A thyroid scan of the highly agitated hyperpyretic critically ill patient in thyroid crisis is not undertaken. As the patient improves, the scan is usually done and may reveal an unsuspected substernal goiter or hyperactive ("hot") nodule.

8. A *nonstimulating environment* is particularly important for this patient. Hyperpyrexia renders a cool room necessary; if oxygen is needed, it may be given by tent since this can further cool the patient. As these patients are emotion-

ally labile and their nervous system is quite excitable, they should be kept in a quiet, somewhat darkened atmosphere, and loud or sudden noises should be prevented if possible.

The disturbing effect of visitors is strictly avoided. The nursing personnel should aid the physician in helping the family understand that the patient's irritability and frustration are the result of his illness. The patient's tremendous anxiety may be somewhat alleviated by the calm demeanor and quiet reassurance of the nursing personnel.

9. A *diet high in protein, carbohydrates, and vitamins* is ordered. Most patients have a voracious appetite although an occasional patient may need to be encouraged to eat. The patient may need help with his eating, especially his liquids, if he is unusually tremulous; this assistance is given in an unobtrusive manner.

The high protein content aids in preventing the body from using its own protein for energy, while the high carbohydrate content aids in protecting the liver, since liver glycogen tends to be depleted. The reason for the high vitamin content has already been mentioned.

Stimulants of all types, such as coffee, tea, chocolate, or carbonated beverages, are avoided; however, if the patient becomes more agitated by being denied access to these liquids, it is better therapy to give him limited amounts.

Another nursing measure that may need to be taken is protection of the eyes if exophthalmos is so severe that the eyelids fail to close. This excitable patient may not tolerate eye patches, and eye drops or ointments of some type may be ordered to keep the eyes moist.

The critical period for this patient usually lasts only a few days, but close medical supervision may be required for many months until he returns to the euthyroid state.

Chapter **33**

Adrenal insufficiency
and addisonian crisis

Typical initial orders include

1. Intravenous infusion
2. Steroids
3. Pressor agents
4. Salt tablets and high-salt diet
5. Antibiotic
6. Laboratory studies

CLINICAL FINDINGS

The patient having adrenal insufficiency may have his precarious balance disrupted by infection, gastrointestinal disturbance, trauma, or surgery. He comes for treatment with symptoms of weakness and sweatiness that may progress to prostration with profound hypotension. He may also have nausea, vomiting, diarrhea, abdominal pain, headache, and hypovolemia. His temperature may be either elevated or subnormal; cyanosis and pulmonary edema may occur.

This syndrome may take place as an initial episode, or it may occur in a patient known to have chronic adrenal insufficiency who has not taken his hormones or who has been subjected to unusual stress or exposed to infection.

In addition to these findings, the most obvious sign of true addisonian adrenal insufficiency is increased pigmentation. The skin of the Caucasian appears to have a good suntan; yet the coloring will be present on portions of the body not ordinarily exposed to sunlight. Heavy pigmentation will be noted in the body folds and at pressure points, such as the knees, elbows, belt line, knuckles, palmar creases, and crural folds. Hyperpigmentation in these locations is almost pathognomonic of Addison's disease. These patients may also have multiple black freckles, sparse body hair, and, rarely, bluish black mucous membrane pigmentation. Most of them have small hearts and low blood pressure.

PATHOGENESIS

True Addison's disease, or chronic adrenal insufficiency, is an uncommon condition; but relative adrenal insufficiency occurs with some frequency.

Adrenocortical insufficiency is the result of incapability of the adrenal cortex to produce cortisone and other metabolically active steroids in response to stress. This inability may be caused by atrophy, organic destruction of the glands, or failure of ACTH production by the pituitary gland.

The classic patient with Addison's disease has symptoms brought on by destruction of the adrenal cortex by tuberculosis. While only a small percentage of the occurrences originate from tuberculosis at the present time, the spontaneously occurring disease is usually one of idiopathic adrenocortical atrophy.

The *symptoms* of Addison's disease include weight loss in an asthenic individual, muscular weakness, and easy fatigability. Complaints referable to the gastrointestinal system may arise such as anorexia, nausea, vomiting, abdominal pain, or diarrhea. The blood pressure is low, and the patient may have difficulty with dizziness or syncope or both due to postural hypotension. Because there is a deficiency of the hormones necessary to aid the conversion of protein into glucose, the patient may undergo episodes resembling hypoglycemia with symptoms of insulin shock (symptoms, page 211).

Severe insufficiency. Severe adrenocortical insufficiency results from the hemorrhagic destruction of the adrenals as seen in the Waterhouse-Friderichsen syndrome. The meningococcus is the causative organism in the majority of the cases; however, the staphylococcus, pneumococcus, and streptococcus have also been isolated. Overdosage with anticoagulants has been implicated as well.

The signs of *Waterhouse-Friderichsen syndrome* include nausea, vomiting, abdominal pain, headache, and petechiae that may progress to purpura. The petechiae result from capillary and arteriolar destruction, while extravasation of blood from the damaged vessels accounts for the purpura. The more extensive the purpura, the greater is the likelihood that the adrenals are involved. Meningococci fairly commonly invade the adrenal glands. A gram stain of petechial fluid may reveal the meningococcic organisms. The patient's temperature usually rises extremely high, and then vascular collapse ensues. Death usually occurs within from 24 to 48 hours of the appearance of the purpura.

Relative insufficiency. Relative adrenocortical insufficiency is of greater importance than true Addison's disease because it occurs much more frequently. It results from pituitary-adrenal suppression brought about by adrenal hormones exogenously administered usually over a long period of time, although it may occasionally occur after as short an administration as three weeks. The exogenous cortisone, acting on the pituitary gland, inhibits ACTH production and atrophies the adrenal cortex. This mechanism of endogenous suppression by exogenous administration of adrenocortical steroids is so efficient that it is used to treat adrenocortical hyperplasia. Absence of hyperpigmentation in the patient with relative adrenal insufficiency secondary to suppression of function from exogenous hormones is a major differential point from the patient with true Addison's disease.

This suppression is commonly seen in patients who have taken steroids over a long period of time for such conditions as rheumatoid arthritis or chronic pulmonary disease. When this patient is placed in a stressful situation, his adrenals are unable to respond adequately and the patient suffers vascular collapse. It is predicted that relative adrenal insufficiency will take place with greater frequency. Increasing amounts of steroid hormones are components of many compound prescriptions, and these compounds are being used to treat a diversity of conditions.

TREATMENT

Specific treatment is restoration of fluid volume and electrolyte balance and replacement of hormone.

1. An *intravenous infusion,* begun immediately after blood has been drawn for laboratory studies, may be initiated with normal saline solution or 5% glucose in saline solution. The patient is usually hypovolemic with a disproportionate decrease in sodium content because of the body's inability to conserve sodium. Small increments of hypertonic saline may be required. If there is marked hypotension and shock, plasma expanders or blood may be necessary.

2. *Adrenocorticosteroids* are administered, for specific treatment consists of replacement of deficient adrenocortical hormones by the use of injectable preparations. These may be added to the intravenous infusion or injected intramuscularly. If the patient's condition is not critical, these hormones may be given orally. Hydrocortisone and dexamethasone are frequently used.

For the patient in acute adrenal insufficiency, amounts considerably larger than the usual physiologic doses of steroids may be required. The patient who has primary adrenal insufficiency may require an equivalent of only 5 mg. of prednisone daily for fairly adequate maintenance, but the patient in acute adrenal insufficiency or crisis may need the equivalent of 100 mg. during the first 24 hours to counteract the shock and low-salt syndrome. Oral steroids, usually prednisone, are administered as soon as the patient is able to take medications by mouth; then the oral dose is gradually reduced until maintenance levels are reached.

3. *Pressor agents,* such as phenylephrine (Neo-Synephrine) or metaraminol (Aramine) may be required to treat the state of advanced vascular collapse. However, the patient is uniformly refractory to pressor agents without the concomitant use of adrenocorticosteroids.

4. *Sodium chloride* is given orally as soon as the patient is able to swallow. It may be added to oral fluids or food or given in tablet form. A high-salt diet is needed to offset the patient's inability to conserve sodium.

5. *Antibiotics* are almost routinely used as the acute episode is frequently precipitated by an infectious process. Respiratory tract infection is a common causative factor. In the absence of contraindications, an antibiotic such as penicillin is usually started initially.

6. Several *laboratory studies* may be helpful in establishing the diagnosis. These include electrolyte, urea nitrogen, and glucose determinations, complete blood count, roentgenogram of the chest, tuberculin skin test, survey of the abdomen, and adrenal hormone assays.

Electrolyte determinations classically reveal the serum sodium to be quite depressed, possibly as low as 120 mEq./liter. The serum potassium is classically elevated more than 5 mEq./liter. Some physicians have found it useful to establish a sodium-potassium ratio of the serum electrolytes, with a ratio of less than 30 suggestive of adrenal insufficiency.

The *blood urea nitrogen* (BUN) may be elevated, and the blood *glucose* may be low. The *complete blood count* usually reveals a significant eosinophilia with a tendency to lymphocytosis; the normochromic and normocytic anemia is accentuated as the patient receives adequate fluids. *Roentgenogram of the chest* may make evident past or present tuberculosis, and the tuberculin skin test may be positive. A *survey film of the abdomen* may reveal evidence of adrenal calcification, which occurs in approximately one fourth of all patients; but this finding is not pathognomonic of chronic adrenal insufficiency.

Adrenal hormone assays, including the determination of hydroxycorticoid and 17-ketosteroid output in the urine over a 24-hour period, aid in diagnosis. The adrenal cortex secretes a number of hormones performing slightly different functions. Portions of these hormones are normally excreted in the urine. Although the two just mentioned are not the only adrenocortical hormones produced, the depression or absence of these hormones in the urine is strong confirmation of inadequate adrenal function.

These determinations may be impossible in the patient critically ill with severe adrenal insufficiency, for treatment will be required before the specimens can be collected.

The nursing care for this patient is supportive. Since he is especially hypersensitive to stress, a calm environment must be maintained, and all procedures should be explained. One should carefully check the vital signs frequently and watch for signs of hypoglycemia (page 212) and hyponatremia (see page 184). The patient should be protected from all sources of infection since he is especially susceptible. He should be at complete bed rest, with all activity assisted until the acute episode has ended.

RELATED FILM

Addison's disease, Color, 32 minutes, available from Audio-Visual Film Library, Dept. M-497, Eli Lilly and Company, Indianapolis, Ind. 46206.

This film helps toward understanding this disease entity.

The obstetric patient

Chapter 34

Obstetric complications

Although the obstetric patient is rarely placed in the intensive care unit, there are four groups of complications for which she may require intensive care: (1) acute toxemia, (2) hemorrhage, (3) infection, and (4) those complications resulting from a preexisting disease, such as diabetes.

ACUTE TOXEMIA

Some degree of toxemia occurs in approximately 5% to 10% of all gravidae; it is responsible for a large number of maternal deaths and an even larger number of perinatal deaths, primarily because of prematurity. The basic etiology of toxemia is unknown, although it appears to be related to the products of conception and is probably hormonal. The clinical syndrome closely resembles the hypernatremic state (see page 185).

Toxemia of pregnancy can be almost eliminated by careful observance and control at the first signs of difficulty, which include *edema, hypertension,* and *proteinuria.* A pregnant woman may begin retaining sodium and then water, becoming edematous. Arteriolar spasm may develop, producing hypertension, which can reduce the blood supply to all parts of the body and may subsequently damage the major organs, such as the brain or kidneys; uterine ischemia is especially dangerous to the fetus. Proteinuria or albuminuria may be a consequence of the renal ischemia and diminished kidney function and may progress to severe protein deficit and hypoalbuminemia. The low osmotic pressure of the protein-deficient plasma further contributes to extravascular fluid retention. The excessive fluid in the body can produce severe complications. Cerebral edema can cause confusion, irritability, convulsions, and coma; congestive heart failure may develop and culminate in pulmonary edema.

Although toxemia is a continuum varying from mild to lethal, the acute toxemias can be classified as preeclampsia, mild or severe, and eclampsia.

Preeclampsia. Preeclampsia is characterized by a rather sudden change in the patient who had previously been normal in respect to blood pressure, urine, and lack of edema. This syndrome, which is more prone to occur in young primagravidae, usually occurs during the last two or three months of pregnancy. The height of the blood pressure is not as significant as the relationship it bears to previous determinations and to the age of the patient.

The most constant sign of preeclampsia is the sudden onset of excessive weight gain due to accumulation of sodium (and water) in tissues. This *edema* almost always precedes the visible face and finger edema in the more advanced stages. Although *albuminuria* usually occurs after the onset of *hypertension* and weight gain, it may occasionally precede them.

These signs may be in evidence without the patient's knowledge, for she may feel well; but as the process continues she gets symptoms that usually include a severe continuous *headache, edema* of the face and fingers, blurred or dim *vision,* persistent *vomiting,* and *oliguria.*

Mild preeclampsia. The diagnosis of mild preeclampsia is established when any one of three criteria is met: (1) a gravida of 20 weeks or more who has previously been normal develops a blood pressure elevation with systolic reading 140 mm. Hg or more, or 30 mm. Hg above her usual blood pressure, or a diastolic pressure of 90 mm. Hg or more, or an increase in diastolic pressure of 15 mm. Hg or more, which elevations must be observed on two occasions at least six hours apart; (2) edema of the hands and face in the morning; and (3) mild proteinuria on two or more successive days.

Severe preeclampsia. Severe preeclampsia is present if one or more of the following signs is present: (1) systolic blood pressure of 160 mm. Hg or more or diastolic of 110 mm. Hg or more on at least two occasions while the patient is at bed rest, (2) proteinuria, (3) oliguria, (4) cerebral or visual disturbances, and (5) pulmonary edema or cyanosis.

Early *treatment* includes increased *rest,* a *diet* low in sodium and calories but with increased protein, and *fluid intake* between 2,000 and 2,500 ml. or more during hot weather.

Eclampsia. Eclampsia is diagnosed when the preeclamptic patient becomes comatose or convulsive or both. Convulsion may occur before the onset of or during labor or, more rarely, after the delivery. Fever is present in about half of the cases. The patient may show many of the manifestations of hypertensive encephalopathy (see page 74). She may be combative and resistive due to increased intracranial pressure.

Preeclampsia and eclampsia may also be present in a patient with preexisting hypertensive disease. Toxemia may be seen at any time during this patient's gestation, but it is more prone to occur after the twenty-fourth week. Its treatment is the same as for preeclampsia.

Treatment. The treatment for each patient with preeclampsia and eclampsia is individualized regarding all aspects of the condition. Generally, the management is twofold: (1) individual medical control of the edema, hypertension, oliguria, and convulsions, for which no single drug is ideal; and (2) obstetric management of the pregnancy.

The *edema* may be treated with diuretics, such as the thiazides. By her excreting water and sodium, the patient's hypertension may also be reduced to a degree when the circulating fluid volume decreases. Since potassium is also excreted, potassium supplements may be necessary. Allowed foods that are high in potassium should be included in the diet, such as tomato juice, bananas, oranges, grapefruit, lean beef, and salmon.

Hypertension may be regulated with a variety of drugs, such as reserpine.

Because hypertension may be an adaptive mechanism to compensate for arteriolar spasm of the cerebrum or placenta, marked reduction of the blood pressure is avoided.

If rauwolfia alkaloids are given to the mother in large quantity immediately before delivery, stuffiness of the nasal passages of the baby may result; and the infant, a nose breather, may die from asphyxia.

The treatment of *oliguria* or *anuria* may include use of extreme osmotic diuretics, such as mannitol; approximately 200 to 500 ml. may be injected intravenously in an attempt to stimulate renal activity. If renal failure is prolonged, peritoneal dialysis may be mandatory as an emergency measure (see page 195).

Convulsions may be controlled with magnesium sulfate, which acts as a vasodilator and sedative when given either intravenously or intramuscularly. It should be given slowly when administered intravenously and the blood pressure carefully monitored. If convulsions persist or the blood pressure remains elevated, magnesium sulfate may be repeated as often as at four- or six-hour intervals as long as the patellar reflex (see Glossary) is present and urinary output is adequate (from 20 to 25 ml. per hour). Intravenous calcium gluconate is a specific antidote for magnesium sulfate and should be immediately available. Since convulsions may continue to occur as long as 48 to 72 hours into the postpartum period, increments of magnesium sulfate may be given during this time.

Sedatives may be prescribed, such as phenobarbital; injectable amytal may be necessary in more severe cases. Morphine is frequently used for hospital patients who are not in labor. If delivery occurs soon after sedatives have been given, one must watch for their depressing effects on the neonate's respiration. *Oxygen* is frequently given to increase the level in the mother's blood in an attempt to provide an adequate supply for the fetus. Administration by nasal cannulae may be the easiest method to use.

The leading *cause of death* in toxemic patients is pulmonary edema with congestive heart failure (see pages 21 and 24). Other causes of death include acute renal failure (page 191), cerebral hemorrhage (page 149), anoxia (page 101), aspiration followed by pneumonia (page 118), or lung abscess.

Since there are no drugs ideal for prolonged use in the convulsive patient, it is desirable that she be in the best possible condition with vital functions under control and then be delivered, either vaginally or by cesarean section. These patients tolerate anesthesia poorly, both spinal and general, and blood pressure must be continually monitored. It is almost mandatory that there be no anesthesia, either general or conductive, within from eight to ten hours after a convulsion caused by eclampsia. If she has convulsed, a cesarean section may be done after the abdomen has been infiltrated locally. Some patients react satisfactorily to a slow intravenous administration of an oxytocic substance and artificial amniotomy.

The danger of prematurity must be weighed against the possibility of damage to both the mother and infant if the pregnancy is allowed to continue. There is general agreement that there is a close correlation between the duration (rather than the severity) of severe preeclampsia and the subsequent development of chronic hypertension.

Nursing care. Nursing care of the patient includes very careful monitoring of the vital signs, especially the blood pressure. Scrupulous attention should be paid to the fluid intake and output, and the physician should be notified immediately of diminishing urinary output. An indwelling catheter may be necessary if the patient is sedated and there is doubt about adequate urinary output.

The patient should rest as much as possible in a quiet, slightly darkened, nonstimulating environment. She should be protected from injury with padded side rails, and a mouthpiece of some variety should be immediately available in case of convulsions (but in a drawer out of sight if she is conscious or family members are present). The patient should be questioned about visual disturbances or a headache, which may be premonitory symptoms of a convulsion (care of the convulsing patient, page 134).

Airway patency *must* be assured at all times. It should be remembered that asphyxiation is the leading cause of death of the obstetric patient. An airway is inserted if necessary, and suctioning equipment should be immediately available. If secretions are excessive, the patient is placed on her side in such a manner that secretions will drain from her mouth and lessen the likelihood of aspiration.

Since this mother is hypersensitive to stimuli and also needs rest, she should be disturbed as little as possible with necessary nursing care if she is not in active labor. Treatments and nursing care should be combined to provide longer periods of uninterrupted rest. For example, maternal vital signs and fetal heart tones can be checked at times medications are given; at the same time, one can watch closely for signs of labor.

After the labor begins and the contractions occur at close intervals, one should observe the patient closely and place a hand on her abdomen to note the strength, frequency, length, and character of uterine contractions. Since intrauterine bleeding is a complication of toxemia, one must watch for its signs (page 233). An obstetric set and fibrinogen should be available, for the patient may have a cataclysmic labor with sudden delivery.

Since convulsions may occur as long as from 48 to 72 hours after the birth of the infant, close postpartum observation is essential. The oxytocic substances should be avoided as they have a vasopressor effect.

HEMORRHAGE

The causes of hemorrhage during pregnancy are generally considered in relation to the stage of gestation. The most frequent causes of *bleeding during the first half of pregnancy* are ectopic pregnancy and abortion, while placenta praevia and abruptio placentae are the common causes of *hemorrhage during the second half of gestation. Postpartum hemorrhage* may occur from hypofibrinogenemia, uterine atony, lacerations, or retained placental fragments.

Ectopic pregnancy. An ectopic pregnancy occurs about once in every three hundred pregnancies when the fertilized ovum does not implant in the endometrium but becomes lodged elsewhere, as on an ovary, in the cervix, or in the abdominal cavity. The most common site is a fallopian tube which may be stenosed from prior inflammation, or the narrowing may be congenital.

The patient, who is usually aware of being in the first trimester of pregnancy, generally experiences sudden knifelike pain in either lower abdominal quadrant produced by the rupturing of the tube and release of its contents into the peritoneal cavity. This may or may not be accompanied or soon followed by vaginal spotting or bleeding, and the patient develops shock out of proportion to the external bleeding. This shock, which may be due to blood loss into the peritoneal cavity, accompanies symptoms of peritonitis with abdominal tenderness and rigidity; progressive hypotension; tachycardia; rapid, shallow respirations; and cold, clammy skin. The patient is usually quite apprehensive, and, if the shock progresses, cerebral ischemia may render her unconscious.

Treatment. The treatment is immediate surgery. An intravenous infusion is begun immediately and fluids and plasma expanders administered. Blood is infused as soon as it is available if there has been marked loss. An indwelling catheter is inserted to ascertain the degree of shock by the amount of urinary output (see page 17). Vasopressor drugs may be necessary if shock is severe (see page 260). ACTH may also be necessary.

Abortion. The aborting patient likely to be admitted to an intensive care unit is one with severe hemorrhage to the point of shock.

Treatment. The treatment is dilatation and curettage as soon as possible in addition to treating the shock by means of intravenous infusions of fluid, plasma expanders, and blood, an indwelling catheter to determine the degree of shock, vasopressor agents, and adrenal steroids if the shock is severe. The vital signs are monitored frequently. Recommended is the supine position in which the legs are elevated; the Trendelenburg position is not suggested since the pressure of the abdominal viscera increases pressure on the heart and lungs.

Placenta praevia. In placenta praevia, the placenta attaches in the lower uterine segment instead of at the usual site of implantation in the uterine body. A *low implantation* is located near the internal cervical os but does not cover any part of it, while it partially covers the os in *partial placenta praevia;* it completely covers the cervical os in *total placenta praevia* (Figs. 34-1 and 34-2).

Since this condition occurs more frequently with multiparity, especially if the pregnancies are in rapid succession, it has been theorized that the ovum is seeking a richer vascular bed. Placenta praevia will occasionally occur when the placenta is normally attached in the uterine body; however, the placenta will be larger than usual, apparently attempting to compensate for the decreased vascularity of the uterine body.

The *primary symptom* of placenta praevia is *painless bleeding* during the last trimester caused by dislodgement of a portion of the placenta. Additional symptoms include an abnormal fetal presentation due to low placental implantation, and the placental souffle (see Glossary) may be heard below the umbilicus.

Although a vaginal examination is desirable to establish the diagnosis, it is usually deferred if bleeding is minimal and if the fetus is premature for fear of increasing hemorrhage and damaging both the fetus and the mother.

Fig. 34-1. Partial placenta praevia.   **Fig. 34-2.** Total placenta praevia.

If the obstetrician thinks it is imperative to do a vaginal examination, special precautions are taken. Since the examination may precipitate massive hemorrhage, it is done in the operating room equipped with a double setup and readied for the delivery, either vaginally or by cesarean section.

When the diagnosis is confirmed or fairly well substantiated by clinical findings, each case is treated individually, and the type of therapy will depend on various factors. These include the condition of the mother (amount of bleeding and degree of shock), condition of the fetus (viability and degree of prematurity), stage of labor (absence of signs of labor or presence of mild contractions, cervical dilatation, or ruptured membranes), and the presence of infection.

If bleeding is minimal, if the fetus appears satisfactory but premature, and if there is no evidence of infection, the obstetrician may elect to observe the patient closely and attempt to let the pregnancy continue. The mother is hospitalized, instructed to rest in bed, and closely observed.

If the hemorrhage is severe and threatening to the life of the mother, immediate delivery is performed, usually by cesarean section since this is safest for both mother and infant.

Related nursing care. A cardinal rule: The nurse must never examine a bleeding pregnant patient rectally or vaginally. *Only* the physician performs these examinations since there is grave danger of precipitating major hemorrhage.

If the patient is bleeding severely, immediate treatment for shock is begun (see page 231). There are usually standing orders so that immediate treatment of bleeding patients can be initiated. These include orders to start intravenous infusion with a large-bore needle (18 gauge so that blood can be given later from the same venipuncture), to collect blood for immediate typing and cross matching, then to begin intravenous fluids if the patient arrives before the physician.

The fetal heart tones are checked at frequent intervals; the vaginal opening is inspected often since there is increased danger of a prolapsed cord because of the low placental implantation if the membranes have ruptured. If prolapse should occur, while auxiliary personnel are notifying the physician, the patient is immediately placed in the knee-chest position if she can cooperate. If she cannot, she is placed in marked Trendelenburg position. These positions allow the fetal head to gravitate away from the maternal pelvis.

In the postpartum care of this patient, particular emphasis is placed on sterile perineal care since there is more danger of infection from the low implantation; antibiotics are usually ordered.

Abruptio placentae. In abruptio placentae the placenta, which is usually implanted normally in the uterine body, is prematurely separated from the uterine lining after the twentieth week of gestation. (If it separates before the twentieth week, it is classified as an abortion.) The separation may be partial or complete.

The cause is unknown, but it occurs much more frequently in the toxemic patient; it may follow trauma.

The detachment may occur over a period of time, separating minutely initially and then continually increasing due to the pressure of the collected blood. Bleeding may not be evident externally if the placental separation is centrally located and the placental margins are still intact, or if the blood breaks through the amniotic membrane into the amniotic sac. It is also concealed if the fetal head is positioned low and blocks the internal cervical os. Concealed hemorrhage, which generally accompanies complete separation, is frequently associated with toxemia and is a grave hazard for both mother and fetus. External bleeding, which occurs more commonly, usually accompanies partial separation (Figs. 34-3 and 34-4).

Symptoms. The classic symptoms include the sudden onset of a painful uterus (due to separation of the placenta) with or without vaginal bleeding. The uterus is tender and extremely hard, and asymmetric enlargement may be observed at the area of hemorrhage. The abdomen becomes rigid and boardlike. Shock is present and may be out of proportion to the amount of bleeding. Symptoms of shock include tachycardia, increased respiration, hypotension, pallor, dizziness, and apprehension. Fetal heart tones may be increased, decreased, or not heard at all; the fetus may become unusually active.

Treatment. Treatment is immediate delivery by cesarean section to protect the mother and attempt to save the fetus. The continued separation of the placenta further increases hazard to both. An amniotomy may be done immediately, for the release of the amniotic fluid may immobilize the fetal head against the separated portion of the placenta and promote hemostasis. An oxytocic drug may be added to the intravenous infusion to stimulate mild contractions.

Abruptio placentae may occur while the patient is in active labor and has had no prior signs of difficulty. It would be detected by the appearance of

Fig. 34-3   Fig. 34-4

Fig. 34-3. Abruptio placentae without external bleeding.

Fig. 34-4. Abruptio placentae with vaginal bleeding.

vaginal bleeding or the change in character of labor with the uterus remaining in a constantly contracted state. Other signs would be present (page 233).

Complications. In addition to the danger of hemorrhage, other complications are likely to accompany abruptio placentae, such as hypofibrinogenemia, uteroplacental apoplexy, and acute renal failure.

Hypofibrinogenemia arises from a blood coagulation defect. This occurs in about 10% of the cases of severe abruptio placentae; it can also happen with postpartum hemorrhage, septic abortion, and missed abortion or the retention of a dead fetus, or it may be due to amniotic fluid embolism (see Glossary).

Symptoms include uterine bleeding, lack of response to usual measures to stimulate uterine contractions, hematuria, melena, gingival bleeding, ecchymoses, and bleeding from venipuncture sites.

Treatment consists of rapid administration of fibrinogen intravenously after the fibrinogen level is determined to be low. In addition, aminocaproic acid (Amicar) is available, a potent drug that aids in the clotting mechanism. It is stressed that a positive diagnosis of hypofibrinogenemia be made before administration since the drug can cause intravascular clotting. Blood may also be transfused, but massive amounts are necessary to raise the fibrinogen level.

Uteroplacental apoplexy, resulting from widespread infiltration of blood into the uterine musculature and under the uterine peritoneum, occurs in from 10% to 20% of cases of abruptio placentae, with the highest incidence being in the more severe cases. The uterus remains flaccid and fails to contract. A hysterectomy may be necessary.

Acute renal failure may follow abruptio placentae (see page 191). The longer

Fig. 34-5

Fig. 34-6

Fig. 34-5. Nurse checking height of fundus in abdominal cavity after delivery.

Fig. 34-6. Correct way of massaging fundus after delivery. First, the side of one hand is placed firmly above the symphysis pubis to prevent descent of the uterus. Second, the nurse places the flat of the other hand on the patient's fundus and firmly massages in a circular motion. After she feels the fundus tightening under her hand, while still keeping her other hand placed as indicated, she presses downward to express clots from the uterus. If there are conditions that cause uterine atony such as prolonged induction labor, toxemia, large baby, multiple deliveries, or general anesthesia, this massage is done vigorously every ten or fifteen minutes or more often as is necessary.

the delivery is delayed following onset of placental separation, the greater the likelihood of hypofibrinogenemia and acute renal failure.

Postpartum hemorrhage. Postpartum hemorrhage may result from *hypofibrinogenemia, uterine atony, lacerations,* or *retained placental fragments.*

Uterine atony, in which the uterus feels boggy, may be overcome by firm massage of the fundus (see Fig. 34-6) and the use of oxytocic drugs. Lacerations require sutures, and a dilatation and curettage is usually performed to remove retained placental fragments.

Related nursing care. The postpartum patient must be closely followed for signs of hemorrhage by means of observation of the vaginal opening and frequent check of the vital signs. If there is hemorrhage, one should note the type (bright red bleeding indicates fresh bleeding while dark blood indicates old hemorrhage), amount (if hemorrhage is excessive, the pads and sheets are saved for the physician, rendering estimating the amounts unnecessary), and *how* it is discharged (a building up and gushing with clots usually indicates bleeding within the uterus; a constant trickle generally indicates cervical bleeding or a vaginal laceration).

The height of the fundus is noted. Immediately following delivery, the fundus should be between the umbilicus and symphysis pubis, but then it rises above the umbilicus in twelve hours (Figs. 34-5 and 34-6). It may be pushed to one side by distended intestines or the position of the patient. A full bladder can also push the fundus into the epigastrium and tends to promote atony.

INFECTION

The patient having infection most likely to be admitted to an intensive care unit is one with *septic abortion*. The patient appears critically ill. Her symptoms usually include profuse odorous vaginal bleeding, chills, fever, exquisitely tender abdomen and reproductive organs, and symptoms of shock.

Treatment. The treatment is a dilatation and curettage as soon as the patient is able to tolerate the procedure. Massive antibiotic therapy is usually instituted intravenously, and steroids may be necessary.

Complications. Complications may result from septic abortion, such as peritonitis if the uterus has been lacerated or if the infection traverses the entire length of the fallopian tubes. The infecting organism can gain entrance to the blood supply through the uterine veins and produce femoral or pelvic thrombophlebitis, or septicemia may result.

PREEXISTING DISEASES

Two major disorders that may cause difficulty for the pregnant patient are diabetes and heart disease. See page 209 for a discussion of diabetes. The most likely complications for the patient with heart disease would be congestive heart failure (page 21) and abnormal rhythms (page 45).

Miscellaneous conditions

Chapter 35

Anaphylactic shock
and snakebite

Typical initial orders include

1. Maintenance of adequate ventilation
2. Intravenous infusion
3. Epinephrine
4. Maintenance of blood pressure and urinary output
5. Adrenal steroids
6. Antihistaminic

ANAPHYLAXIS

Clinical findings. The patient with anaphylaxis presents one of the more pressing problems encountered in medical practice. Typically the patient is in a reasonably stable condition until he comes into contact with an antigen to which he is hypersensitive. Frequently this is a medicinal compound administered by injection. Within a few seconds to a few minutes after the contact he begins experiencing itching of the eyes, ears, or nose and difficulty in breathing that may be progressive; and there may be onset of edema. Hypotension and tachycardia may advance to unconsciousness, and death will ensue if the situation is not reversed.

Pathogenesis. Anaphylaxis is a severe sudden allergic reaction occurring in a person who has previously been sensitized. This prior exposure may or may not be ascertainable, for example, penicillin exposure through milk containing small amounts of penicillin that had been injected into the cow. The exact mechanism of the reaction is poorly understood; however, it is presumed to occur on an allergic basis.

Histamine is present in almost all organs and tissues and is released when tissues are damaged. It relaxes smooth muscles and greatly increases capillary permeability, thus permitting edema formation. This substance seems to constrict arteries and dilate arterioles, thereby producing a significant or even hazardous hypotension, as blood pressure is maintained primarily by arteriolar tone.

In anaphylaxis, it is believed that the sudden release of large amounts of histamine causes a great pooling of blood in the vascular tree (arterioles, capillaries, and veins) excluding the arteries and heart. Because capillary permeability is increased by the release of histamine, serum leaves the blood stream to enter the interstitial spaces and causes edema notable around the eyes, lips, face, or tongue; it is most dangerous when it produces laryngeal edema, which can obstruct the air passages.

The hypovolemia that occurs produces faintness, pallor, and sweatiness. The patient may become more hypotensive because of loss of fluid from the blood stream. In response to the lowered blood pressure, the heart rate increases and may become arrhythmic. If the patient is conscious, he is usually very apprehensive. If the situation is not reversed, the patient may die from decreased blood supply to his heart, brain, or kidneys.

Histamine causes the smooth muscles of the bronchioles to constrict, producing bronchospasm. Secretion of mucus is also increased. These two factors, plus capillary permeability, may allow the exudation of protein-rich serum into the alveoli, producing respiratory embarrassment and coughing. This protein-rich hyperosmotic exudate may pull additional fluid into the alveoli and bring on frank pulmonary edema.

Unfortunately, there is no adequate method of eliminating the possibility of anaphylactic reactions. Several precautions, however, can be taken to reduce or warn of the likelihood of anaphylaxis.

A patient's history of allergy to specific drugs or foods should be accepted and heeded, since people with allergic histories are more likely to have anaphylactic shock.

While anaphylaxis may occur as the result of a skin or conjunctival test for sensitivity, it still appears safer to do these tests as a precautionary measure before administering larger amounts of the more hazardous potential allergenic agents, such as horse serum preparations.

To check for sensitivity to serum, 0.1 ml. of the serum is injected intradermally on the forearm and the same amount of sterile saline in the same manner in the other forearm to act as a control. Erythema or pruritis occurring within five or ten minutes at the site of injection is interpreted as a positive reaction. If there is no history of a previous reaction and the intradermal test is positive, the serum may possibly be given in divided doses with the preliminary administration of an adrenocorticosteroid. Epinephrine and an antihistaminic should be in readiness. Epinephrine from 0.3 to 0.5 ml. may be given for less severe reactions.

If there is a generalized reaction with respiratory symptoms, **the serum should not be given.** In addition, one should watch the patient closely for progressive symptoms.

If there is a history of reaction to a serum, it is best to avoid the substance unless its use is considered life saving. In this case preliminary measures of giving an antihistaminic and an adrenal steroid should be taken.

In the conjunctival test, one drop of serum is placed in the conjunctival sac; the test is positive if there is redness and tearing within five or ten minutes.

Patients may also experience anaphylaxis with the injection of intravenous contrast media containing iodides. As prophylaxis, an antihistaminic or adrenal steriod or both may be given subcutaneously from 15 to 30 minutes before the dye is instilled into the vein. In addition, epinephrine 1:1,000, levarterenol (Levophed), and an injectable adrenal steroid should be available.

In spite of all these precautions, patients have been known to have no re-actions following trial of a small dose of the intravenous dye but then have a severe reaction when the larger doses were given. They may also experience vascular collapse one or two hours after the dye was injected although no acute initial ill affects had been apparent. Therefore, the patient needs to be watched closely, and any early signs of an allergic response should be reported immediately.

The major offenders producing anaphylaxis are animal serum and drugs by injection, especially penicillin. However, anaphylaxis has been noted after ingestion of foods or medications, including acetylsalicylic acid (aspirin) which is considered to be an innocuous drug by the laity.

Allergic symptoms may vary from being mild to anaphylactic. They may be manifest in only one system, as the integumentary, or may produce symptoms in all systems. Symptoms may be limited to the system contacted, as nausea, vomiting, and diarrhea from ingested food; or gastrointestinal symptoms may progress to pernicious vomiting or explosive diarrhea. Skin symptoms may vary from itching and erythema localized to the area of contact to generalized urticaria. Respiratory symptoms from inhaled antigen may be mild such as sneezing, itching of nose, or rhinorrhea with catarrhal discharge. If bronchospasm is present the patient has the feeling of chest tightness, for the bronchi dilate somewhat with inspiration and are smaller with expiration; the lungs become overinflated and the chest continues to expand. He experiences expiratory dyspnea that can rapidly worsen. The most severe respiratory symptom, laryngeal edema, can obstruct the respiratory passageway and is recognized by the patient's crowing respiration.

If anaphylaxis arises from an insect sting or injection of a drug into an extremity, a tourniquet should be placed immediately above the site, hopefully delaying entrance of the antigen into the general circulation until the drugs have time to be effective. As the tourniquet is gradually released, one watches for recurrence of the symptoms. Such a situation as this is an excellent reason for doing allergy sensitivity tests on the arms rather than the back.

Treatment. Speed is of the utmost importance in treating anaphylaxis, and all orders have to be followed almost simultaneously.

1. *Adequate ventilation* must be maintained. It is imperative that the air-way be patent in this patient, especially if he becomes unconscious or is vomiting. He must also be watched for increasing edema of the respiratory passageway which would be detected by increasing dyspnea and cyanosis, increased respiratory rate with less gas exchange, or a crowing respiration. Mouth-to-mouth resuscitation, if used, is generally more effective when accompanied by thoracic pressure on expiration to aid in decompression of the overinflated lungs.

Oxygen may be administered to compensate for the poor tissue oxygenation caused by inadequate circulation. This should be started before cyanosis occurs. If there is laryngeal edema with crowing respiration that does not improve with injections of epinephrine, an emergency tracheostomy is usually necessary.

2. An *intravenous infusion* with 5% dextrose in water or Ringer's lactate solution is begun; this aids in supporting circulation and provides a ready

access to the circulatory system for the administration of medications since the patient may be approaching profound shock.

3. *Epinephrine* is the drug of choice in treating anaphylaxis, for it seems to have an antagonistic effect on histamine, thus combatting the allergic reaction. It also elevates the blood pressure by vasoconstriction and is a bronchodilator. A dose of from 0.3 to 0.5 ml. may be ordered intramuscularly immediately and repeated every three to five minutes until the symptoms begin to abate. If they are fulminating, the epinephrine 1:1,000 may be diluted in 10 ml. of sterile saline solution; between 0.5 and 1 ml. may be given intravenously at 30- to 60-second intervals until he experiences relief. Injections may have to be repeated for as long as 24 hours in severe cases.

The pulse should be checked closely because epinephrine produces tachycardia, and an overdose predisposes the patient to ventricular fibrillation. The blood pressure should also be followed closely. These vital signs should be especially watched as circulation improves and there is better absorption of the epinephrine.

4. *Maintenance of blood pressure and urinary output* is usually achieved by increasing peripheral vascular resistance by use of vasopressor agents, such as levarterenol (Levophed) or metaraminol (Aramine) by intravenous drip. The precautions mentioned on page 260 should be observed. Blood pressure should be checked very frequently, and these agents should be discontinued as soon as the blood pressure can be maintained without them.

Adequate urinary output is desirable as many offending agents are excreted by way of the urinary tract. The urinary output can also be used to determine the degree of shock (see page 17).

5. *Adrenal steroids* are valuable as concurrent or supportive treatment. The soluble, rapidly-acting adrenal steroids are used, both by single large dose and by intravenous drip. For example, dexamethasone (Decadron), 4 mg. immediately and 12 mg. in the fluid containing levarterenol (Levophed), may be used in extreme cases. The blood pressure should be checked frequently, for the adrenal steroids potentiate vasopressor agents.

Adrenocorticosteroids are usually continued for several days to prevent recurrence of a reaction, and then they are gradually discontinued.

6. *Antihistaminics* may be ordered intravenously initially. After the acute reaction they may be given intramuscularly for the next 24 hours and then orally for several days.

The patient must be watched extremely closely because the shock of anaphylaxis may be a recurring phenomenon, especially if materials are injected that are slowly excreted from the body, such as repository forms of penicillin. Control of the reaction may of necessity be titrated through the period of time required for the drug to be removed from the body.

These patients must also be observed for ischemic or anoxic damage. Congestive heart failure is a common late complication of prolonged anaphylaxis. There is also more tendency toward thromboembolism because of the sluggish circulation. The urinary output should be carefully followed over the next several days to be sure that ischemic necrosis of the tubules has not occurred.

SNAKEBITES

Since snakebites frequently present a syndrome similar to anaphylaxis, a discussion of treatment will be given in this chapter.

Snakebites of two general types are seen in the United States and may require intensive care: the bites of the coral snake and of the viper family.

Bite of coral snake. The coral snake's bite produces rapid and advancing neurotoxicity that affects the spinal cord, brain stem, and vital centers. The respiratory center seems to be particularly susceptible to this neurotoxicity.

Symptoms. Shortly after the coral snakebite, there is dizziness, excessive salivation, difficulty in phonation and swallowing, somnolence, flushing, weakness, or motor paresis especially likely to involve the respiratory muscles. Muscles supplied by the cranial nerves may be obviously involved as suggested by ptosis, diplopia, incoordination of eye movements, and dilation of the pupils. In the fatal case the symptomatology progresses to coma, convulsions, and respiratory failure.

Treatment. Treatment is both specific and supportive. *Specific* treatment includes the use of antivenin; while there is no specific antivenom for a coral snakebite, the cobra antivenin is effective. Package directions should be followed closely.

Supportive treatment includes venous occlusion by placing a tourniquet immediately above the bitten area if the bite is on a limb. The tourniquet should be tight enough to prevent venous return but not so constricting that it occludes all circulation. One should check to see that the pulse is still felt in the tied extremity. If swelling continues, a second tourniquet should be applied above the edematous area and then the first tourniquet released.

Additional treatment may include cooling of the area with an ice pack to diminish circulation, and mild sedation may be needed.

If the individual is bitten by a snake of unknown type, equipment should be readily available to support respiration should it become necessary.

Bite of pit viper. The *rattlesnake,* a member of the viper family, causes the largest number of bites and greatest number of deaths from snakebite in the United States. Its bite produces a syndrome similar to anaphylaxis in addition to a severe hemotoxicity. The red cell membrane is damaged, leading to hemolysis and sludging. Coagulation is initiated by venom and intensified by the sludging. Simultaneously, capillary permeability is increased and hemorrhage becomes extensive as clotting factors are destroyed.

Symptoms. Systemic symptoms include shock, shortness of breath, cyanosis, numbness and tingling of the face, and severe muscle spasms that can progress to convulsions. The hemolysis, the extent of which is probably a reliable indication of the intensity of the injury, leads to hematuria and hemoglobinuria. There may be early and progressive jaundice.

Treatment. *Specific* treatment is use of polyvalent antivenin that is effective for all pit-viper bites. Package directions should be followed closely.

Supportive treatment includes venous occlusion above the bite, ice packs over the bite, and efforts to maintain blood volume and oxygen-carrying capacity with intravenous fluids, plasma expanders, and whole blood transfusions as needed. In addition, since hemoglobin is more soluble in an alkaline solution, efforts should be made to maintain alkaline urine output because the presence of free hemoglobin within the serum produces hemoglobinuria which is likely to result in renal tubular damage. To accomplish this, sodium bicarbonate or sodium lactate may be given intravenously.

Antibiotics are almost routinely used. The possible contamination of the fangs, in addition to the tremendous local edema and extravasation of blood, is quite likely to produce infection.

Moderate doses of adrenocortical hormones are used in an effort to suppress histamine release and hemolysis and exert a suppressing effect on the altered capillary permeability.

Blood to be typed and cross matched should be drawn when the initial intravenous infusion is begun as the hemolysis may be rather sudden in onset and devastating in its extent. Symptoms suggesting hemolysis and anaphylaxis may appear immediately following the bite or may be delayed for a few hours.

Since relapse of the patient following the initial treatment is common, he should be closely watched for the next several days.

Chapter 36

Poisonings

Cardinal principles of care include
1. Maintenance of adequate ventilation
2. Maintenance of access to circulation
3. Evacuation of stomach
4. Monitoring of vital signs
5. Check of urinary output

A detailed chronicling of all the poisonings and drug overdoses by accident or suicide attempt would require much more space than is here available; however, the poisoned patient is frequently seen in a general hospital, and his situation often demands intensive management. Specific treatment of drug over-dosage depends upon drug identification. A detailed review is available in Dreisbach's *Handbook of Poisoning*, which should be readily accessible in emergency rooms and intensive care departments.

Since there are more than five hundred poison control centers in the United States, the telephone number of the one nearest each hospital should be prominently placed in each emergency room and intensive care unit. Personnel are constantly available in these centers to answer specific questions about poisonings.

In many cases the offending agent is not immediately identifiable, but making use of certain cardinal principles may save the lives of a large number of these patients. There is considerable variation in the clinical findings, depending on the drug or chemical by which the patient has been intoxicated. A few of the more common representatives will be discussed later in this chapter.

CARDINAL PRINCIPLES OF CARE

The cardinal principles that should be observed when caring for the victim of any poisoning or overdosage include the following:

1. *Adequate ventilation* must be maintained by any means necessary. Airway patency may necessitate suctioning, an oropharyngeal airway, an endotracheal tube, or a tracheostomy (see page 100).

Oxygen may be required, as many of these drugs are respiratory depressants and anoxia is a prominent feature. If ventilation is inadequate, assisted ventilation may be necessary using expired air ventilation or a portable resuscitator until some type of respirator can be used. Assisted ventilation may actually be the specific treatment of choice for certain intoxications, such as kerosene or carbon monoxide poisonings, since these chemicals are excreted through the respiratory tract (see page 248). Page 88 supplies further discussion of respiratory support.

2. An *intravenous infusion* with 5% dextrose in water is begun early in the treatment primarily to provide ready access to the circulation and also to ensure adequate hydration and urinary output. If circulation is impaired by venous dilatation and shock, circulation must be supported by the use of vasopressor agents.

3. The *stomach should be evacuated* in almost all cases of suspected poisonings or drug overdosage even if some period of time has passed since the suspected ingestion of the overdosage of the agent; for the depressing effect of most toxins is such that general metabolism is depressed, including gastric emptying and intestinal absorption. Consequently, a moderate amount of toxic material may remain in the stomach even hours after the ingestion of toxic doses.

Most physicians prefer gastric lavage to production of emesis for these reasons: (1) There is considerably less likelihood of aspiration with use of the Levin tube. (2) The procedure is probably less traumatic to a perhaps already irritated esophageal lining; it is especially important to withdraw caustic material through a Levin tube rather than subject the esophageal mucosa to a second exposure to the corrosive material. (3) Many patients are comatose, and there is danger of aspiration. (4) Many of these patients may convulse, which also increases the danger of inhalation of vomitus. The stomach can be evacuated by means of suction after a Levin tube is inserted, and then lavaged with irrigations of normal saline solution, sodium bicarbonate, or water, depending somewhat on the suspected ingested agent.

4. *Vital signs are monitored frequently* during the early phases of treatment. It is seldom possible to tell from the initial appearance of the patient the degree of drug exposure; consequently respiratory depression or vascular impairment may occur at any time.

The heart rate and rhythm are electronically monitored for the same reason. An increasing heart rate or abnormal rhythm may indicate anoxia, or it may signify exposure to a cardiotoxic drug. Abnormal rhythms may require additional specific treatment (see page 45).

5. *Fractional urinary output* is watched closely since many drugs are nephrotoxic. At the slightest indication of decreasing urinary output, mannitol or urea diuresis is used (see page 272). In addition, increasing fluid intake presents a greater amount of material available to the kidneys for excretion of the toxic material. Occasionally the presence of severe nephrotoxicity or severe poisoning with a dialyzable agent will be adequate indication for dialysis by means of either the simpler and somewhat longer peritoneal dialysis (page 195) or hemodialysis with one of the kidney machines.

Additional measures may be required to treat specific conditions that are likely to arise. Specific *antidotes* are given when such are available. *Antibiotics* are necessary to combat the pneumonia that is likely to follow aspiration of vomited material or the pneumonitis following kerosene or gasoline ingestion.

COMMON POISONINGS

As space is limited, no attempt will be made to detail the many types of drugs that can intoxicate. However, a brief review of the specific findings in several of the more common situations and the special therapeutic endeavors available, in addition to the routine management, is considered worthwhile.

Sedatives and hypnotics. Sedatives and hypnotics account for the greatest number of severe drug overdosages, especially from suicide attempts. The barbiturates are the most common offender in this group and depress the central nervous system, seemingly progressing from the cortex to the lower centers. The vital centers are only depressed later and with exposure to fairly large doses.

Symptoms. The common findings may include a progression of the following: sleepiness, confusion, unsteadiness, coma, respiratory depression, hypore-flexia, and vascular collapse.

Treatment. The most important therapeutic measures include adequate support of respiration and adequate fluid intake, as many of these drugs are excreted through the kidneys. If adequate circulatory and respiratory support is available, a patient may recover from a phenomenally large overdose of barbiturates. *Methylphenidate (Ritalin)* by injection has been suggested as a somewhat specific antidote for the barbiturate overdosage, but its use should in no way preclude the cardinal rules of management previously listed.

Opiate overdosage. Opiate overdosage differs slightly from barbiturate overdosage in that spinal cord stimulation with cortical and medullary depression is usually a feature.

Symptoms. Signs of toxic doses of narcotics include pinpoint pupils, unconsciousness, severe respiratory depression, cyanosis, and hypotension.

Treatment. Nalorphine (Nalline) in from 5 to 10 mg. doses intravenously and repeated as necessary is almost specific treatment for most narcotic overdosages. Again, the drug treatment should not be permitted to supplant the standby of respiratory and circulatory support.

Tranquilizers. The phenothiazine group of tranquilizers is frequently used, and severe overdosage is occasionally seen in suicide attempts since the drugs are frequently prescribed to the depressive patient who is more susceptible to suicide. These drugs also seem to potentiate the effect of narcotics, barbiturates, and alcohol so that an occasional accidental overdosage may be seen by a combination of tranquilizers with those substances.

Symptoms. Clinical findings in these patients are very similar to those present during barbiturate overdosage except for the fact that many of these drugs have a rather marked anticholinergic effect. This results in dryness of the mouth, hypotension, tachycardia, nausea, and ataxia; some of these agents are also hepatotoxic. The patient may have convulsions resulting from anoxia.

Treatment. No specific treatment is available other than the general measures previously mentioned on page 245.

Amphetamines. Intoxication with the amphetamine type of drug, which is similar to epinephrine and is therefore an adrenergic agent, is occasionally seen from an accidental overdosage in the individual taking the drug for "kicks." It is also seen in the asthmatic who has taken repeated doses of ephedrine-like agents for relief of bronchial asthma. These drugs stimulate the muscles and glands innervated by the sympathetic branch of the autonomic nervous system.

Adrenergic crisis. Acute intoxication with the amphetamine drugs produces symptoms also present in adrenergic crisis. The same symptoms are also produced by overdosage of the sleep-inducing drugs containing scopolamine offered to the public without a prescription.

Symptoms. These findings include nervousness, irritability, fever, tachycardia, muscle spasms, dilated pupils, blurred vision, nausea, vomiting, convulsions, hypertension, and cardiac arrhythmias.

Treatment. Treatment includes use of sedation and the adrenergic-blocking agents, such as propranolol (Inderal) or phentolamine hydrochloride (Regitine), with the choice depending on the dominant symptoms.

Cholinergic crisis. Cholinergic crisis is a syndrome occasionally seen in the patient taking neostigmine salts in large doses for assistance with urinary retention or control of myasthenia gravis. It is also seen in exposure to cholinesterase-inhibiting insecticides, some of which are absorbed through skin contact.

Symptoms. The clinical findings in cholinergic crisis are anorexia followed by headache, dizziness, weakness, tremors, salivation, nausea, vomiting, abdominal cramping, bradycardia, diarrhea, pulmonary edema, convulsions, coma, heart block, and death.

Treatment. In addition to the general supportive measures, *atropine* or atropine derivatives in large parenteral doses repeated frequently is an almost specific *antidote* for the cholinergic crisis.

Arsenic poisoning. Arsenic poisoning is rather typical of heavy metal poisoning.

Symptoms. Arsenic poisoning is characterized by violent gastroenteritis, diarrhea which usually contains blood and mucus, circulatory collapse, convulsions, and coma.

Treatment. In addition to the general supportive measures mentioned, dimercaprol (BAL, British anti-lewisite) may be used to combine with the heavy metal and render it physiologically inactive. It should be used promptly, for administration six hours after exposure is probably of little effect. Specific details of dosage and mode of administration are available in the package's information and in various poisoning handbooks, including that of Dreisbach.

Petroleum distillates. Petroleum distillates, such as kerosene, fairly frequently cause poisoning. When these agents are ingested, they are absorbed into the bloodstream and then partially excreted through the lungs.

Symptoms. Pulmonary irritation is the major manifestation and may progress to frank pulmonary edema.

Treatment. In addition to the general supportive measures and treatment of specific complications, the patient may be given mineral oil to retard absorption. Adrenal steroids may help to reduce the postaspiration pneumonia. Positive pressure breathing may mechanically assist in control of pulmonary edema since this type of edema is refractory to digitalis or diuretics.

Carbon monoxide. Carbon monoxide poisoning is exposure of hemoglobin to carbon monoxide through inhalation. This results in the formation of carboxyhemoglobin which is incapable of carrying oxygen, and internal anoxia results. As the carboxyhemoglobin is actually redder than oxyhemoglobin, the patient will not appear cyanotic.

The *immediate toxic effect* is that of cerebral anoxia, which may cause the patient's death. Carbon monoxide poisoning is usually effected by inhalation of fumes from internal combustion engines. In the past it has been considered to be a complication of winter driving in autos whose faulty exhaust systems permitted leakage of exhaust fumes into the automobiles. This has been the principle cause in the past other than suicide attempts. However, two individuals suffering carbon monoxide poisoning have recently been seen at the Baldwin County Hospital, Milledgeville, Ga., whose difficulty occurred during the summer because of leakage from a faulty exhaust system into a closed, air-conditioned automobile.

Symptoms. The symptoms of carbon monoxide poisoning are closely related to the dosage and the period of exposure. The symptoms can be very light; or there may be a severe syndrome with impaired judgment, confusion, fainting, headache, nausea, irritability, and unconsciousness with progressive respiratory failure. Symptoms are notoriously insidious in their onset and progression.

Treatment. Modes of treatment include artificial hyperventilation and exchange transfusions. Recovery is quite gradual because the toxic manifestations of this condition are largely the result of intracranial pathology. The use of mannitol or urea may reduce cerebral edema significantly (see page 272).

Cyanide intoxication. Cyanide intoxication results in a syndrome very similar to that of carbon monoxide poisoning.

Symptoms. It permanently reduces hemoglobin and renders it incapable of carrying oxygen. However, as this hemoglobin is of a darker color, cyanosis will be characteristic of cyanide exposure.

Treatment. Treatment includes measures to improve the oxygen-carrying capacity of the blood by oxygen administration and exchange transfusions.

Salicylate intoxication. Salicylate or aspirin intoxication is one of the more common accidental poisonings. Salicylates have significant effects, both locally in the gastrointestinal tract and systemically.

Local effects. The local effects of excessive salicylate intake is primarily severe gastroenteritis. The gastritis may be severe enough to produce gastric hemorrhage. *Symptoms* include nausea, vomiting, hematemesis, and melena. *Treatment* is gastric evacuation and administration of an alkali, both as sodium bicarbonate which is absorbed and as a nonabsorbable alkali, such as aluminum hydroxide. If hemorrhage is significant, transfusions may be required.

Systemic effects. *Systemically* salicylate intoxication affects either metabolism by producing acidosis or the central nervous system directly. The *symptoms* of metabolic acidosis include Kussmaul breathing, acidemia, reduced carbon dioxide—combining power, and acetonuria. This is *treated* by intravenous alkali, such as sodium bicarbonate or sodium lactate. Fluid administration is increased to the point of producing diuresis.

Salicylates, directly toxic to the central nervous system, have their earliest effect on the vestibular apparatus, producing vertigo. At increased levels, the salicylates produce central nervous system irritability evidenced by altered states of consciousness, muscular twitchings, convulsions, and coma; progression of toxicity can produce death.

The large doses of salicylates also have a direct effect on the clotting mechanism and may produce bleeding syndromes. Supplemental vitamin K may be required.

If salicylism is not adequately controlled by gastric lavage, administration of fluid to the point of diuresis, and alkalinization, peritoneal dialysis is indicated.

RELATED NURSING CARE

In addition to the measures already mentioned, the nurse should examine the patient's mouth for evidence of burns or any remaining chemicals. Any vomitus should be saved for further study.

One should ask the person who brought the patient if he is aware of any medicine or poison container that was near the patient.

If it is suspected that overdosage was a suicide attempt, all articles that could be used for a second attempt, such as glassware and silverware, should be removed, and the patient should constantly be attended. A second attempt is quite likely, for the primary problem still remains and is compounded by failure of the suicide attempt.

Equipment and drugs

Chapter 37

Intensive care unit: physical plan, equipment, and supplies

Many factors must be taken into consideration in the planning and equipping of an intensive care unit. In addition to personnel, who were discussed in Chapter 1, these elements include the physical plan, equipment, and supplies.

These factors will vary somewhat with the purpose of the unit and the type of patient to be attended. For example, the requirements for a general intensive care unit caring for all types of critically ill patients might vary somewhat from a coronary care unit or a cardiovascular surgery unit. The possibility of care of infectious patients necessitates a facility in which isolation technique is possible.

This discussion regards a general unit that might be incorporated into a 150-bed to 300-bed general hospital, although many of the generalizations would apply to the specialty units as well. Hospitals smaller than 150 beds may not find it feasible to have a separate unit, but they may want to equip one or two rooms for intensive care near the nurses' station.

When hospitals have multiple units, their proximity enable sharing of certain equipment as well as personnel in periods of peak activity.

PHYSICAL PLAN

An intensive care unit should encompass a relatively small area, but it should afford critically ill patients a measure of privacy while simultaneously permitting their constant surveillance by personnel. Most hospitals have found some variation of the half-circle arrangement to be quite effective, with a nursing station at the center of the half circle.

If at all possible, the unit should have individual rooms or cubicles. These should be well lighted, individually air conditioned, and soundproofed, insofar as possible. The wall and door adjacent to the nurses' station should be half glass with curtains over the glass area that may be drawn when privacy is desired. The head of the bed should be visible from the nursing station (Fig. 37-1).

Each room should have a lavatory, a small closet, an overbed light, and a night light. A generous supply of electrical outlets is mandatory as is an electrical system adequate to supply several pieces of equipment simultaneously.

INTENSIVE CARE UNIT
Baldwin County Hospital

Fig. 37-1. Floor plan of five-bed intensive care unit at the Baldwin County Hospital, Milledgeville, Ga., showing visual lines.

Wall-mounted equipment is recommended when possible, for it interferes little with direct patient care activities. Wall-mounted television sets with pillow speakers are desirable. The television programs may be enjoyed by the patient admitted for close observation who is not seriously ill and also by the patient recuperating from a critical illness while still requiring close observation. The patient seems less lonely and less disconcerted at the restricted visiting hours and closeness of the walls of his room when he has this contact with the rest of the world.

EQUIPMENT AND SUPPLIES

(As an aid to those hospitals anticipating an intensive care unit, the following equipment and supplies were needed to open the five-bed unit at the Baldwin County Hospital in Milledgeville, Ga.)

Each patient's room contains the following:

Bed—the most satisfactory bed is easily movable, preferably of the recovery room stretcher type, and can be readily changed to place the patient in any desired position. It is more suitable if it is narrow enough so that nursing personnel can reach any portion of the patient from one side of the bed; this also permits its easier passage through a doorway.

Bedside table

Overbed table

Footstool

Wall-mounted oxygen outlet with gauge

Wall-mounted suction outlet with gauge

Wall-mounted mercury sphygmomanometer

Wall-mounted intravenous stands

Clock with second hand

Cardiac board for immediate use in case of cardiac arrest

All five rooms are wired to the console at the nurses station and have a wall rack for an oscilloscope and pacemaker. Four rooms have oscilloscopes and pacemakers that may be moved as necessary.

Various pieces of equipment and certain supplies should be readily available so that a trip to another part of the hospital will not be necessary during an emergency.

The mandatory equipment for an intensive care unit includes the following: (1) mechanical means of supporting respiration, (2) electronic equipment, (3) specific sterile supplies, and (4) certain drugs.

Mechanical means of supporting respiration. *Portable respirators* (also known as bag and mask ventilators) should be immediately available for the patient who needs assisted ventilation for a short period of time.

An *automatic cycling mechanical respirator,* such as the Bird, is necessary for supporting respiration over a prolonged period of time.

Additional equipment for respiratory support includes oxygen masks, catheters, cannulae, airways, endotracheal tubes in various sizes, and a laryngoscope with blades of assorted sizes.

Electronic equipment. Electronic equipment, which is imperative, includes *monitoring units, pacemakers,* and a *defibrillator.* This equipment is discussed in Chapter 8.

Desirable but not mandatory equipment includes a *rotating tourniquet machine,* which is recommended. It provides even pressure to the extremities and releases this pressure at set intervals. Most importantly, it frees the nurse to perform other pressing duties for the patient whose critical condition makes using this machine necessary.

Another piece of desirable equipment is a battery-powered portable pacemaker with external and catheter electrodes to be used if transfer of the patient is required.

Auxiliary electrocardiographic equipment and a high quality portable x-ray machine are desirable but not mandatory equipment. The necessity for these machines would depend on the proximity of the unit to the heart station and radiology department in each hospital.

Sterile supplies. Certain sterile supplies are necessary. Essentials include one of each of the following: (1) venous cutdown tray; (2) tracheostomy tray with clean-up kit; (3) thoracotomy tray with bottle, stopper, tubing, and solution; (4) spinal tray with manometer; and (5) catheter tray with extra Foley catheters and drainage bag. At least four pairs of each of the standard sizes of sterile gloves should be available.

Additional sterile supplies include dressings, knives and knife blades, suturing material, Levin tubes, sump tubes, towels, basins, and syringes and needles in assorted sizes. Flasks of sterile solutions, such as water and normal saline solution, are needed for irrigations.

Drugs. Certain drugs, such as the following, are necessary for immediate use:

Adrenergic agents (vasopressors)
Ephedrine sulfate
Epinephrine (Adrenalin)
Isoproterenol (Isuprel)
Levarterenol (Levophed)
Metaraminol (Aramine)
Methoxamine (Vasoxyl)
Adrenergic-blocking agents
Phentolamine (Regitine)
Adrenocorticosteroids
Dexamethasone (Decadron)
Hydrocortisone (Solu-Cortef)
Analgesics
Acetaminophen (Tylenol)
Acetylsalicylic acid (aspirin)
Anileridine (Leritine)
Codeine
Dihydromorphinone (Dilaudid)
Meperidine (Demerol)
Morphine
Oxymorphone (Numorphan)
Antidote: nalorphine (Nalline)
Antiarrhythmic agents
Procaine amide (Pronestyl)
Propranolol (Inderal)
Quinidine gluconate
Anticholinergic agent
Atropine
Anticoagulants
Heparin sodium
Warfarin (Coumadin)
Anticoagulant antidotes
Phytonadione (AquaMephyton, Mephyton)
Protamine
Anticonvulsant agents
Diphenylhydantoin (Dilantin)
Magnesium sulfate
Antihistaminics, antiemetics, psychotherapeutic agents
Amitriptyline (Elavil)
Chlorpheniramine (Chlor-Trimeton)
Chlorpromazine (Thorazine)
Dimenhydrinate (Dramamine)
Diphenhydramine (Benadryl)
Hydroxyzine pamoate (Vistaril)
Prochlorperazine (Compazine)
Promazine (Sparine)
Promethazine (Phenergan)
Antihypertensive agent
Reserpine (Serpasil)
Bronchodilator
Aminophylline (theophylline ethylenediamine)
Central nervous system stimulants
Caffeine and sodium benzoate
Methylphenidate (Ritalin)
Nikethamide (Coramine)
Coronary vasodilator
Nitroglycerine
Digitalis preparations
Digoxin (Lanoxin)
Lanatoside C (Cedilanid)
Diuretics
Ethacrynic acid (Edecrin)
Furosemide (Lasix)
Hydrochlorothiazide (Esidrix)
Mannitol
Meralluride (Mercuhydrin)
Mercaptomerin sodium (Thiomerin)
Electrolyte solutions
Calcium gluconate
Dextrose in saline
Dextrose in water (5%, 10%, 50%)
Isotonic saline
⅙ Molar sodium lactate
Plasma protein fraction (Plasmanate)
Potassium chloride
Ringer's Lactate
Sodium bicarbonate
Sodium lactate
Sedatives
Amobarbital (Amytal)
Pentobarbital (Nembutal)
Phenobarbital sodium (Luminal Sodium)
Secobarbital (Seconal)

Other needs. Various additional pieces of equipment are needed. These include adult and pediatric sphygmomanometers, stethoscopes, otoscope-ophthalmoscope combination, Clinitest and Acetest tablets, Miget urinometers (for measuring specific gravity), Uri-meters (for measuring hourly urine output), disposable prep tray, water-soluble jelly, linen savers, and an ample supply of linens, charting forms, and necessary stationery supplies. Other supplies needed include an intermittent suction machine (for gastrointestinal decompression), bedside commode, and portable intravenous stands.

Emergency cart carries *defibrillator* with synchronizer and the following:
Portable resuscitators
Electrode paddles and electrode paste
Airways and endotracheal tubes
Intracardiac needle
Arm boards, tourniquets, alcohol sponges
Cardiac arrest tray (for opening the chest)

Tray of emergency drugs:

Aminophylline
Caffeine and sodium benzoate
Diphenylhydantoin 100 and 250 mg. (Dilantin)
Epinephrine (Adrenalin)
Glucose 50%
Hydroxyzine pamoate (Vistaril)
Isoproterenol (Isuprel)
Lanatoside C 0.4 and 0.8 mg. (Cedilanid)
Levarterenol (Levophed)
Lidocaine 1% and 2% (Xylocaine)
Magnesium sulfate
Meralluride (Mercuhydrin)
Metaraminol (Aramine)
Methoxamine (Vasoxyl)
Procaine amide (Pronestyl)
Propranolol (Inderal)
Quinidine gluconate
Theophylline

GENERAL POLICIES

The following general policies have proved to be helpful and are presented to the family of each patient:

Admission to the intensive care unit is arranged directly by the physician with the nurse in charge of the unit; she will notify the admission office.

All patients in the intensive care unit have two attending physicians listed on the chart at the time of admission.

Private duty nursing is not permitted in the unit.

Visitors are permitted one at a time for ten minutes every two hours or at the discretion of the nurse. Visitors may wait in the solarium. The unit has direct communication with the solarium for conversation.

The unit is staffed with registered nurses, licensed practical nurses, and nurses aides.

Flowers are not permitted in the unit and the patient's personal articles should be kept at a minimum while he is in the unit.

ROUTINES

The following routines have proved to be satisfactory and are offered as suggestions:

Temperature, pulse, respiration, and blood pressure are taken routinely every four hours or more frequently, depending on the condition of the patient and the physician's order.

A fluid intake and output record is kept concerning each patient and totalled every eight hours. A 24-hour total is recorded by the night nurse at 7 A.M. The amount of all irrigating solutions used is subtracted from the total amount of drainage to give the true drainage.

The following information concerning each patient admitted to the unit is recorded in a census book: name, age, physician, diagnosis, date and time of admission, and date and time of transfer or discharge.

Supplies, emergency trays, and emergency drugs must be maintained at a proper level at all times by being replaced as soon as possible after they have been used.

All equipment is properly cleaned after use and kept in working order. Operation manuals are kept readily available.

When patients are being monitored, a 6-inch electrocardiograph strip is taped to the nurse's note at the beginning of each shift and whenever it is necessary.

If shock is apparent, 1,000 ml. of 5% dextrose in water is begun intravenously by means of an 18-gauge needle and a Foley catheter inserted.

Intensive care beds are not to be used for convenience, and utilization shall depend only on the patients' needs. In the event that all beds are filled, priority of discharge is decided by the Intensive Care Committee after review and consultation with the attending physician.

Chapter 38

Drugs used during intensive care

Nursing personnel charged with the care of the critically ill patient should have thorough knowledge of and experience with certain groups of drugs and some specific medications. In reviewing drugs, it may be helpful to classify them as (1) those having specific pharmaceutical effect, (2) those depressing some normal body function, or (3) those potentiating some normal body function. A large number of drugs can be at least superficially understood by reference to this classification.

Some representative drugs needed in the intensive care situation will be generally discussed in regard to their major classification, mode of action, therapeutic use, and toxicity. The user of the drug must read package inserts and reference books for further information. These drugs are listed by both generic and trade names according to these major classifications beginning on page 250. Each drug is also cross indexed so that information regarding it can be found quickly.

In addition to being alert for the appearance of known side effects of each drug, the nurse must **watch for symptoms of hypersensitivity in all drugs given.** These symptoms include skin eruptions, angioneurotic edema, fever, respiratory embarrassment that can be progressive, cyanosis, nausea, vomiting, and diarrhea. Thrombocytopenic purpura can also result from drug usage.

ADRENERGIC DRUGS

Adrenergic drugs have an effect similar to that of epinephrine. As a group, these drugs produce peripheral vasoconstriction, cardiac acceleration, increased myocardial irritability, and bronchodilation. *Potent vasoconstriction* is the primary effect of some of the adrenergic drugs; therefore, they are used for supporting blood pressure in the event of vascular collapse. This action is mediated by the alpha adrenergic receptors.

Toxicity and side effects are the result of sympathetic nervous system stimulation, and overdoses bring about frank *adrenergic crisis*. Symptoms include severe headache, delirium, dilatation of the pupils, hypertension, tachycardia, and abnormal cardiac rhythms. In addition, there may be precordial pain, pallor, nausea, and vomiting.

These drugs are *contraindicated* for patients with hypertension, hyperthyroidism, and heart conditions other than when bradycardia or heart block is prominent.

Since there are important differences in various drugs in this group, several will be discussed individually.

Epinephrine. Epinephrine (Adrenalin) is the parent substance. It stimulates (and probably mediates the effect of) a major portion of the sympathetic nervous system. It is primarily used by injection for bronchodilation. It is usually given in dosages of a fraction of a milligram subcutaneously for relief of bronchospasm, or it may be administered in somewhat larger doses in an oil base for more prolonged effect.

Because of its intense myocardial stimulation, epinephrine may be injected directly into the heart while the heart is simultaneously massaged as a part of resuscitative efforts during cardiac arrest.

Isoproterenol. Isoproterenol (Isuprel) is an adrenergic drug that is primarily used for bronchodilation and administered sublingually or nasally. The latter administration has a local adrenergic effect that seems to be fairly well confined to the respiratory tract; for this reason it has fewer side effects. In larger sublingual dosages, the patient may experience anxiety, tachycardia, and some degree of hypertension.

Isoproterenol is used by injection to stimulate the ventricles and to control some of the bradycardiac abnormal rhythms of extremely slow rates or high degrees of heart block, such as the Adams-Stokes syndrome. When used in this manner, it is frequently given by slow dilute intravenous drip, heart rate and rhythm being continuously monitored. It may also be used occasionally to maintain adequate circulation in preparation for the use of an electronic pacemaker, or when one is not available if the heart rate is too slow to support normal function.

Metaraminol. Metaraminol (Aramine) is readily absorbed from an intramuscular injection and is usually given in fractional doses until the desired blood pressure is reached. It may be diluted in glucose in water or normal saline solution and administered by intravenous drip to the patient with severe hypotension.

Side effects include hypertension, headache, tachycardia, and abnormal rhythms.

Levarterenol. Levarterenol (Levophed), the most potent vasoconstrictor in common use, causes such intense vasoconstriction that it can be administered only intravenously. It is used when the need for peripheral vasoconstriction is extreme. Local instillation or infiltration results in such severe vasoconstriction of the local vasculature that tissue necrosis almost uniformly takes place.

Because of the intense vasoconstriction and possibility of extreme hypertension, patients receiving levarterenol drip must be monitored very closely. A transient headache may indicate overdosage. Prolonged use produces such vasoconstriction that peripheral damage, especially to the kidneys, may result.

The patient may receive blood or plasma and levarterenol simultaneously; however, the drug is diluted in other fluids and injected at another site, for the natural plasma enzymes may destroy its effect if levarterenol is added to the plasma or blood.

Related nursing care. The blood pressure must be monitered at very frequent intervals when the patient is receiving vasopressor agents.

When *levarterenol* is being administered, the injection site must be observed very frequently. This is especially important if the patient is restless or has to be moved for any reason. *Phentolamine (Regitine)* and a syringe should be immediately available in case of tissue infiltration.

The nurse should be especially careful to note that the correct dosage is given by the correct route since these are extremely potent drugs.

Since these drugs are usually kept on an emergency tray, they are to be restocked as soon as possible after use.

ADRENERGIC-BLOCKING AGENTS

Phentolamine (Regitine) is primarily used for its vasodilatory and hypotensive effects. It is most frequently used to prevent local ischemic necrosis following infiltration of an infusion containing levarterenal. It is diluted and infiltrated through multiple sites into the ischemic area. It is also occasionally used to counteract the hypertensive effect of adrenergic crisis from vasopressor overdosage.

Phentolamine was initially introduced as a test for pheochromocytoma, a tumor that produces epinephrinelike hormones capable of bringing on hypertensive syndromes. In this test the drug is given intravenously, and an immediate significant drop in blood pressure suggests the presence of this tumor.

The primary *side effect* is hypotension.

ADRENOCORTICOSTEROIDS

The adrenocorticosteroids are a group of related compounds normally produced by the adrenal cortex (epinephrinelike hormones are produced primarily in the adrenal medulla). Several of these hormones are similar in action, yet they have slightly different effects physiologically.

Mode of action. The myriad of therapeutic uses of corticosteroids is related to their many physiologic and pharmacologic activities that affect almost all metabolic patterns. The *primary actions* of the corticosteroids are (1) to increase catabolism by increasing protein breakdown and glucose formation, (2) to stimulate glucagon breakdown to form glucose, (3) to suppress histamine release and effect, (4) to produce sodium retention and potassium loss, (5) to suppress pituitary ACTH production, and (6) to increase virilization.

Therapeutic use. Corticosteroids are frequently useful in the critically ill patient. Their mode of action is poorly understood; nonetheless, as with all hormones they serve as catalysts in various physiochemical reactions. This particular group of compounds is most useful in supporting the body's stress reactions.

The *primary uses* of these compounds include (1) replacement in adrenocortical insufficiency for which rather small doses are required; (2) usefulness in the physiologic exhaustion states, as with septicemia and septicemic shock; (3) lessening the hypersensitivity reactions in severe allergic syndromes such as acute asthma, anaphylaxis, and intense allergic skin conditions; (4) suppression of the autoimmune syndromes, such as lupus erythematosus, hemolytic anemia, and thrombocytopenic purpura; and (5) suppression of all of the manifestations of inflammation, including redness, pain, fever, and swelling, and suppression of the acute arthritic syndromes and rheumatic carditis.

Side effects. Side effects and complications are largely related to pharmacology. Edema, characteristic moonface, and hypertension may be evidence of the sodium-retaining effect, which may also precipitate congestive heart failure. The anti-inflammatory effects may lead to breakdown of arrested tuberculosis or failure of local control in other infections. The catabolic effect of long-term use may eventuate in marked protein wasting, even of the protein matrix of the bone. This produces osteoporosis and accompanying hypercalcemia which may result in formation of calcium urinary stones as well as susceptibility to pathologic fractures. Corticosteroids also produce central nervous system effects of headache, vertigo, increased intracranial pressure, and occasionally frank psychosis. They are also ulcerogenic, either precipitating or producing peptic ulcers.

Long-term administration suppresses pituitary ACTH production which, with stress, may lead to relative adrenal insufficiency and vascular collapse, as mentioned on page 220. This insufficiency may also occur following abrupt withdrawal of the corticosteroids. The slight androgenic effects of these compounds may produce acne and virilization.

Due to their effect on glucose metabolism, these drugs may worsen diabetes and occasionally appear to precipitate diabetes.

Related nursing care. The nurse must watch for side effects and toxicity when a patient is receiving any of these drugs.

If a critically ill patient has been receiving corticosteroids and then his dosage is reduced or discontinued, one must watch for signs of adrenal insufficiency (page 220).

ANALGESIC DRUGS

Analgesic drugs, which are primarily used for relief of pain, help to allay anxiety and decrease peristalsis, and some have antitussive action. Codeine and dihydromorphinone (Dilaudid) are commonly used in oral cough preparations because of their specific depressing effect on the cough center.

They are generally given by subcutaneous injection, and the less potent medications may be given orally. On occasion they may be given intravenously if the patient is in severe pain or experiences marked hypotension with decreased perfusion of tissues.

Because of their tendency to produce euphoria and the body's ability to become chemically dependent, use must be carefully controlled and long-term administration avoided to prevent addiction.

Side effects. Toxicity and side effects are related to their therapeutic action of depressing the central nervous system. Signs include excessive somnolence or dizziness, depressed respiration, hypotension, pinpoint pupils, bradycardia, and constipation; certain analgesics cause nausea and vomiting in some patients. Bladder sphincter spasm can lead to urinary retention.

Related nursing care. If a patient is in shock when an analgesic is given, the nurse must watch for the depressing effects of the drug as his condition improves and the medication is more fully absorbed.

One should use other nursing comfort measures, such as a back rub or change of position, if these can relieve the patient's discomfort without drug therapy.

The patient's being informed that an analgesic is being given seems to increase the drug's effectiveness.

ANTIARRHYTHMIC DRUGS

Antiarrhythmic drugs, which have their effect upon the cardiac conduction system, are used primarily for the control of ectopic rhythms. The following drugs *depress* the myocardium. Drugs that *increase* cardiac rhythm are listed among the *adrenergic drugs* or the *anticholinergic drugs*.

It should be remembered that mural thrombi may be dislodged from the atria when atrial fibrillation reverts to normal rhythm.

Lidocaine and procaine amide. Lidocaine (Xylocaine) is a local anesthetic agent; procaine amide (Pronestyl) is a derivative of procaine. Both drugs produce a cardiac effect that is mediated primarily by depressing the conduction system and decreasing myocardial irritability. When they are given intravenously, the patient should be simultaneously monitored and his cardiac rhythm, electrocardiographic complexes, and blood pressure followed.

Procaine amide is usually injected intravenously in a single dose in emergencies. It is given slowly at a rate not exceeding 50 mg. per minute; it may be given to a maximum dose of 2 gm. It may also be given by mouth for the treatment of any abnormal rhythms that result from ectopic foci or irritability. Extrasystoles, atrial fibrillation, atrial flutter, and tachycardia are indications for its use, as is ventricular tachycardia.

Toxicity is related to a specific myocardial depression suggested by widened QRS complexes; it can also produce hypotension.

Quinidine sulfate. Quinidine sulfate is a specific depressant of the myocardium and the conduction system; it lengthens the period during which the heart is refractory to stimuli. Initially it is usually given as a single 200 mg. tablet for treatment of any of the ectopic rhythms, and then the dosage is progressively increased until desired therapeutic effect is achieved or symptoms of toxicity occur. It is also available as an injectable preparation in the form of a gluconate for treatment of the critical abnormal rhythms, such as ventricular tachycardia.

Toxicity is suggested by bradycardia, reduced contractile force, and reduced impulse conduction manifested electrocardiographically by QRS widening and evidence of heart block. As quinidine is a myocardial depressant, congestive heart failure may be aggravated by its use.

Gastrointestinal *side effects* include nausea, vomiting, abdominal cramps, and diarrhea. Tinnitus and visual disturbances may also be signs of toxicity.

Propranolol. Propranolol (Inderal) is a recently available potent beta adrenergic–blocking agent that has proved to be relatively safe to the present time. It is used when it is desirable to counteract the naturally occurring beta adrenergic effect of epinephrine (which is the primary effect of epinephrine on the myocardium and the cardiac conduction system). In blocking this type of adrenergic effect, the drug represents a valuable tool for the control of the rapid abnormal rhythms.

Propranolol is available for oral and parenteral use. It is probably the drug of choice in the rapid arrhythmias associated with digitalis intoxication. It has also demonstrated effectiveness against most rapid arrhythmias of both atrial and ventricular origin, as well as being an aid in control of severe angina; but it has not yet been licensed for use in the latter situation.

Contraindications and side effects are related to the adrenergic blockage. It tends to worsen bronchospasm in asthma. Since it is thought to have the direct effect on the myocardial fibers of weakening the force of contraction, it should be used with caution in the patient with congestive heart failure. Diabetics should be watched for signs of insulin overdosage since propranolol masks some of the early indications of hypoglycemia.

Related nursing care. The electrocardiographic complexes are observed carefully while the patient is receiving these drugs. The physician is to be notified if a marked decrease or change in the rhythm occurs, especially if there is a simultaneous decrease in the blood pressure.

The blood pressure is checked and the pulse counted before each dose is administered. One should note the quality of the pulse as well as the rate and rhythm.

The nurse must check the apical-radial pulse at regular intervals and notify the physician of a marked pulse deficit.

The patient should be discreetly questioned regarding side effects.

ANTICHOLINERGIC DRUGS

Anticholingeric drugs counteract cholinergic effect (cholinergic drugs, page 269) and depress the parasympathetic nervous system. They are also referred to as vagal blocking agents because much of their action is mediated through the vagal system.

Action. Anticholinergics produce the following (due to unopposed sympathetic effect): dilated pupils, reduced secretions from the nose and throat, decreased salivation, depressed intestinal motility, and lessened gastrointestinal fluid production. They reduce sweating and have an antispasmodic action in the biliary tract. Bladder atony and lack of sphincter relaxation may result in urinary retardation or urinary retention.

Concerning their effect on the cardiovascular system, these drugs permit unopposed activity of the cardio-accelerator forces that are under sympathetic (adrenergic) control, hence tachycardia. Atropine is occasionally used intravenously in very large doses for the patient with heart block in an effort to permit the accelerator forces to increase the rate.

Belladonna alkaloids, especially *atropine,* are typical members of this group; *methantheline bromide* (Banthine) is a typical synthetic agent. Their effect is one of depressing parasympathetic nervous function and thereby permitting an increase in sympathetic function as the sympathetic efforts go unbalanced. These drugs seem to have a cumulative effect in some individuals.

Scopolamine, which produces somnolence and amnesia, is a major ingredient in the sleep-producing products that are available without prescription.

Therapeutic use. The most common therapeutic use of the anticholinergic agents is for reducing the intestinal motility and gastrointestinal secretory activity of the patient with peptic ulcer or functional gastrointestinal disease. They are also used preoperatively to reduce secretions in the respiratory tract. Relief of biliary colic may be obtained by their use.

Side effects. Toxicity and side effects include tachycardia, dryness of secretions of the mouth and nose, flushed skin due to decreased sweating and vasodilation; photophobia and blurred vision may result because pupils are dilated, and the decreased intestinal muscle tone can produce constipation. Urinary retardation and retention can result from the bladder atony and increased sphincter tone.

Related nursing care. When side effects from these drugs are predictable, such as dryness of the mouth and flushing of the skin when atropine is given subcutaneously, the patient should be informed of these effects at the time the drug is given, for this obviates his concern.

One should note the early signs of side effects that could become a major difficulty for the patient, such as an increasing pulse rate or urinary hesitation. The physician should be informed of these symptoms.

The nurse must be certain of correct dosage since small amounts of these drugs are ordered.

ANTICOAGULANT DRUGS

Anticoagulant drugs are frequently used in the critically ill patient since he is especially prone to thromboembolic complications. Therapy with anticoagulants is generally used for treatment of venous thrombosis, pulmonary and cerebral embolism, and congestive heart failure. It has been frequently used in the treatment of thrombotic arterial disease, both cerebral and coronary. The commonly used anticoagulants are of two types: heparin sodium and coumarin compounds.

Contraindications to use of anticoagulants are a patient known to have bleeding tendencies, such as hemophilia, or one who is hemorrhaging. It is also contraindicated or used with caution in the patient with peptic ulcer, ulcerative colitis, or continuous intestinal intubation (due to lack of absorption of vitamin K).

Heparin sodium. Heparin sodium, usually derived from animal lungs, prolongs clotting time; it also seems effective in reducing platelet adhesiveness. As its action is immediate, it is used when prompt anticoagulation is desired.

The average adult patient will require approximately 10,000 U.S.P. units every six to eight hours. It can be given intravenously; if longer action is desired, it is given intramuscularly or into the deep subcutaneous tissues, as in the fat of the abdominal wall. The last two routes prolong its rate of absorption but increase the likelihood of hematoma formation and may also cause the drug to be irregularly absorbed.

The United States Pharmacopeia requires that heparin concentration be expressed in units of activity. For a long period of time, 10,000 units were roughly equivalent to 100 mg. However, with some improvement in purification in recent years, somewhat less than 100 mg. may be equivalent to 10,000 units; therefore, the preferred measurement for ordering the drug at the present time is units.

Heparin is usually injected at regular intervals intravenously, intramuscularly, or subcutaneously, but it may be used regionally in vascular surgery. For example, it may be injected into a peripheral artery that is temporarily obstructed distally. In regional use, its action is usually counteracted by injection of protamine sulfate, which specifically blocks the heparin effect as soon as circulatory integrity is reestablished.

Heparin has the distinct advantage that its anticoagulant effect can be almost instantaneously reversed by the intravenous injection of protamine sulfate, or blood transfusions can be administered to supply necessary clotting factors. Heparin has the disadvantage of requiring parenteral administration at frequent intervals because of its short-term action. The anticoagulant effect is estimated by clotting time determinations that are usually made daily.

Coumarin derivatives. The coumarin derivatives act by interfering with prothrombin production. They are usually given by mouth, a large initial loading dose being required. An interval of from approximately 24 to 72 hours is usually necessary to achieve a prothrombin time that is two to three times the control; this is considered adequate therapeutic range. Patients vary greatly in their maintenance dose.

The physician frequently orders administration of the initial doses of heparin and coumarin preparations simultaneously, for the heparin effect will have disappeared by the time the coumarin preparations have prolonged the prothrombin time.

The coumarin drugs have their effect by interfering with vitamin K metabolism. Patients lacking or unable to absorb vitamin K are particularly susceptible to anticoagulant effect. This includes patients with diarrhea, liver disease, malabsorption syndrome, and gastrointestinal intubation.

Numerous commonly used drugs affect coumarin anticoagulation by potentiation. The prothrombin time must be checked often when anticoagulants are used concurrently with antibiotics (which interfere with intestinal flora and vitamin K absorption) or salicylates (which are very weak coumarin-type anticoagulants). Mineral oil is contraindicated since it binds vitamin K and prevents its absorption. In addition, phenylbutazone (Butazolidin) greatly potentiates the effect of anticoagulants.

Bishydroxycoumarin (Dicumarol) requires an initial loading dose of from 300 to 800 mg. in the first 72 hours; then maintenance dosage may vary from 25 to 150 mg. daily as regulated by prothrombin time determinations.

Warfarin (Coumadin) is probably the most popular current anticoagulant. The loading dose is approximately 50 mg. initially by mouth with maintenance dosages varying from 2.5 to 25 mg. daily as determined by prothrombin time levels. This drug is also available for injection. Prothrombin time determinations are initially made daily and then several times a week while the patient is in the hospital.

ANTICOAGULANT ANTIDOTES

Excessive anticoagulation is treated by administration of vitamin K preparations, but this process may take several hours. Blood transfusions may also decrease the prothrombin level.

Phytonadione. Phytonadione (Mephyton) appears to be the most effective vitamin K preparation for the antagonism of coumarin anticoagulation; it seems to be more effective orally than parenterally.

Protamine sulfate. Protamine sulfate is the specific antagonist of heparin anticoagulation. It has no other significant use and no major side effects; 100 mg. counteract 10,000 units heparin.

Related nursing care. The patient must be observed carefully for any evidence of hemorrhage, such as hematomas on the body, and any evidence of hematuria or melena.

If the patient hemorrhages from excessive effect of heparin, further absorption of the drug may be slowed by placing an ice bag over the injection site.

Protamine sulfate and vitamin K should be readily accessible.

ANTICONVULSANT DRUGS

Diphenylhydantoin. Diphenylhydantoin (Dilantin) is used primarily for the control of convulsions. It is probably the most effective drug for the control of grand mal seizures and has been used for years for this purpose as an oral preparation. It is chemically akin to the barbiturates, and its mode of action is its depressing effect on the cerebral cortex.

Diphenylhydantoin is also available for either intramuscular or intravenous use. The parenteral form is frequently used in the treatment of status epilepticus. It has also been used for control of ectopic cardiac rhythms. Its effectiveness in depressing the cardiac conduction system is apparently similar to its depressing effect on the central nervous system.

Side effects. Toxic effects are rather rare except for gingival hypertrophy with prolonged administration and occasional skin reactions. Ataxia may occasionally occur.

Since diphenylhydantoin is mildly vasodilatory, it is capable of producing a significant but transient hypotension when given intravenously. For this reason the blood pressure should be monitored during administration by this route. The cardiac rhythm should also be followed closely because of the drug's effect on the conduction system. When used to treat abnormal rhythms, observation should include electrocardiographic monitoring.

Related nursing care. Since diphenylhydantoin affects the cardiac conduction system and may produce peripheral vasodilation, the blood pressure and pulse should be followed closely when the drug is given parenterally in the treatment of either convulsions or ectopic rhythms.

Magnesium sulfate. Magnesium sulfate, used parenterally for control of convulsions in hypertensive encephalopathy and eclampsia, is both antihypertensive and depressant to the cerebral cortex. It is usually given intravenously slowly to the point of controlling symptoms. It is available in 10 ml. vials as a 10% solution.

Magnesium sulfate is also specifically depressant to muscle, both smooth and skeletal. This effect on the uterus may be used therapeutically when uterine tetany is produced by large doses of an oxytocic drug.

Side effects. Side effects and toxicity include hypotension and somnolence. Respiratory depression and cardiac arrest may also occur.

Calcium gluconate. Calcium gluconate is the specific antagonist to magnesium sulfate. Additional uses for calcium gluconate are (1) to treat respiratory alkalosis, (2) to neutralize the citrate anticoagulant in transfused blood, and (3) to treat hypocalcemic tetany caused by hyperventilation or disturbance of the parathyroid glands.

Calcium gluconate is used with caution in digitalized patients, as it potentiates digitalis and seems to produce arrhythmias of intoxication.

ANTIHYPERTENSIVE DRUGS

Antihypertensive drugs are thought to act by reducing the number of sympathetic nerve impulses, by producing direct vasodilation by relaxing the smooth muscles of the blood vessels, or by promoting sodium and water excretion.

These drugs can be divided into three major classifications: (1) rauwolfia alkaloids, (2) ganglionic blocking agents, and (3) diuretics (discussed on page 271). Although it is not clearly understood how diuretics lower blood pressure, it is thought this may partially result from a decrease in the volume of the circulating fluid.

Rauwolfia alkaloids. Reserpine (Serpasil), a rauwolfia alkaloid, is primarily used as an antihypertensive agent, although it is also a psychotherapeutic agent. Its exact mode of action is unknown, but it is thought to be mediated through the central nervous system, probably through the brain stem. Several other rauwolfia alkaloids have similar effects.

In the treatment of mild to moderate hypertension, reserpine is usually given orally and is frequently combined with the thiazide diuretics. In the treatment of severe hypertension or hypertensive crisis, it may be given intramuscularly; it is extraordinary in that approximately ten times the usual oral dosage is needed by intramuscular injection. Effects tend to be slowly cumulative.

Side effects. Toxic effects include drowsiness from central nervous system depression and nasal congestion due to vasodilation. It frequently produces unpleasant dreams and occasionally precipitates psychotic states. A parkinsonian tremor is occasionally produced. Reserpine can increase gastrointestinal secretions and motility; therefore, it is sometimes considered to be ulcerogenic by either producing or precipitating peptic ulcer disease.

Related nursing care. Since patients react differently to drugs, the nurse must watch for signs of postural hypotension, such as dizziness and light-headed feeling upon sitting erect or standing. If the patient has a history of long-standing moderate hypertension, these symptoms may occur when the blood pressure is in a range considered normal; however, this would be hypotensive for this patient. Additionally, higher blood pressure is needed for elderly patients to force blood through arteriosclerotic vessels.

Ganglionic blocking agents. Ganglionic blocking agents, such as guanethi-dine (Ismelin), are useful for treatment of the patient with severe hyperten-sion. Other drugs of this type are mecamylamine (Inversine), pentolinium (Ansolysen), and trimethaphan camphorsulfonate (Arfonad). These drugs block transmission of impulses through the autonomic nervous system ganglia, and most of these drugs block both sympathetic and parasympathetic nerve cells. This chemical denervation of the vascular tree results in loss of vasoconstrictor tone and, hence, hypotension.

Most of these drugs are available as both oral and injectable preparations, and dosages required vary considerably. Because of their potency, they must be used with extreme caution as reduction of necessary perfusion pressure to vital organs such as the brain, heart, and kidneys is possible.

Side effects. Side effects vary but may include postural hypotension, blurred vision, urinary retention, constipation, and impotence.

Related nursing care. The nurse must watch for signs of hypotension and note each patient's reaction to drug therapy. The physician should be notified when the blood pressure is beginning to range in normal limits as he may want to decrease the dosage to prevent hypotension.

To avoid postural hypotension in an ambulatory patient, he is instructed to first sit on the side of the bed a few seconds before he stands; this allows his circulatory system to adjust to the upright position.

BRONCHODILATORS

Bronchodilators, such as *aminophylline (theophylline ethylenediamine)*, have their major therapeutic effect in relief of bronchospasm and vasospasm. Prepa-rations are available for intravenous, rectal, and oral use. Although amino-phylline may occasionally be ordered to be injected intramuscularly to prolong its effectiveness, it causes local tissue irritation and prolonged pain.

Side effects. The major side effect is hypotension due to vasodilation. Nausea and vomiting may result from oral administration, while rectal irritation may be due to administration by that route.

Related nursing care. Blood pressure should be checked very frequently if aminophylline is given intravenously since it can produce hypotension. The nurse should be aware that anorexia, nausea, and vomiting may be brought about by administration of this drug, while rectal irritation may be due to the rectal suppositories containing aminophylline.

One should encourage the patient with bronchospasm to take fluids to aid in liquefying secretions.

CHOLINERGIC DRUGS

The parasympathetic portion opposes and balances the sympathetic portion of the autonomic nervous system in those organs that receive innervation from both portions. The parasympathetic nerve impulse is mediated by acetylcholine, a neurohormone thought to aid in transmission of nerve impulses at synapses and myoneural junctions. Drugs that potentiate this effect of acetylcholine, either directly or indirectly, are referred to as *cholinergic agents*.

Action. The action of these drugs is one of increasing gastrointestinal peristalsis and secretion, increasing muscular tone of the urinary bladder, and relaxing the bladder sphincter. In addition, they may slow the heart, increase bronchial musculature tone and secretions, and cause increased sweating and some degree of peripheral vasodilation.

Therapeutic use. The most frequent use of this group of drugs is to counteract the paralytic ileus and bladder atony that frequently follow abdominal surgery and the urinary retention following delivery. Drugs of this group, such as *pantothenyl (Ilopan)* and *bethanechol (Urecholine)*, are usually initially given by injection and then administered orally as the patient improves.

Side effects. Toxic effects include increased gastrointestinal secretions and hyperperistalsis causing nausea, belching, abdominal cramps, flatulence, and diarrhea; bradycardia and heart block may occur in severe cases. Hypotension and flushing are also symptoms of toxicity. Asthma can be precipitated in susceptible individuals.

Atropine is the best antagonist and should be readily available.

Related nursing care. As the patient improves, the dosage is usually decreased, and the drug is discontinued when it is no longer needed. The physician should be alerted to symptoms indicating the necessity for decreasing or discontinuing the drug.

If the patient mentions having had asthma or a peptic ulcer, the nurse should make sure this information is known by the physician.

DIGITALIS PREPARATIONS

Digitalis preparations are an important drug group frequently used in the critically ill patient. Specific drugs commonly used include digoxin, gitalin, digitoxin, and lanatoside C (Cedilanid).

Action. The mode of action of digitalis is (1) by directly affecting the myocardial fibers to strengthen the force of contraction and (2) by slowing the conduction system.

To digitalize the patient, digitalis preparations may be given initially in dosages as great as ten times the maintenance dose, depending on the individual preparation and the patient's response. The maintenance dose of digitalis will vary in different individuals and depends on both total body content and daily excretion.

When it is unknown if the patient has been taking digitalis, fractional doses are given. In an emergency situation, such as pulmonary edema, lanatoside C is usually used. One half to three fourths of the full digitalizing dose may be administered initially and be followed by fractional doses at later intervals of from one to three or four hours, depending on the patient's condition. This medication is usually administered intravenously in an emergency situation for two reasons: (1) It is the most rapid method of obtaining effect; and (2) since the patient usually has a degree of shock, the effect obtained from oral or intramuscular administration would be unreliable.

Therapeutic use. The major therapeutic use of digitalis is in treatment for congestive heart failure. It is occasionally used to control the ventricular rate in rapid abnormal rhythms when congestive heart failure is not present.

Side effects. Digitalis toxicity is manifested by bradycardia and gastrointestinal symptoms such as anorexia, nausea, vomiting, and diarrhea. There may also be visual disturbances such as blurring or tinted vision, usually yellow. It can produce heart block of any degree; and almost any abnormal rhythm, including the rapid arrhythmias, may be a complication of digitalis intoxication.

The effect of digitalis is potentiated by hypokalemia, and intense diuresis in a digitalized patient may result in hypokalemia precipitating digitalis intoxication.

Related nursing care. Pulse rate is checked before each dose is administered. If the radial pulse is less than 60, the apical-radial pulse is checked. If there is a difference, the physician should be questioned concerning the administration of the drug.

Early onset of gastrointestinal manifestations of digitalis intoxication, such as anorexia, nausea, or diarrhea should be noted.

The nurse should discreetly question the patient about other signs of intoxication, such as visual disturbances.

DIURETICS

Diuretics are used in situations of sodium and fluid retentions, such as edema, ascites, pleural effusion, or cerebral edema of numerous etiologies. Generally, although not always, sodium and water are retained together.

The most common use of these drugs is as an adjunct in the management of congestive heart failure and hypertensive vascular disease. Numerous endogenous hormones (and administered exogenous hormones), such as progesterone and cortisone, produce edema, which diuretics may help in removing. Diuretics are sometimes helpful in the fluid retention associated with chronic liver disease but are usually avoided during edematous states produced by primary renal failure.

Basically there are three types of diuretics: (1) those that inhibit fluid and electrolyte reabsorption from the tubules, (2) those that block the effect of antidiuretic hormone or aldosterone, and (3) those that produce diuresis by hyperosmolarity.

Tubular inhibitors. The mercurial diuretics, thiazide diuretics, ethacrynic acid, and furosemide all have their effect by tubular inhibition. This permits a greater portion of the glomerular filtrate to progress through the tubules into the renal collecting system. Normally only approximately 1% of the material filtrated passes to the collecting tubular system; a much larger percentage, perhaps from 5% to 6%, of the glomerular filtrate may be excreted when these diuretics are given.

Mercurial diuretics. The mercurial diuretics, which are available for injection, produce their effect in the renal tubule; they may be used in cases of severe edema.

Side effects and toxicity include stomatitis, skin eruptions, and gastrointestinal irritation. Prolonged administration may produce permanent tubular damage, and the intense diuresis may bring about electrolyte abnormalities.

Thiazide diuretics. The thiazide diuretics are effective by interfering with tubular reabsorption of sodium, potassium, and water. They are usually effective orally, are fairly well tolerated, and are used in any situation in which edema is present. Some preparations are available for injection.

The *major side effect* is related to electrolyte deficiencies, especially hypokalemia (page 185). When a thiazide diuretic is used concurrently with digitalis preparations, the hypokalemia has a potentiating effect upon the status of digitalization, and patients with hypokalemia are quite susceptible to digitalis intoxication. For this reason, potassium supplements may need to be administered concomitantly with this group of diuretics.

Ethacrynic acid and furosemide. Ethacrynic acid (Edecrin) and furosemide (Lasix), which have their major effect in the renal tubules, are the most potent diuretics currently available and may be obtained for both oral and parenteral administrations.

The primary advantage of these compounds over other diuretics is their almost instantaneous effect, for demonstrable diuresis begins within a few minutes of intravenous injection and within half an hour of oral administration.

Side effects and toxicity are related to profound diuresis with severe electrolyte depletion. They differ from other diuretic drugs in this major point: When significant deficiencies are produced by the usual diuretics, the effect of the drugs is self limited; however these compounds may continue their diuretic effect even in the face of severe depletion states. They may also produce diarrhea.

Spironolactone. Spironolactone A (Aldactone A) is another tubular diuretic, but it has its effect in a manner slightly different from the previously mentioned drugs affecting the renal tubules, for it blocks aldosterone. Aldosterone is the adrenal hormone that exerts a controlling effect on the renal tubular reabsorption of sodium. Spironolactone competes with this hormone for tubular effect, thus partially blocking the sodium-retaining and antidiuretic effect of aldosterone.

Spironolactone has the advantage of tending to decrease the excretion of potassium. Spironolactone and the thiazides are sometimes used together when the need for diuresis is extreme; they are additive in effect.

Toxicity can occur if renal function is depressed and excessive potassium is retained, thus producing hyperkalemia.

Osmotic diuretics. *Mannitol* and *urea,* classified as osmotic diuretics, are nontoxic compounds of such a molecular weight that they remain largely in the intravascular space but are passed with glomerular filtrate. When injected intravenously, they cause interstitial fluid to move into the vascular system and thus increase renal blood flow and glomerular filtration, resulting in diuresis.

Preparations are available for intravenous injection, usually in concentrations between 5% and 20%. They are given over a fairly short period of time.

These agents are employed for several diuretic purposes, including their use (1) for restoring glomerular filtration following periods of renal ischemia; (2) as a therapeutic test in states that may have caused tubular damage; (3) for reducing the pressure from edema in interstitial tissue, especially cerebral edema following neurosurgery and head trauma; and (4) for diluting the toxic substances in poisonings as they are excreted.

Toxicity includes the potential for producing vascular overload and worsening congestive heart failure by the marked shift of fluid from the extravascular to the intravascular space. By means of profound diuresis these compounds may produce significant systemic dehydration (as when used to treat cerebral edema).

Related nursing care. Signs of electrolyte depletion should be noted (page 184) as should the effect of these drugs on pulse and blood pressure.

Since these patients are frequently weighed daily, accurate weights (on the same scales, in the same amount of clothes, at the same time of day) should be recorded.

The patient should be told to expect diuresis when the drug is given since copious urination may be alarming. His calls should be answered promptly and a container should be immediately available for urination.

Accurate record of fluid intake and output should be kept.

The physician should be notified of marked decrease in urinary output, which might indicate kidney failure.

Bibliography

Abelson, D. M.: Hyperthyroidism, Med. Sci. **19**:41, Feb. 1968.

AHA Committee on cardiopulmonary resuscitation: A manual for instructors, American Heart Association, 1967.

Anthony, C. P.: Textbook of anatomy and physiology, ed. 7, St. Louis, 1967, The C. V. Mosby Co.

Barbata, J. C., Jensen, D. M., and Patterson, W. G.: A textbook of medical-surgical nursing, New York, 1964, G. P. Putnam's Sons.

Beeson, P. B., and McDermott, W.: Cecil-Loeb Textbook of medicine, ed. 12, Philadelphia, 1967, W. B. Saunders Co.

Beland, I. L.: Clinical nursing, New York, 1965, The Macmillan Company.

Bendixen, H. H., et al: Respiratory care, St. Louis, 1965, The C. V. Mosby Co.

Bergerson, E. S., and Krug, E. E.: Pharmacology in nursing, ed. 11, St. Louis, 1969, The C. V. Mosby Co.

Bissell, G.: Nondiabetic endocrine emergencies, Hosp. Med. **3**:39, Jan. 1967.

Bookman, R.: Emergencies in allergy, Hosp. Med. **1**:18, Nov. 1965.

Bordicks, K. J.: Patterns of shock, implications for nursing care, New York, 1965, The Macmillan Company

Brener, J. L.: Clinical features of benign and malignant goiter, Hosp. Med. **3**:58, Mar. 1967; **3**:18, Apr. 1967.

Bryant, R., and Overland, A.: Woodward and Gardner's Obstetric management and nursing, ed. 7, Philadelphia, 1964, F. A. Davis Co.

Cooper, L. F., et al: Nutrition in health and disease, ed. 14, Philadelphia, 1963, J. B. Lippincott Co.

Davis, C. C.: Eclampsia, Hosp. Med. **3**:41, Apr. 1967.

Davis, J. E., and Rubin, R.: Obstetrics for nurses, Philadelphia, 1963, W. B. Saunders Co.

Dickens, M. L.: Fluid and electrolyte balance, Philadelphia, 1967, F. A. Davis Co.

Dison, N.: An atlas of nursing techniques, St. Louis, 1967, The C. V. Mosby Co.

Dreisbach, R.: Handbook of poisoning, Los Altos, Calif., 1966, Lange Medical Publications.

Egan, D. F.: Management of acute pulmonary edema, Hosp. Med. **2**:20, Feb. 1966.

Englert, E., Jr.: Pancreatitis, Diagnostic criteria, Pearl River, N. Y., Lederle Laboratories, June 1967.

Erwin, G. Y.: Coronary care units in a small hospital, J. Med. Ass. Georgia **57**:65, 1968.

Fitzpatrick, E., Eastman, N., and Reeder, S.: Maternity nursing, ed. 11, Philadelphia, 1966, J. B. Lippincott Co.

Forsham, P., editor: Endocrine system and selected metabolic diseases, Summit, N. J., 1965, Ciba Pharmaceutical Co.

Francis, C. C.: Introduction to human anatomy, ed. 4, St. Louis, 1964, The C. V. Mosby Co.

Goldman, M. J.: Principles of clinical electrocardiography, Los Altos, Calif., 1964, Lange Medical Publications.

de Gutierrez-Mahoney, C. G., and Carini, E.: Neurological and neurosurgical nursing, ed. 4, St. Louis, 1965, The C. V. Mosby Co.

Ingalls, A. J.: Maternal and child health nursing, St. Louis, 1967, The C. V. Mosby Co.

Jackson, F.: The treatment of head injuries, Summit, N. J., 1967, Ciba Pharmaceutical Co.

Johnston, D.: Total patient care, ed. 2, St. Louis, 1968, The C. V. Mosby Co.

Jude, J. R., and Elam, J. O.: Fundamentals of cardiopulmonary resuscitation, Philadelphia, 1965, F. A. Davis Co.

Kaiser, T. F.: Immediate management of injuries of the lower urinary tract, Hosp. Med. **3:**53, Feb. 1967.

Lyght, C., ed.: Merck manual, ed. 11, Rahway, N. J., 1966, Merck, Sharp and Dohme Research Laboratories.

Meltzer, L. E., Pinneo, R., and Kitchell, J. R.: Intensive coronary care, a manual for nurses, Philadelphia, 1965, Coronary Care Unit Fund.

Metheny, N. M., and Snively, W. D.: Nurses' handbook of fluid balance, Philadelphia, 1967, J. B. Lippincott Co.

Netter, F. H.: Endocrine system and selected metabolic diseases, vol. 4, Summit, N. J., 1965, Ciba Pharmaceutical Co.

Physicians' desk reference, ed. 22, Oradell, N. J., 1968, Medical Economics.

Plum, F.: Axioms on coma, Hosp. Med. **4:**20, May 1968.

Ports, A. E.: Abnormalities of the placenta, Columbus, Ohio, Ross Laboratories, 1963.

Rodman, M. J., and Smith, D. W.: Pharmacology and drug therapy in nursing, Philadelphia, 1968, J. B. Lippincott Co.

Shafer, K., et al: Medical-surgical nursing, ed. 4, St. Louis, 1967, The C. V. Mosby Co.

Smith, D., and Gips, C.: Care of the adult patient, ed. 2, Philadelphia, 1966, J. B. Lippincott Co.

Sovie, M. S., and Israel, J. S.: Use of the cuffed tracheostomy tube, Amer. J. Nurs. **67:**1,854, 1967.

Stacy, R. W., and Santolucito, J. A.: Modern college physiology, St. Louis, 1966, The C. V. Mosby Co.

Stedman's Medical dictionary, ed. 20, Baltimore, 1961, The Williams & Wilkins Co.

Sutton, A. L.: Bedside nursing techniques, Philadelphia, 1968, W. B. Saunders Co.

Taber, C. W.: Cyclopedic dictionary, ed. 10, Philadelphia, 1965, F. A. Davis Co.

Trainex corporation. Tracheostomy care, Garden Grove, Calif., 1967.

Tuttle, W. W., and Schottelius, B. A.: Textbook of physiology, ed. 15, St. Louis, 1965, The C. V. Mosby Co.

Weiner, M. M., Marks, J. L., and Padovano, C.: Coronary care unit nursing manual, Hackensack, N. J., 1967, Nursing Manual Fund.

Winter, C. C., and Roehm, M. M.: Sawyer's Nursing care of patients with urologic diseases, ed. 2, St. Louis, 1968, The C. V. Mosby Co.

Glossary

acidosis a condition of excessive hydrogen ion concentration in body fluids with serum pH less than 7.35.

acinus the smallest division of a gland.

Adams-Stokes syndrome a syndrome of unconsciousness or convulsions resulting from inadequate cerebral blood flow associated with a high degree of heart block or transition from one rhythm to another, as with the onset of ventricular tachycardia.

adrenergic crisis a condition of extreme overactivity of that portion of the sympathetic nervous system mediated by epinephrine, producing epinephrine intoxication. Symptoms are hypertension, tachycardia, arrhythmias, dry mouth, decreased intestinal motility, dilated pupils, anxiety, and psychotic behavior.

alkalosis condition of excessive concentration of hydroxide ions, or a deficit of hydrogen ions in body fluids with blood pH greater than 7.45.

alveolus terminal microscopic air sac of the lungs; the actual site of blood-gas exchange.

amniotic fluid embolism embolus that enters the mother's venous sinuses and carries amniotic fluid, vernix, or meconium into pulmonary capillaries; occurs during abnormal or traumatic labors. Generally death ensues within one or two hours, and the embolism is diagnosed at necropsy. Symptoms are similar to those of pulmonary edema and include uterine relaxation and postpartum hemorrhage. There is no specific treatment.

amplify to increase the size of; commonly used in reference to electronic magnification of electrical currents produced by physiologic activity of the body.

anaphylaxis extreme sensitivity reaction characterized by shock and marked increase in capillary permeability producing soft-tissue edema.

anasarca diffuse increase in body interstitial fluid; generalized edema.

anastomosis the connection of two hollow vessels or organs.

aneurysm a saclike bulging of a vessel wall either weakened by disease or abnormal at birth.

angina pectoris (*angina*, choking, *pectoris*, pectoral muscle) a condition in which the heart muscle receives insufficient blood supply (ischemia), causing chest pain.

ankylosis pathologic fixation of a joint so that movement is markedly limited.

anoxia literally, without oxygen; a condition of inadequate oxygen supply to tissue because of inadequate blood supply or inadequate oxygen content of the blood; results in tissue injury or death.

anticholinergic agent a drug or chemical that blocks the transmission of impulses across the parasympathetic ganglia or blocks the effect of acetylcholine; antivagal effect. Atropine is such an agent.

aorta the major artery leading away from the heart.

aphasia inability to transmit ideas by language in its various forms, such as speaking, reading, writing.

apnea without respiratory activity.

arrhythmia abnormal rhythm, usually of the heart; a term used generally to describe all forms of heart abnormalities including disturbances in rate, rhythm, and conduction.

arteriography roentgenography of an artery that has been injected with radiopaque media.

arteriosclerosis stiffening and hardening of the arteries. Atherosclerosis is generally a major factor.

ascites a collection of serous fluid within the abdominal cavity.

asphyxia a state of being without air, or a decreased oxygen content in the body.

asthma a clinical condition manifested by wheezing and produced by bronchiolar constriction and inflammation, usually allergic in origin.

atelectasis a condition involving collapse of a portion of lung tissue.

atherosclerosis a condition of hardening of arterial vessel walls usually produced by subintimal collection of lipid material; commonly used synonymously with arteriosclerosis.

atrioventricular (AV) node small mass of neuromuscular fibers in septa located at the junction of the atria and ventricles which conduct electrical impulse from atria to bundle of His.

atrium either of the two collecting chambers of the heart. The right atrium receives blood from vena cavae, and the left atrium receives blood from the pulmonary veins.

bacteremia the presence of viable bacteria in the bloodstream. It may be transient, and does not necessarily denote blood stream infection (or septicemia).

bellows a machine capable of expanding and contracting so as to move air. The respiratory bellows are the rib cage, diaphragm, intercostal muscles, and accessory respiratory muscles that enable to chest to expand and contract in order to move air into and out of the lungs.

bifurcate to divide into two branches.

bigeminal pulse a paired rhythm. Beats are in pairs followed by a pause.

bilirubin a breakdown product of hemoglobin after salvage of the iron content; secreted in bile. Elevation of blood's bilirubin content produces jaundice.

Biot's respiration a type of abnormal breathing frequently occuring during central nervous system disturbances; characterized by totally irregular respiratory activity varying in frequency and volume.

bradycardia a slow heart rate with fewer than 60 beats per minute.

bronchiectasis a condition with bronchiolar dilatation, usually accompanied by odorous pus formation.

Brudzinski's sign present when flexion of the neck produces flexion movement of the lower extremities; indicates meningeal irritation.

bruit an abnormal sound from the eddying currents produced by the passage of blood over an irregular surface or through a narrow portion of a vessel.

bundle of His group of neuromuscular fibers in the ventricular septum that convey an electrical impulse from the AV node to the right and left branches of Purkinje fibers to stimulate ventricular contraction.

calibrate to compare in measurement (relative to time, distance, weight, pressure, or energy) to a known standard.

cardiac cycle the electrical and mechanical activity encompassed in the period of time from any given point of heart activity to the same point in the next beat.

cardiac output quantity of blood pumped by the heart per minute.

cardiospasm a persistent contraction of the sphincter between the esophagus and the stomach (cardiac sphincter); frequently produces a substernal pain easily mistaken for cardiac pain.

cardioversion a method of countershock of the heart at such a time in the cardiac cycle so as to interrupt an abnormal rhythm and permit resumption of a normal rhythm.

carotid artery one of the principal arteries supplying blood to the head and neck; arises from the aortic arch on the left and the innominate artery on the right.

carotid sinus (or body) collections of sensory cells near the bifurcation of the carotid artery that are sensitive to pressure and carbon dioxide content of the blood. These bodies aid in the reflex control of heart rate, blood pressure, and respiration.

catecholamine one of a group of hormones produced largely but not exclusively by the adrenal medulla. They have an adrenergic effect for they produce tachycardia, hypertension, sweating, anxiety. Epinephrine is the best known of these compounds.

cephalad in the direction of the head.

cephalin flocculation test a test of liver function based on flocculation or clumping by abnormal proteins; generally considered to be indicative of hepatocellular disease as opposed to obstructive liver disease.

chemoreceptor nerve cell sensitive to concentrations of certain chemicals.

Cheyne-Stokes respiration a type of cyclic respiratory activity characterized by a period of apnea, followed by gradually increasing rate and depth of respiration until a peak is reached, and then a gradual or sudden decrease to another period of apnea.

cholangiogram roentgenogram of the bile ducts.

cirrhosis a liver disease characterized by destruction of liver tissue with replacement by fibrous tissue and distortion of liver architecture.

claudication pain produced by action and resulting from ischemia; relieved by rest.

clonus repetitive, regular, rapid contractions of a muscle group once it has been stimulated; usually indicates central nervous system disease and affects the arms and legs.

coalesce to fuse or run together.

coarctation (of the aorta) a congenital incomplete constriction of the aorta, commonly at the site of the ligamentum arteriosus. The increased resistance increases cardiac activity and causes hypertension limited to the portion of the body above the obstruction.

collateral an alternate path; commonly used to refer to circulatory paths that increase in caliber when obstruction to the usual path of blood flow is present.

coma unconsciousness during which there is no response to stimuli.

concussion of brain soft tissue injury to the brain resulting from a sudden blow to the head; results in momentary loss of consciousness but no demonstrable, immediate damage.

contractile power strength of contraction produced by shortening of a muscle.

contralateral pertaining to the opposite side.

contusion a bruise; an injury to tissue without a breaking of the skin.

coronary pertaining to the arteries supplying the cardiac muscle.

cor pulmonale heart disease resulting from right ventricular strain produced by pulmonary disease with pulmonary hypertension.

cortical referring to the cortex, the superficial layer of the brain, kidney, or adrenal gland.

crepitation a crackling feeling or sound.

crural pertaining to the thigh.

cyanosis a bluish hue imparted to the skin and mucous membranes by excessive concentrations of reduced hemoglobin in the small vessels.

debilitated wasted or weakened, as by chronic illness.

decompensation failure, as cardiac decompensation or heart failure.

defibrillator an electric machine used for interrupting ventricular fibrillation by shocking the heart. The same equipment slightly modified is used for interrupting other abnormal rhythms (cardioversion).

depolarization loss of electrical charge or polarity.

diaphoresis marked or excessive perspiration.

diastole period of relaxation of the heart during which the cavities fill with blood.

diplopia double vision.

diuretic an agent that increases urine production.

dorsiflexion contraction toward the back, especially in joints capable of flexion in more than one direction, such as the wrist.

dyspnea labored or difficult breathing.

ecchymosis a superficial collection of blood under the skin.

eclampsia toxemia of pregnancy accompanied by coma, convulsions, hypertension, edema, and proteinuria.

ectopic of abnormal location or origin.

edema collection of abnormal amounts of fluid in the interstitial spaces.

egress an outflow. To go out.

electrode a contact, usually metallic, for introduction of or detection of electrical activity.

electrolyte a chemical which, when dissolved, dissociates into an electrically charged particle capable of conducting an electrical current; also used as a generic term in reference to electrically charged particles (ions).

embolus an abnormal material floating free in the bloodstream until it lodges in some branch too small to permit its passage; usually thrombotic material but may be fat, air, or amniotic fluid.

emphysema a chronic lung condition produced by overdistention and destruction of alveoli by air entrapped behind partially obstructed bronchioles.

encephalitis inflammation, usually viral, of the brain.

encephalopathy condition of abnormal brain function without pathologic abnormalities, as from toxins or edema.

endarterectomy the surgical removal of material from the intima of an artery by stripping away the endothelial lining and adherent material.

endocardium the endothelial lining of the heart; continuous with the endothelial lining of the vascular tree.

endogenous originating from within.

epicardium the fibrous, serous membrane covering the heart; the visceral pericardium.

epidural over the dura.

epilepsy a group of conditions resulting in ectopic foci of cerebral cortical activity that produce episodic abnormalities of function, such as convulsions.

eructation belching.

eschar scab; an early protective covering of injured tissue formed by serum protein and fibrin precipitation with fibroblastic proliferation and inclusion of cellular debris.

exacerbation worsening of a disease.

exogenous originating outside of.

exsanguination blood deprivation.

extraneous outside and unrelated.

extrasystole a premature beat or contraction.

exudate a liquid discharge or weeping.

fibrillation rapid muscular twitching.

flaccid without tone.

flail not fixed or anchored.

focus a specific location.

fusiform tapered at both ends.

gastrectomy removal of all or part of the stomach.

gastrostomy creation of an opening into the stomach for the purpose of feeding or decompression when esophageal obstruction is present or the esophageal route is undesirable.

grand mal epilepsy a generalized convulsive seizure that may be accompanied by tongue biting and loss of sphincter control.

heart block interference with conduction of electrical impulses at any point in the cardiac conduction system; usually further defined by location.

hematemesis vomiting of blood.

hematocrit the percentage of blood composed of cellular (largely erythrocytes) elements.

hemianesthesia loss of sensation in one half of the body.

hemiparesis muscular weakness of one half of the body.

hemiplegia paralysis of one half of the body.

hemodynamics the factors in blood flow, related to the force of the circulating blood.

hemolysis alteration or destruction of blood cells by physical or chemical means or because the cells are fragile.

hemopericardium a collection of blood within the pericardial sac, capable of markedly altering cardiac efficiency by means of interference with ventricular filling.

hemothorax accumulation of blood within the thorax, usually in the pleural cavity.

hepatization the stages of lobar pneumonia in which the lung has the appearance of liver tissue.

hepatomegaly enlargement of the liver.

homeostasis maintenance of equilibrium in the internal body chemistry or environment.

homolateral referring to the same side.

hydrocephalus condition of increased cerebrospinal fluid within the cranium.

hyperkalemia (hyperpotassemia) excessive potassium content of the blood (greater than 5.5 mEq./liter).

hyperkinesia excessive muscular activity.

hypernatremia excessive serum sodium content (greater than 150 mEq./liter).

hyperosmolarity having a greater concentration of solutes than normal blood; has characteristic of drawing fluid from an area of less solute concentration.

hyperpnea increased respiratory rate and depth.

hypertrophy enlargement of or increase in bulk of a part.

hyperuricemia increased uric acid in the blood (greater than 5 mg. per 100 ml.); characteristic of gout.

hypochloremia decrease of chloride in serum; occurs during prolonged gastric suctioning.

hypoglycemia blood sugar below normal, less than 60 mg. per 100 ml. true glucose.

hypokalemia serum potassium lower than normal (less than 3.5 mEq./liter).

hyponatremia depression of serum sodium content (less than 130 mEq./liter).

hypothalamus the highest center in the brain stem having to do with autonomic function.

hypovolemia diminished blood volume.

ictal convulsive.

idiopathic condition of unknown cause.

idioventricular originating in the ventricle.

infarct an area of necrosis produced by interference with blood supply.

inspissate to harden, especially by drying.

interstitial the area between the cells and the intravascular area.

intima the cellular lining of the vascular tree; endothelium.

ischemia temporary anemia of a part due to inadequate blood supply.

isoelectric the electrical base line in an electrocardiogram.

jacksonian epilepsy a specific type of convulsion that begins as a repetitive contraction of a single muscle group and then spreads first cephalad then caudal.

Kernig's sign absence of the ability to extend the leg when the thigh is flexed on the abdomen; a sign of meningeal irritation.

ketosteroids a group of adrenal and gonadal hormones with a ketone attached (usually at the 17 position of the steroid nucleus). These hormones have anabolic and masculinizing effects.

Kussmaul respiration a specific type of respiration characterized by rapid, deep, unlabored, forceful respiratory effort, commonly seen in acidosis.

labile subject to much variation; unsteady.

Leriche syndrome syndrome of occlusion of the aorta at the aorto-iliac bifurcation; classically produces claudication, impotence, and decreased or absent femoral pulses and is commonly caused by atheromatous occlusion.

leukocytosis an increase in white blood cells to more than 10,000/cu. mm.

leukopenia an abnormally low white blood cell count (fewer than 3500/cu. mm.).

loculation division into pockets.

lues syphilis.

mannitol a low molecular weight, poorly metabolized sugar.

mediastinum the median space in the thoracic cavity bounded anteriorly by the sternum, posteriorly by the vertebrae, laterally by the lungs, and inferiorly by the diaphragm.

mediate to go between or transfer.

melena digested blood in the stool, usually tarry and foul smelling.

meningitides plural of *meningitis*.

mesentery peritoneal fold that suspends the intestinal tract from the dorsal spine.

millivolt measure of electrical pressure; 0.001 volt.

monitor an electronic device that can transmit the signal of each heart beat. To watch continuously.

mucolytic tending to dissolve or liquefy mucus.

mural against or on a wall of a cavity, as a mural thrombus on the interior wall of the heart.

murmur a heart sound, usually abnormal, produced by eddying currents set up by blood flow through abnormal channels, such as a resistant stenosed valve cusp or regurgitant streams of blood through incompetent valves. The timing and characteristics of murmurs give considerable information concerning underlying heart conditions.

myocardial insufficiency inadequate contractile power of cardiac muscle. If progressive, it results in cardiac decompensation or congestive heart failure.

myocardium muscular structure of the heart.

myxedema the classic findings of chronic thyroid deficiency: puffiness, lethargy, hypotension, diminished reflexes.

necrosis death of tissue.

nonviable nonliving.

nuchal pertaining to the neck.

occlusion obstruction to flow through a vessel; usually refers to blood vessels.

occult hidden.

orthopnea condition in which the most adequate oxygenation is obtained in the erect position. The supine position produces increased dyspnea.

oscilloscope a vacuum tube with a coated, fluoresced surface on which is projected a beam of electrons causing fluorescence of the area on which the beam is focused. By being subjected to a magnetic field, the beam may be bent. If this magnetic field is controlled from the amplified current produced by cardiac contraction, the oscilloscope may be adjusted to trace a continuous electrocardiogram.

osmosis the physiochemical phenomenon characterized by the passage of fluid from an area of lesser concentration to an area of greater concentration.

P wave that portion of the electrocardiogram produced by the electrical activity of atrial contraction.

pacemaker that area, organ, instrument, or individual which initiates activity.

palliative relieving slightly; ameliorative as opposed to curative.

palsy interference with normal function, as of a nerve.

papilledema swelling of the optic disc or nerve head produced by interference with venous drainage through the central retinal vein; usually from increased intracranial pressure.

paradoxical pulse pulse that decreases or disappears during inspiration.

paralytic ileus intestinal paralysis without organic obstruction.

parasympathetic nervous system that portion of the autonomic nervous system consisting of ganglia having their origin in the cervical and caudal autonomic ganglia, mediated by acetylcholine (cholinergic) and generally balancing and opposing the sympathetic nervous system.

parenteral administration by any route other than the digestive tract.

patellar reflex a deep tendon reflex of contraction of the quadriceps femoris elicited by sharply striking the relaxed patellar tendon.

pathognomonic strongly indicative or diagnostic.

perfusion the supplying of tissue with fluid.

pericardicentesis needle-tapping of the pericardial sac for the purpose of removing fluid.

pericardium the membranous sac enclosing the heart; the parietal pericardium.

peripheral on the surface or away from the center.

peripheral resistance the resistance to blood flow offered by the muscular tone and diameter of vessels.

peritoneal dialysis use of the peritoneum as a semipermeable membrane for removal of solutes from the body by repetitive introduction into and drainage of fluid from the peritoneal cavity. The fluid has an electrolyte composition similar to that of tissue fluid except it is without those solutes whose removal is desired.

petechia a very small extravasation of blood resulting from abnormally fragile capillaries.

petit mal epilepsy disease characterized by momentary loss of awareness and contraction of a small muscle or group of muscles. There is no preceding warning or aftereffect.

phagocytosis the property which some cells possess of engulfing foreign material; one of the body's defense mechanisms.

pheochromocytoma a chromaffin cell tumor usually in the adrenal medulla. These tumors are capable of producing epinephrinelike hormones that may be responsible for hypertensive syndromes.

phlebothrombosis the accumulation of a thrombus or blood clot within a vein without significant inflammation.

phlebotomy an opening artificially produced in a vein for the purpose of removal of blood.

placental souffle a murmur synchronous with the mother's pulse heard over the placenta in the pregnant uterus. It is produced by the large, localized blood flow as the blood enters the dilated uterine arteries.

plaque an abnormal area or patch on a part of the body.

pleura serous membrane lining the lung (visceral pleura) and the thoracic cavity (parietal pleura).

plexus a fine network of vessels or nerves.

pneumonia bacterial, chemical, viral, or rickettsial infection of the lung.

pneumothorax a collection of air in the pleural cavity.

polarity the property of having electric potential or charge, one area being negative with reference to another area.

potential an electric charge.

potentiate to increase the activity of.

P-R interval the period of time on the electrocardiogram between the onset of atrial activity (P wave) and the onset of ventricular activity; normally from 0.10 to 0.20 second.

premonitory coming before, warning; commonly used to describe minor symptoms preceding major difficulty from injury.

pressor an agent or drug used to increase blood pressure, usually by increasing peripheral resistance.

prognosis outlook; commonly used in reference to anticipated outcome of patient suffering from a specific condition or complication.

prophylaxis prevention; activities intended to prevent disease or complications in distinction to activities designed to treat disease.

psychomotor epilepsy a disease characterized by loss of awareness although performance of a simple motor action is continued.

pulse differential (or pulse deficit) the difference between peripheral pulse rate and heart rate. At rapid or irregular rates the heart may contract again before there has been adequate filling with inadequate systolic ejection to produce a palpable pulse.

Purkinje fibers modified neuromuscular fibers that distrtibute impulses throughout the myocardium; usually located immediately under the endocardium.

QRS complex that portion of the electrocardiogram produced by ventricular depolarization.

Q-T interval that period on the electrocardiogram from the onset of depolarization (first QRS deflection) to the end of repolarization (T wave), normally less than 0.40 second.

rale an abnormal breath sound heard over the chest and caused by partial obstruction.

recannulate to make another opening through (as an occluded vessel).

refractory resistant to treatment.

repolarization electrical recharge or return of polarity.

respiratory acidosis increased hydrogen ion concentration produced by carbon dioxide retention, usually from inadequate ventilation.

retrograde in a reverse direction.

rhonchus a coarse, abnormal breath sound, as snoring.

rubor redness.

saphenous pertaining to a major venous system that drains most of the superficial tissue of the leg and is prone to develop varicosities. It empties into the femoral system.

sarcoidosis a disease of unknown etiology characterized by nontubercular granuloma formation and having special affinity for lymphoid tissue.

septicemia active bacterial infection of the bloodstream.

septum a dividing wall between parts of an organ.

serotonin a compound released from certain tissue cells with a strong epinephrine activity; produced in increased amounts from carcinoid tumors resulting in much of the symptomatology of these tumors.

sino-atrial (SA) node a small collection of neuromuscular tissue near the junction of the superior vena cava and right atrium; serves as the normal pacemaker.

spastic having exaggerated muscle tone, usually with stronger muscles involved in a state of almost continuous contraction.

ST segment that portion of the electrocardiogram from the end of ventricular depolarization (last deflection of QRS complex) to the beginning of repolarization (or the T wave), normally isoelectric.

stenosis a narrowing or constriction of an opening.

steroid a group of compounds that have a basic 4-ring chemical structure resembling cholesterol. Many of these compounds have strong hormonal activity.

stertorous strenuous or struggling respiratory effort.

stroke volume the amount of fluid ejected by any pump with a single cycle, usually used in reference to the heart.

stupor unconsciousness during which the individual responds only to painful stimuli.

subarachnoid under or beneath the arachnoid or meningeal membrane, adherent to the brain surface.

subdural beneath the dura or outer fibrous membrane covering the brain.

subintimal under or beneath the intima or membrane lining blood vessels, usually arterial vessels.

subphrenic beneath or under the diaphragm.

sulfobromophthalein (BSP) test a test of liver function based upon the ability of the liver to remove the abnormal dye from the blood.

supernatant the top layer of a suspension separated by centrifugation or gravity.

sympathetic nervous system that portion of the autonomic nervous system whose impulses are mediated by epinephrine, therefore having an epinephrinelike effect; normally opposed to and balancing parasympathetic activity.

syndrome a group of symptoms seen together.

systole the period of cardiac contraction.

T wave that portion of the electrocardiogram written during ventricular repolarization.

tachycardia rapid heart rate (more than 100 beats per minute).

tamponade use of a plug. A cardiac tamponade interferes with ventricular filling because of the pressure of fluid collected in the pericardium.

thrill an abnormal vibration produced by eddying currents from obstruction, narrowing, or irregularity to blood flow; a murmur or bruit felt rather than heard.

thrombus a stationary blood clot.

torsion twisting.

toxicity potential for harm; poisonous quality.

tremulous with tremors; shaking.

trephine to open the skull by drilling.

trophic pathologic tissue changes from chronic ischemia.

turbid cloudy.

turgor normal cellular tension.

U wave an inconstant electrocardiographic deflection resembling and following the T wave but of less amplitude and duration, generally of no significance.

unilateral on one side only.

urca one of the end products of protein metabolism.

urobilinogen a breakdown product of hemoglobin.

Valsalva's maneuver forceful expiratory effort against a closed glottis, as in straining during defecation.

varices saccular abnormalities of a vein usually produced by the combined factors of increased venous pressure and disruption of venous valves.

vasoconstrictor an agent that produces contraction of the smooth muscles in the walls of blood vessels, decreasing their diameter and increasing resistance.

vasodilator an agent that produces relaxation of the smooth muscles of blood vessels walls permitting their expansion, increasing their diameter, and decreasing their resistance to flow.

vasopressor see *vasoconstrictor*.

vena cavae the major veins returning blood to the right atria. The superior generally drains the blood above the heart, while the inferior drains blood below the heart.

ventricle

of the brain the four fluid-filled cavities within the brain.

of the heart the two muscular cavities that propel blood into the systemic and pulmonary arterial trees.

viable living or capable of living.

voltmeter an instrument with two electrical contacts that is used to measure the electrical potential between two points.

Waterhouse-Friderichsen syndrome a syndrome of acute catastrophic adrenocortical insufficiency occuring most commonly as a complication of adrenal hemorrhage in meningococcic meningitis.

water intoxication a syndrome produced by inadequate electrolyte intake to replace losses without concomitant restriction of water. Symptoms primarily result from hyponatremia and include headache, irritability, psychoses, cramps, and convulsions.

Wenckebach phenomenon an unusual cardiac arrhythmia produced by progressive AV block resulting in progressive prolongation of the P-R interval. During progressive block, periodically an impulse arrives at the ventricle during the refractory period and no ventricular response occurs.

Index

---

*Italicized numbers indicate main discussion of
topic.